Healing Poisoned Medicine

Medicine That Heals vs. Medicine That Kills

Reed T. Sainsbury, N.D.

iUniverse, Inc.
New York Bloomington

Healing Poisoned Medicine
Medicine That Heals vs. Medicine That Kills

Copyright © 2008 by Reed T. Sainsbury, N.D.

All rights reserved. No part of this book may be used or reproduced by any means, graphic, electronic, or mechanical, including photocopying, recording, taping or by any information storage retrieval system without the written permission of the publisher except in the case of brief quotations embodied in critical articles and reviews.

iUniverse books may be ordered through booksellers or by contacting:

iUniverse
1663 Liberty Drive
Bloomington, IN 47403
www.iuniverse.com
1-800-Authors (1-800-288-4677)

Because of the dynamic nature of the Internet, any Web addresses or links contained in this book may have changed since publication and may no longer be valid. The views expressed in this work are solely those of the author and do not necessarily reflect the views of the publisher, and the publisher hereby disclaims any responsibility for them.

ISBN: 978-0-595-47183-6 (pbk)
ISBN: 978-0-595-91462-3 (ebk)

Printed in the United States of America

Contents

Acknowledgements	xi
Dedication	xiii
Foreword by Rashid A. Buttar, D.O.	xv
Introduction	1
Disclaimer	5

Chapter 1: The Pulsation of Life — 7
- You are a Self-Healing Organism
- The Cell is Immortal
- Thomas Edison's Wisdom
- How Your Body Heals - One Cell at a Time
- Warning at the Zoo
- Don't Mess with Mother Nature
- Cyanide – Friend or Foe?
- Graviola
- Identifying the Problem with My Car
- Radio Signals and Energy
- Kirlian Photography
- CEDSA (Computerized Electrodermal Stress Analysis)
- Benjamin Franklin

Chapter 2: Health Care or Disease Maintenance — 37
- America's Disease Maintenance System
- Eliminating Competition
- A Cure for Cancer – Outlawed in the USA
- Americans Have the Most Expensive Health Care, But Not the Best
- Horse Urine for Health?
- Dr. Semmelweis - Killed for Teaching the Truth
- Murder by Prescription
- Vioxx – A Killer Drug
- Terrorists Among Us
- Americans Demand Justice
- The Truth Hurts
- The Paradox of Modern Medicine
- Hippocratic or Hypocritical?

Chapter 2: Health Care or Disease Maintenance (cont.)
    Heroes in the Emergency Room
    Insanity
    The Cancer Industry
    Healing Cancer
    Poison for Health?
    Cats: Created by God to Kill Mice
    Without Herbs We Would Die

Chapter 3: Healing the Cause of Dis-Ease   87
    The Lymphatic System
    Rebounding (Lymphasizing)
    Finding the Cause of Dis-ease
    Mother Nature's Food Chain
    Own Your Dis-ease and Be Healed
    Weight Loss Without Trying
    High Cholesterol or Sluggish Thyroid?
    Losing Weight and Keeping It Off
    Stevia – Mother Nature's Sugar Substitute
    Nutrition and Detoxification
    Skin Lesions Healed
    Your Spleen - The Septic Tank of Your Body
    Don't Ignore Your Body's Warning Signs
    Diarrhea
    Fever
    Colds

Chapter 4: Healers or Drug Dealers?   119
    Epilepsy Healed
    You Only Find What You are Looking For
    The Right Fuel
    You Reap What You Sow
    Is Your Car Worth More Than Your Health?
    Words of Wisdom
    Ask the Right Person
    Motivation to Win
    My First Eye Opener to Health
    Living Foods for Living People
    Healing Energy of Plants

Chapter 4: Healers or Drug Dealers? (cont.)
Mother Nature's Intelligence
Digestion and the Bowels
A Headache Healed
Remodeling Your House

Chapter 5: Your Amazing Body   **161**
The Incredible Miracle Of Birth
The Eyes
The Ears
Smell
Taste
Blood
The Lungs
The Bones
The Muscles
The Skin
The Digestive System
The Nerves
The Brain
DNA

Chapter 6: Medical Myths Exposed   **181**
Gallbladder – A Necessary Organ or Bio-trash?
Liver/Gallbladder Flush For Stones
The Cholesterol Myth
Deadly Hydrogenated Oils
The Appendix
No Incurable Diseases
Crohn's Disease Healed
Dis-ease: Your Body's Way of Filing Bankruptcy
Earning Your Cancer Trophy
The Antibiotic Paradox
Acidosis – The Terrain That Favors Dis-ease
Neutralizing Acids in the Body
Mother Nature's Foods – Healing Light Energy
Let's Be Practical
Dr. Sainsbury's Health Plan
The Awakening

Chapter 6: Medical Myths Exposed (cont.)
- Courage to Wield the Sword of Truth
- Confessions of a Medical Heretic
- Toxic Metals
- Mercury Facts
- Root Canals
- Autism – A Symptom of Heavy Metal Poisoning

Chapter 7: Vaccinations - Wolves in Sheep's Clothing   231
- Polio
- Measles
- The Origin of Vaccinations
- Vaccinations Weaken Your Immune System
- Chickenpox and Shingles
- What Doctors Have to Say About Mass Vaccinations
- Vaccination Ingredients
- Homeopathy – An Alternative to Vaccinations
- Vaccine Exemption Affidavit

Chapter 8: Never Surrender   263
- Chiropractic Adjustments Allow Me to Compete
- Motorcycle Accident Crushes My Football Dreams
- Controversy in the Doctor's Office
- My Struggle
- Back to Gold's Gym
- Powerlifting

Chapter 9: Master of Puppets   271
- How Much Do Your Drugs Actually Cost?
- If We Could Patent the Sun
- The Drug Business
- Money Equals Power
- Rockefeller Oil Interests and I.G. Farben
- The Big Drug Deal
- Restructuring Medicine in the USA
- Who Owns Insurance Companies?
- The FDA - A Pawn in the Game
- Money Handlers
- Medical Ghost Writing
- Paying to Squash Competition

Chapter 9: Master of Puppets (cont.)
No Honest Opinions in the Media
How are Doctors Educated About Drugs?
Your Doctor is Not God
Hypocrites

Chapter 10: Your Health Under Attack   291
Balancing the Body
Circulation
Why Do Arteries Get Blockages but Veins Don't?
Enzymes for Health
Diabetes
Chiropractic Adjustments
The Healthiest People in the World
Mineral Functions and Deficiency Symptoms
U.S. Senate Document #264
Water
Chlorine
Poison in Our Drinking Water
Antidepressant Drugs Cause Abnormal Behavior
Headaches
Aspirin
Actions Speak Louder Than Words
Aspartame: The Poison in Our Food
Soft Drinks
Birthing
Hospital Birth vs. Home Birth
Protein
Where Do Cows Get Protein?
High Protein Diets – Not So Healthy
Mother Nature's Healers
Where to Start?
Health Tips

Chapter 11: Healing Secrets Your Doctor Never Told You   337
Health Evaluation
Did You Know…
A Recipe for Dis-ease
Health Books for Seekers of Wisdom

Chapter 12: The Energy in Emotions   **375**

    Healing the Cause of Cancer
    Healing Power of the Mind
    Divine Guidance from on High
    Kinesiology
    The Subconscious Mind
    The NEED to Be Happy
    Love Heals
    Mirrors in Life
    Placebos: A Factor in Your Healing
    Negative Emotions – A Cause of Disease
    The World We Create with Thoughts
    Freedom is a Choice
    Weight Gain – An Emotional Issue
    Love
    Agape Love
    EGO
    Why Relationships Fail
    Children are Great Teachers
    Transforming Your Life
    The Power of the Spoken Word
    Winning
    Conclusion

Index   419

Acknowledgements

I would like to thank the following people who have helped me write this book. Some have been teachers, others have encouraged me to make a difference and some have been my source of strength and blessed me with a desire to write. God being the Creator of all has given me everything I am and everything I have. To the Almighty I am eternally grateful for the abundance with which He blesses me.

I'd like to thank my sweet wife, Bethanne, who always encourages me to reach my goals. She has raked me over the coals in editing this book and it has been a humbling experience. All the pictures and graphics in this book were created by her. Many of them were done late at night after the kids were in bed. Without her help this book wouldn't exist. I'd like to thank the three beautiful children God has entrusted me with; Dallas, Brooklyn (The Great Bibbitusky) and Rockman (Rocko - The Magnificent). To come home from work and see them drop what they are doing and come running to their daddy, is worth more than all the gold in the world.

I want to thank my parents, especially my father who has taught me to always seek the truth and to remember there is always two sides to every story. A special thanks goes to my mother for always being the most unselfish person I have ever known. Her silent example of serving has taught me a priceless secret to happiness.

I'd like to thank Marijah McCain N.D., Max Skousen, Larry Bristow N.D., Scott Forsyth, Amazon John Easterling and my brother Scott Sainsbury whose passion for health ignited a spark within me to study alternative medicine and learn how the body truly heals. I want to thank James J. Hawver, N.M.D., President of Standard Enzyme Company for all his support. A special thanks goes to Lowndes Harrison, M.D., and Jane Nelson for all of their editing efforts in making this book a success. I'd also like to thank all of my clients who have allowed me to serve them in whatever way I could. You have been my greatest teachers. You are the true tests to see if what we do at Life Essentials Natural Healing Clinic works. Thank you and may God bless you abundantly.

Dedication

I dedicate this book to everyone who is sick and tired of being sick and tired. This is for medical doctors, health care professionals and most importantly you, the person who is fed up with our current medical system that suppresses symptoms with toxic harmful drugs that maintain disease but never heals. When it's your health, you want the best, you want something that works-because you deserve it. This book is for you. May the innate intelligence within heal you as you provide your body, mind and spirit with the proper environment and tools necessary to experience optimum health.

Foreword

With the impending failure of the current medical system in place, along with the increase in chronic disease the aging population is facing, it is no wonder that the public at large is no longer tolerating the inadequacies of traditional medicine. As a result, there are many books about natural health and holistic healing on the market today. Some of these books give the readers information that they have been searching for while others provide a sense of reinforcement for belief systems the reader may already possess or intuitively are guided towards. However, it has been my experience, that many of the books on the market today which have an integrative or holistic slant, lack a certain component necessary to make a connection with the reader.

Many of the people seeking a book on integrative medicine or holistic healing are doing so because of a personal challenge or the condition of a loved one which has been refractory to conventional treatment. The reason for them reading such a book is a "real" reason, and not merely a curiosity. Some of these people may even be considered "desperate" due to their impending situation or condition. It is truth that the reader seeks and help the reader desires. And so the search goes on for the right book containing the right information that may shed some light on the dilemma the reader is facing.

Despite many of these books containing important information and even information that the reader may be searching for in particular, most of these books lack the passion and conviction behind the words that have been written. I would venture to say that some may even be "dry" and boring. They certainly lack the quality of capturing the interest of the reader to the point that one doesn't want to put down the book. In fact it is rare to find a nonfiction scientifically based health information book that has not been watered-down, edited, re-edited, changed, amended or otherwise completely ruined, to the point where the original intention of the author has been completely lost and the emotion and passion have been virtually dissected out.

It would be analogous to the white bread we see in the food markets which have had all the nutrient value removed from the flour used to make the bread, and then re-fortified with vitamins and minerals that are considered to be good for the body. The question is, why remove these nutrients from the flour in the first place? Similarly, the good information is removed or changed when edited or amended for the final printing of most books and in the process, the passion of the author and the conviction of his or her beliefs is lost to the reader.

This is a frustration that I have personally experienced while writing my own books where the editors have changed the content to such a degree that the meaning and intention behind my words was changed to a degree that sometimes I didn't even recognize the words as ever having been mine. The only solution seemed to be either not to write the book or self publish the manuscript in order to retain the original intention.

So it was with great pleasure that I read the manuscript I was asked to review when requested to write this forward. I found myself becoming engrossed in the personal story of Dr. Sainsbury, how he began his journey and what led him on the path that eventually found him writing a book on natural health. The varied topics presented in a strong and zealous manner with tangible examples and engrossing stories made for a book that was as entertaining as it was informative. Some may find it "too extreme" to one side but I would disagree. It is the nature of most health books to avert being too extreme, when in reality, it is in fact, exactly what is needed. Remember that truth is on one side and a lie is on the other extreme. For those who feel that ANY book on health that is biased to one side lacks a balanced perspective, I would counter that those who write in this manner, have seen the light and can not step back into the darkness, for being "balanced" would require keeping one foot in the darkness.

For the novice, this book is a raw look at the reality of what many of us know to be the truth regarding medicine and healing. It is an unapologetic and passionate presentation that will help initiate those who are first learning of this subject. For the veteran, it provides a refreshing point of view that will often put a smile on your face because you know exactly the emotion that the author is experiencing as he wrote the words. This book will help open many eyes and will be a contribution to the cause of awakening the collective consciousness that no longer will tolerate the inadequacies and failure of traditional medicine.

Rashid A. Buttar, DO
FAAPM, FACAM, FAAIM

Introduction

Unable to sleep, I laid in bed next to my wife who was slumbering through the night peacefully. I looked up on the dresser to see the red-lighted digits of my alarm clock glowing in the blackness of the night read 2:17 A.M. Something within woke me with a desire to write this book for people who are searching for an alternative to prescription drugs and surgery. Sick people everywhere pray to God for help and deliverance from their illness. Why? Because the prescription drugs are not working and the adverse side effects are making them sicker.

Most of us at one time or another in life have spent a miserable night or two hunched over the toilet puking our guts out. We've experienced having "the flu" and it is hell. There is nothing in this world that is worth as much as your health. After being sick, to be able to sleep peacefully and then to wake up feeling refreshed and full of energy so that you can work and play pain free causes a humble man to fall on his knees and thank God for blessing him with health. Good health is worth more than any amount of money.

> **"The health of the people is really the foundation upon which all their happiness and all their powers as a state depend."** Benjamin Disraeli – Former Prime Minister of the United Kingdom (1804-1881)

I went into the computer room and began writing this book as fast as I could type. I typed nonstop for hours as this book unfolded like someone else was dictating it and I was just the scribe. I didn't have to stop and think, it flowed from my fingers like magic.

The sun came up over the trees and a beam of light came shimmering through the window reminding me it was morning time. I walked out into the living room and the sun was sending another magic ray of light through the window perfectly illuminating just the picture of Christ hanging on our wall. It was stunning. Was it coincidence?

I had over twenty pages typed on the computer and when I read it through, it was perfect. I couldn't believe I had just written that. I left for work that morning excited about the book I was writing and the potential to give something to the world. I couldn't wait for the next chance to write more. I truly felt that Divine Intelligence was manifesting through me now. Infinite wisdom from on high was illuminating my mind. I was on fire, accepting my call to serve others by teaching them how to heal. This wasn't my work, it was God's. I was merely allowed to be part of, *"...He that believeth on me, the works that I do shall he do also; and greater works than these shall he do," St. John 14:12.* I was then and still am humbled, honored and determined to accomplish this assignment from on High.

The next morning I woke up early. I was eager and anxious to see what would be written today. When I went to pull my manuscript up on the computer there was an error. After having computer experts try to retrieve my file, I was forced to face the facts. All of it had been lost. Immediately after hearing that news, I knew that the adversary, the powers of darkness, didn't want this manuscript to get out. I was reminded of what my father had taught me growing up; *the truth is always persecuted, whether it is health, history, politics, or religion.* The forces of darkness are in full operation to destroy, twist, and distort light.

With that understanding, I acknowledge that there will be some who oppose what I say in this book. That is perfectly alright. This book has been written to empower those who choose to experience true health.

Through the grace of God and his love I have witnessed miracles in my life and the lives of my clients. It has been said that truth is stranger than fiction and, as odd as it sounds, I have learned that, the more I give, the more I have.

God has blessed me and I choose to give back to the world a fraction of what has been given to me. I cannot sit silently by as good people poison their bodies with drugs and mutilate their bodies through unnecessary surgical procedures. I am compelled to make a difference.

When Jesus Christ went into the temple with a whip and overthrew the money-changers table's and drove out the vendors, the "turn the other cheek" philosophy went out the window. He drove corruption out with power and force. He came to set things straight. This book is written to set things straight in the health care field. People deserve to be healed; not doped up on expensive, toxic drugs to maintain their diseases with for the rest of their lives. What kind of life is that?

Like Robert Frost once said, "Two roads diverged in a wood, and I took the one less traveled by, and that has made all the difference." Americans deserve to know the truth about how the body heals and the corruption taking place in modern medicine. I choose to make a difference by taking the road less traveled.

Some day I will vacate this tabernacle of clay we call a body. I will go back to the dust from whence I came. I only have a limited time left in my mortal existence to give what I have to give and then I will move on to bigger and better things and leave it with my posterity and all those who want empowerment. I hope and pray what I have to share will be a blessing to you and everyone with whom you choose to share this light and healing wisdom.

> "The last suit that you wear, you don't need any pockets."
> Wayne W. Dyer, Ph.D.

As a naturopathic doctor I must admit that I do not have all the answers. The complexity and healing intelligence of the human body is humbling to study. I am a student willing to learn all that I can to help others heal. The day I stop learning is the day I cease to exist in this mortal life.

Most of our clients come in after medical doctors and prescription drugs have failed to help and their doctor has told them that they will just have to learn to live with their disease. They come in out of desperation because mainstream medicine has no hope or cure to offer them. Intelligent people are not satisfied with just maintaining disease with drugs. They will not settle for that.

Subtle whisperings from within, also known as intuition or "the Spirit," teaches most people that there is a way to heal and be made whole. The spirit of truth is given to everyone who comes into this world. To maintain your disease with drugs is a mockery of the divine intelligence and life-force that governs your body, all of life, and the entire universe.

When a symptom presents itself, it is because something in your body is out of balance. When you detoxify the body and balance it nutritionally you fix the problem! Don't sit there like a poor helpless victim taking addictive and harmful drugs whose side effects may be worse than the actual symptom you are trying to cover up. Just say no to drugs. You deserve better. Your body is a temple. It's hard for the Spirit to be there when your God-given senses are dulled with chemical drugs.

The intelligence that knew how to create you in the womb knows how to heal you now. However, the stressors must be removed so that it can work. Drugs fail to address the true cause of disease, which are the stressors (toxins) within, interfering with normal cellular activity.

Have you ever stopped to wonder why some wealthy people, celebrities and successful business owners, who can afford the best medical care available in the world are turning to alternative medicine? Wise people find what is effective for healing, not necessarily what is covered by insurance.

Like I use to tell my wife when we were young single college students out living life to the fullest in my 1973 Chevy 4x4 at the base of a steep mountain covered in mud, "Hang on, we're going for a ride." Her fingerprints are still engraved in the dashboard of that big blue truck from the intense, white-knuckled "four-wheeling" we did, and although she won't admit it, deep down inside she loved every minute of it. So, hang on because this book is going to take you for a ride on the other side of health, the one your doctor has never addressed. The one that will empower you to heal without man-made chemicals messing things up inside, causing more harm than good, like they often do.

Disclaimer

The author is in no way attempting to treat, diagnose, prevent or cure disease with any of the information contained in this book and accepts no liability for you choosing to follow any recommendations. Consult your physician before following any recommendations in this book.

It is important to understand that the laws in the USA forbid me from being able to treat, diagnose, cure or prevent disease. The AMA has a patent on those words and only a licensed medical doctor can do that. And although it is legal for a licensed medical doctor to violate the Hippocratic oath and prescribe toxic drugs that cause harm and sometimes even kill patients, it is illegal for me to claim I can cure you using natural, nontoxic remedies, even though thousands of people can testify how they have been healed using natural remedies.

I am not a medical doctor. I don't want to be a medical doctor. I am a naturopathic doctor. The word "doctor" means to teach. When you come in to our office we focus on finding the cause of disease. We do not "treat" symptoms or "maintain" disease with drugs.

After we identify the cause of your disease we support the organs, glands and systems with natural nutritional formulas and detoxification therapies that balance the body. When your body is balanced, healing occurs and symptoms go away naturally, just as ants and flies go away when there's nothing for them to eat in a clean trashcan. If your symptoms go away, it's not our fault. We didn't cure you, your intelligent body responded naturally to the environment you chose to provide it. This is called health and it is your God-given birthright to heal any and every disease you may have developed according to the environment you provided for your body, mind, and spirit to dwell within.

Chapter 1
THE PULSATION OF LIFE

> **WARNING:**
>
> IF YOU WANT TO CLAIM IGNORANCE AND BE A POOR VICTIM THEN PUT THIS BOOK DOWN NOW AND DO NOT READ ANY FURTHER. SOME OF THE INFORMATION IN THIS BOOK MIGHT BE UPSETTING AND CAUSE YOU TO FEEL ANGRY FOR THE INJUSTICE BEING INFFLICTED UPON AMERICANS DISGUISED IN THE NAME OF HEALTH CARE.

> **"All truth passes through three stages. First, it is ridiculed; second, it is violently opposed; third, it is accepted as being self-evident."**
> Arthur Schopenhauer – German Philosopher

Are you sick and tired of being sick and tired? This book is for all the people who want to understand the mysteries of health and how the body truly heals. So many people want to understand why they are sick and what they need to do in order to heal but their medical doctor has failed to teach them what is causing their disease and what is needed to heal. They know deep down that the solution to solving their health problems is not a list of more adverse-reaction causing prescription drugs.

When you are fed up with your doctor playing the symptom chasing game with your health and each year the prescription list gets a little longer and your health gets a little worse then it is time to put a stop to the insanity. It is time for a change. THIS IS YOUR WAKE UP CALL. This book will give you what you need to heal. Nature's medicine doesn't harm your liver and doesn't cause symptoms worse then the one you are taking the drug for in the first place.

When your medical doctor starts prescribing new drugs to combat adverse side effects from the first one, then that should be a big flashing warning sign to wake up from your dream drug, fairy tale, health fantasy. It isn't working so let's stop the insanity and do something different, for crying out loud! The medicine that is supposed to be helping you is backfiring and causing more harm then good. My health isn't worth the risk to putting toxic drugs into it and playing Russian roulette in hopes that the side effects are not worse then the symptoms I'm attempting to cover up. What could possibly be more ridiculous then this insane paradox?

> **"Every drug stresses and hurts your body in some way."** Robert Mendelsohn, M.D. 1926-1988 - Former President of the National Health Federation and Author of Confessions of a Medical Heretic

Any one who doesn't have sense enough or intuition to feel and know that this feeble attempt to achieve optimum health is a laughable joke should put this book down now and stop reading. If your brain is so indoctrinated that you can no longer reason with good common logical sense, then you are wasting your time. It's no different than an atheist trying to prove to you that God does not exist as the two of you watch the sunset over the Cascade mountain range in Washington state with the majestic snowcapped Mt. Rainier towering over 14,000 feet high in the blue sky.

We are surrounded by intelligent life activity. Just south of Mt. Rainier is the Columbia River and each year millions of salmon swim from the Pacific Ocean up the Columbia, hundreds of miles to high mountain streams. Many swim up to the Snake River and then turn up the Salmon River where they miraculously find their way back to the very creeks and exact location where they were born. After the long journey back to their birthplace, they lay their eggs to renew the cycle of life. How do they know where to go to get back to their exact birthplace? Science doesn't have an answer. Obviously there is a governing energy field we haven't yet figured out.

> "We don't know a millionth of one percent about anything."
> Thomas Edison

The universe in which we live is governed by intelligent order. It is through this intelligence that we are living along with every other form of life including these amazing salmon.

Corrupt statistics and slick attorneys can prove just about anything, especially if large sums of money for their benefit are involved. We live in a world that is greatly influenced by money and not necessarily what is in your health's best interest. As you turn the pages you'll be met with common sense, health wisdom and natural remedies that have been proven effective. Healing comes on different levels for different people, there is no cure all for everyone. In our clinic we work with what each individual needs, not what works for fifty-one percent.

When someone is diagnosed with a supposedly incurable disease by their medical doctor and his or her plan is to maintain the disease with toxic drugs that suppress the symptoms without ever finding the cause and providing the individual with an opportunity to heal then that is when many Americans demand an alternative. When patients take drugs for many years and begin suffering adverse side effects from the toxic drugs, they become disgusted with modern medicine and demand natural alternatives. Within the pages of this book, you'll find the wisdom to put a stop to that foolish nonsense.

If you have been diagnosed with a disease you have two choices;		
1. Prepare to suffer	or	2. Prepare to heal

You are a Self-Healing Organism

> "Intelligence is present everywhere in our bodies…our own inner intelligence is far superior to any we can try to substitute from the outside." Deepak Chopra, M.D - Author of Quantum Healing

Your body is so intelligent that if you cut fifty percent of your liver out it will grow back again. As a matter of fact, if we keep cutting half of it out, the cells in the remaining half will grow and divide again and again until your liver returns to normal size. Just as your liver knows how to grow back, it knows how to heal.

God created and engineered your body to be self-healing when given the correct nutrients and detoxifiers. The stressors in the body, which we call toxins, must be removed in order for cells to heal. You can't feed your body Fruit Loops, Diet Cokes, Pringles, Twinkies, and Oreos and expect healing miracles. That is about as absurd as putting Kool-Aide in your gas tank and expecting your car to run. Your car requires gasoline to burn in the engine and your body requires living cell food in order to be healthy and run smoothly.

> "...a kind of super intelligence exists in each of us, infinitely smarter and possessed of technical know-how far beyond our present understanding." Lewis Thomas, M.D.

When we bring the body back into balance with whole living foods, addressing the cause with natural plant derived supplements, then we see God's miracles in action and it is called healing. This is how you were created and engineered to function by the Almighty Creator. The power is within you. You have a choice to suppress that intelligent power with drugs or give your cells the tools they need to heal.

> "Each cell is an intelligent being that can survive on its own, as scientists demonstrate when they remove individual cells from the body and grow them in a culture. ...these smart cells are imbued with intent and purpose; they actively seek environments that support their survival while simultaneously avoiding toxic or hostile ones." Bruce Lipton, Ph.D. - Cell Biologist, Stanford University School of Medicine

The Cell is Immortal

An interesting experiment was performed by Dr. Alexis Carrel of the Rockefeller Institute. He proved that the cell is immortal. He was able to keep tissue cells alive indefinitely by nutritious feedings and by washing away tissue wastes. As long as the tissue excretions were removed these cells thrived. Unsanitary conditions resulted in lower vitality, deterioration, and death.

> "Each cell of the blood stream, each corpuscle, is a whole universe in itself." Edgar Cayce - Diet and Health

Dr. Carrel proved how important it is for proper waste elimination by keeping a chicken heart alive for twenty-nine years until someone failed to cleanse its excretions. He concludes, *"The cell is immortal. It is merely the fluid in which it floats which degenerates. Renew this fluid at intervals, give the cell something upon which to feed, and as far as we know, the pulsation of life may go on forever."*

> **"Where there is perfect drainage, there is no death."** P.L. Clark, M.D.

Dr. Carrel was awarded the Nobel Prize for proving the cell is immortal. Why doesn't our current medical system focus on removing waste material from cells through the lymphatic system? Doctors focus on the heart and circulatory system but ignore the lymphatic waste removal system. If we truly had a health care system in this country then medical doctors would be focusing their efforts on the lymphatic system so toxins could drain from the body thus allowing our immortal cells to be healthier and live longer. Unfortunately prescription medication clogs the lymphatic drainage system.

Thomas Edison's Wisdom

> **"The doctor of the future will give no medicine, but will interest his patients in the care of the human frame, in diet, and cause and prevention of disease."** Thomas A. Edison

Many years ago a brilliant inventor, inspired from on high, came to revolutionize the world with his ingenious discoveries, one of which was the light bulb. Thomas Edison's genius and wisdom did not stop with electrical devices, he revealed truths in the field of health as well. Just as he invented the light bulb long ago, which still shines and illuminates homes around the world, he also pointed out to us some important facts about chemical drugs and the way our bodies heal.

> **"Until man duplicates a blade of grass, Nature can laugh at his so-called scientific knowledge. Remedies from chemicals will never stand in favorable comparison with the products of Nature—the living cell of the plant, the final result of the rays of the sun, the mother of all life. When correctly used, herbs promote the elimination of waste matter and poisons from the system by simple, natural means. They support Nature in its fight against disease; while chemicals (drugs), not being assimiliable, add to the accumulation of morbid matter and only simulate improvement by SUPPRESSING the SYMPTOMS."** Thomas A. Edison (1847-1931)

If you don't understand what Edison was trying to say then put this book down and don't waste your time, because you won't understand these profound health facts. Thousands of sick and diseased people have empowered themselves with natural remedies that feed, nourish and cleanse the cells which results in healing and healthy lives. Do you not deserve to live the life you love and love the life you live? Of course you do! It is your birthright. Now is the time to be made whole. Let's heal!

> "Truth wears no mask, seeks neither place nor applause, bows to no human shrine; she only asks a hearing." Eleanor McBean, Ph.D., N.D.

Being an engineering and scientific genius, Thomas Edison understood what it takes to make things work. Viewing the complexity of cells and how awesome the human body is, he knew that no scientist or doctor would ever be able to produce a chemical substance superior to what Mother Nature ingeniously produces in living herbs to nourish and detoxify cells of the human body.

Thomas Edison was able to accomplish so much because he was humble and teachable. He knew he didn't know it all and he was hungry to experiment and learn. With an open mind you can accomplish just about anything. Some doctors have so much education that they think they know it all. Too much education can make you ignorant and stupid if your attitude closes your mind off to other possibilities. Without an open mind there is no learning and without learning there is no progress. If we want to heal cancer we must look in a new direction.

Education is what someone else before you thought to be true and believed and embraced it as the closest thing to "the truth." They wrote it down and now you embrace it as the truth at this time. However, time has an interesting way of revealing our ignorance to us. For example, Christopher Columbus set out to prove "the truth" wrong. Despite the world looking flat and the masses assuming that it was, when Columbus sailed across the ocean he didn't fall off, but he proved the world was round. The truth all of a sudden was no longer believed. What "truth" do we hold on to now, will be proven false in fifty years from now?

Our beliefs change with age and hopefully the evolution of our minds progress upwards. For some this is called wisdom. For example, I once believed Santa flew through the sky in a sleigh and visited everyone in the world every Christmas Eve. Hundreds of years ago most of the world believed the earth was flat. Medical doctors used bloodletting to bleed their patients of bad blood. Why did doctors discontinue bloodletting? Because with time we have realized that bloodletting is ineffective and completely ridiculous. After attempting to bleed bad blood from patients, doctors would then give them a compound of mercury and chlorine called "calomel." Further investigation proved mercury to be a toxic poison. Ironically it's still used in dental fillings, vaccines and other so-called medicines. We believed and did some pretty atrocious and foolish things in the past. At the time, we thought we knew it all just like we do now. Time and experience will hopefully teach us wisdom so that we can let go of foolish practices that keep producing the same disastrous results. Think about it, if drugs really worked diseases would be on the decline not incline, right? Cancer would be on its way out, not increasing like kids with cell phones.

> **"Drugs do not – and cannot – heal, because a body that depends on outside control cannot be considered healthy."** Dean Black, Ph.D. – President of the BioResearch Foundation

Fifty years from now we'll look back and laugh at our foolishness for what we attempt to do now with man-made prescription drugs. If you could look through God's eyes, you would smile and patiently wait for experience to teach us a better way no different than patiently watching a six month old child attempting to crawl or a five year old daughter learning how to read. It is a learning process they are going through and they'll slowly progress with time and do fine. However, wouldn't it be great if we could avoid some of the frustration, bumps, bruises and accidents along the way? We all have our obstacles to overcome, but experience and time are great teachers. Unfortunately, science and medicine progresses funeral by funeral. You get to choose if you want your life to be part of their experimental "practice."

> **"What is attraction? What is repulsion? What makes planets run on scheduled time? Why cannot our scientists even run a train on two rails without accidents and destruction of life and property? What is man at best but a blunderbuss and a terrible sinner? Who knows the secret of the atom? Who has yet penetrated the secrets of a grain of sand? Who has solved the mysteries of a dewdrop? Ask a scientist these questions and in despair he is forced to answer what a kitchen maid would answer, "I don't know."** Dr. V. G. Rocine - Norwegian Homeopath

How Your Body Heals - One Cell at a Time

In the time it took you to read the last paragraph, about ten million red blood cells just died. Every four days you have a new stomach lining. Your body is constantly dying and renewing itself. Ninety-eight percent of the atoms in your body will be replaced within a year.

No doctor has to tell the intelligence within how or when to do this; it just knows and does it automatically–it's called life.

In Paul Bragg's book, *Toxicless Diet,* he explains that every three months you get an entirely new blood stream. Every eleven months every cell in the body has renewed itself, so you practically have a new body every eleven months. Every two years you get an entirely new bone structure, so in three years you really are born again…the renewal process has taken place.

> **"We are all elements of spirit, indestructible and eternal, and multiplexed in the divine."** William A. Tiller, Ph.D. - Department of Material Sciences and Engineering - Stanford University

If every cell within your body dies and is replaced with a new one within a year, then doesn't it make sense that those cells are only going to be rebuilt with what nutrition is found in the food you are eating? You are only as good as the food you eat. In other words, you are what you eat. Actually, it is more accurate to say, you are what you digest. And most of us have clogged colons and grease filled intestinal tracts that don't break down foods very well.

Your cells are like carpenters remodeling a house. Can they remodel if their materials are just as weak as the ones they are trying to replace? Can your arthritic joints become pain free if they never receive the raw ingredients necessary to build healthy tendons, ligaments, muscles and bones? Of course not. Only a fool would remodel his house using termite infested wood, old crumbly wiring and cement for the foundation that cracks and crumbles with the first cold spell.

Your body needs a continual supply of nutrition every day and the elimination channels must remain open for the waste material to come out. Imagine if you told your construction crew that no garbage or waste material could be removed from the house for a month while they labored. Within a short time there would be so much trash built up (scrap wood, sheetrock etc.), it would start interfering with their work progress. Most of our cells are trying to work, but they are loaded with garbage that prevents them from functioning properly. As a result, they become inflamed and this puts pressure on other parts of the body, which creates pain. The solution for pain is not more ibuprofen. Only a fool ignores his body's intelligent alarm system by taking painkillers for long-term use.

> **"Drugs never cure disease – at best they only suppress or alleviate the symptoms. Lasting results can be attained only when a wise doctor assists and supports the body's own healing forces, which institute the health-restoring process and accomplish the actual cure."** Paavo Airola, Ph.D., N.D. - World-leading authority on nutrition and holistic medicine

Warning at the Zoo

A city here in America has a wonderful zoo filled with beautiful, healthy animals of all sorts. The veterinarians are forced to understand health because if their animals aren't healthy, they lose their job. Veterinarians simply can't afford to perform bypass surgery and other expensive surgical procedures on animals like we humans do. They don't have a health care system like we do and they certainly can't tell the veterinarian what's bothering them. So what do they do to keep animals healthy in a zoo? They feed the animals a strict diet of foods that can be utilized at a cellular level. A sign posted near a junk food vending machine at the zoo informs: *"Do not feed this food to the animals or they may get sick and die."* Common sense flashes a red warning sign to alert us that maybe if this artificial food is not safe for chimpanzees and other animals that have similar digestive systems as humans, then maybe we should not consume it either if we want to feel well and experience optimum health.

> **"If you need a good doctor get a veterinarian; animals can't tell him what's wrong, he's just got to know!"** Will Rogers

We humans require living foods in order to continue life. We do not obtain the life force needed from artificial food colorings, preservatives, white flour and sugar. Every other form of life on earth depends upon their diet for health and strength and we humans are no different. Eating an unnatural diet leads to an unnatural lifestyle filled with disease and sickness that eventually ends in death.

Disease is a natural result of an unnatural lifestyle. In order for people to get well they need to take responsibility for the things they put in their mouths. Dr. Reuben exhorts, *"You lock your doors against thieves, don't you? But a thief will only steal your property. Shouldn't you lock your body against bad foods that will steal your life?"*

Don't Mess with Mother Nature

> **"We are part of the earth and it is part of us...for all things are connected."** Chief Seattle - Suquamish Chief 1786-1866

Acetone, acetaldehyde, methyl burrate, ethyl coproate, hexyl acetate, methanol, acrolein and croton aldehyde are all highly toxic poisonous substances. Next time you eat a strawberry it may surprise you to know that you are ingesting all of these poisonous substances. So why don't they poison us when we eat strawberries? Because, all of these substances, taken in a natural organic balanced form created by Mother Nature renders them harmless. The synergy created through nature's intelligence transforms these poisonous isolates into highly nutritious foods. Only when we start isolating certain substances from nature do they become poisons. Isolating ingredients to produce drug compounds which have adverse side effects is Mother Nature's way of shaking her head and cautiously reminding us that she put those ingredients together for a reason. Just because man hasn't evolved enough to comprehend that doesn't justify us tearing apart what she has created.

Carrot juice is high in vitamin A. If you drink a gallon of it, you will not overdose on vitamin A. However, take a whole bottle of man-made vitamin A tablets and you may. Why? One is natural and the other isn't. The body is capable of dealing with an excess of natural plant-foods, but synthesized chemicals can cause you to overdose.

Everything always doesn't necessarily have to be natural in order to be healthy. It just usually turns out that most natural remedies do not harm organs, glands and systems. EDTA (chelation therapy) for example, is not natural. However, it is an effective way to pull heavy metals out of the body and deplaque arteries. It is time to use what works as long as we do not harm the body and its cells in the process.

Cyanide – Friend or Foe?

> **"Amygdalin (Laetrile) appears to neutralize the oxidative cancer-promoting compounds such as free radicals. It's just one more key component for keeping cancer from growing or spreading. Contrary to what people have said about laetrile, amygdalin's former name, it should be considered an effective, entirely safe treatment for all types of cancer."** Robert C. Atkins, M.D. – Founder of the Atkins Diet

Inside the kernels of apricots and peaches is a highly poisonous substance called cyanide. The FDA says cyanide is a poison and has banned its use in most states. They are absolutely right. It is a poison. However, we are only being told half of the story. What they fail to report is that the natural cyanide found in apricot and peach pits is safe for us to ingest and poisonous only to cancer cells in the body. In other words, God created a natural cancer cure that is safe and harmless to healthy cells, but attacks and kills cancer cells. Wow, doesn't that sound like a dream come true? If you and your five-year-old granddaughter could go out to the apricot tree and collect the pits and cure yourself of cancer, then you could imagine what a nightmare that would be for the pharmaceutical company. Be assured they have paid the FDA to dig a hole and bury that information so Americans will keep on using their expensive chemotherapy.

How does the cyanide in the pits know to leave healthy cells alone and only go after cancer? The same way the sun knows how to rise every morning and something is telling your heart to beat this very moment to keep you alive. Just as salmon know where to go to spawn, bees know how to make honey and our skin knows how to knit itself back together and heal cuts because divine intelligence governs the universe. Intelligence in the universe is everywhere. We might make progress in our cancer healing efforts if we could stop thinking about profit margins for five minutes and use what God has already perfectly created in nature. Man comes along and messes everything up because of the almighty dollar.

> "It is still my belief that amygdalin (laetrile) cures metastases." Dr. Kanematsu Sugiura – Sloan-Kettering Institute for Cancer Research

Herbal remedies were designed by nature to be taken just as they are found, whole and perfect. Once they are chemically altered in a lab they become toxic and dangerous. Herbs are nature's medicine cabinet. God knew what He was doing when He gave Mother Nature instructions on how to create the perfect combinations of vitamins, minerals, amino acids, essential fatty acids and enzymes to make in potatoes, carrots, celery, gingko biloba, wheat grass, blue green algae, dandelion root, echinacea, etc. Naturally grown foods and herbs have been ingeniously put together to cleanse, nourish and heal the body. Drugs have no life force, no nutrition, and no enzymes, but herbs have them all. The various ingredients in herbs are placed there by a very wise Mother Nature, who works under the direction of the Almighty. These ingredients compliment each other in a health promoting way. Nature's balancing system is very accurate and when man takes it upon himself to improve upon God's creations, the results can be disastrous. Just look at how many emergency room patients have overdosed on prescription drugs.

> "The medicinal plants, or parts of them, must be used as they are found in nature. Extracts or active elements contained in them should not be isolated and then used, because secondary negative effects may result." Dr. Ernesto Comminotto

Graviola

A good example of how herbs work best when unaltered in a chemistry lab is the Graviola tree from South America's rainforest. Through a series of confidential communications involving a researcher from one of America's largest pharmaceutical companies, the Graviola tree has been studied in more than twenty laboratory tests since the 1970's and has proved to effectively target and kill malignant cells in twelve different types of cancer. It has tested extremely effective in destroying prostate, lung, breast, colon, and pancreatic cancers. The lab tests showed Graviola to be 10,000 times stronger than Adriamycin, a common chemotherapy drug, in killing colon cancer cells. Unlike chemotherapy, Graviola does not harm healthy cells. Much of this research has been done at Purdue University and Catholic University of South Korea. The (NCI) National Cancer Institute included Graviola in a plant-screening program which showed its leaves and stems were effective in attacking and destroying malignant cells.

One of America's largest drug companies tried for nearly seven years to synthesize two of the Graviola tree's most powerful anticancer chemicals. This company was investing a lot of time and money in searching for a cure for cancer while guarding their opportunity to patent it and make a fortune. The research was proving Graviola to be a cancer-killing dynamo. They had dollar signs flashing in their eyes with this potential gold mine. However, their research came to a screeching halt when they failed to create man-made duplicates of two of the tree's most powerful chemicals. Because federal law mandates that natural substances can't be patented, they would never be able to make the killing off of it that they hoped. Subsequently, the company shelved their research and hid it from the world.

One of the researchers couldn't keep quiet about the miraculous anti-cancer herb, Graviola. Understanding the company's goals to make big profits with a patent and their decision to hide the research from the world, he risked his career by reporting the pharmaceutical lab's findings to a company dedicated to harvesting plants from the Amazon Rainforest.

> "For the past fifty years I have been demonstrating that the use of natural nutritional treatment is and must be the most effective form of medicine and that when it is not used and the profession depends solely on the use of toxic drugs the results are abysmal." Abram Hoffer, M.D., Ph.D., FRCP(C)

Identifying the Problem with My Car

I pulled my car into the parking lot of AutoZone. It was sick and I was tired of being stranded when it wouldn't start. Something kept draining my battery and I needed to fix what was wrong. I was fed up with masking the symptoms by having someone jump-start me every time I needed to go somewhere.

The AutoZone man wheeled out a computer device with a meter on it. He hooked it up to my battery and let it sit for a few minutes. He checked my battery and it was good, meaning it would hold a charge. But when he checked my alternator, there was a problem. It wasn't doing its job. It was failing to keep my battery charged and, as a result, draining my battery and leaving me stranded. I bought a new alternator and put it on my car and I was back in business.

Just as a skilled mechanic with the proper tools can identify the problem with a car and fix it, so can a doctor identify the cause of your disease and teach you what is needed to heal. Your health doesn't have to be a mystery. So many medical doctors run test after test and the results come back inconclusive. The disease maintenance system that you pay for is failing to find the cause of your illness, because they are not looking for it. Why? There's no money in cellular detoxification and nutritional therapy. Most medical doctors have no other training besides drugs and surgery. So, when you go into their facility, they will only find something wrong with you that they can treat with a drug or some form of surgery.

The following story will help you understand what I'm talking about when I say modern medicine maintains disease with drugs vs. focusing on healing the cause. Kim sent the following letter to me after working with her for about two months.

Case Study – November, 2006

After going to doctor after doctor I was diagnosed with Multiple Sclerosis in 1997. Most of the doctors I saw in the beginning didn't have any answers and pushed my problems and symptoms aside. After the final diagnosis, I was immediately put on Prozac. When I asked why, they stated that all MS patients are put on an antidepressant medication. I was also prescribed a daily injection of Copaxone (MS medication). I had allergic reactions to this and was taken off the Copaxone and given Avonex (a once a week injection). It had many side effects, the worst being flu like symptoms, leaving me unable to function for twenty-four full hours. Although it was a once-a-week injection, I had one neurologist have me take it twice a week. For a period of about two years on this injection, I was having one MS exacerbation after another. For each exacerbation, I was put on Solu-Medrol and Prednisone. More side effects followed.

This wasn't working, so I was put on another injection, Beta-Serone. Along with the Beta-Serone, I was also taking eight other prescriptions to counteract the adverse side effects and also as precautions for any other symptoms. I slowly took myself off these medications because they weren't helping. They were causing more problems and every time I mentioned those problems, the doctor's answer was just more prescriptions. I eventually built up antibodies to the Beta-Serone.

During all this time, I was also having migraine headaches. Every doctor I went to was willing to write me at least three prescriptions just for migraines. When I asked to be tested to find the cause of the migraines, their responses were, "That will take too long. Just take the medicine prescribed and it will help you sleep off the migraine." No real answers except, "the cause of the migraines could be many things."

I was tired of getting no results and a bunch of prescriptions that would make me feel worse and not help the problem. It was then that I spoke with a friend who told me about Dr. Sainsbury. I set up an appointment immediately.

I had my first appointment with Dr. Sainsbury on September 23, 2006. I was amazed at what he found and the explanations given to me about everything. It all made sense finally.

When I was a child and went for the required school physicals, I was told that I may have a sluggish thyroid, but not to worry, it was nothing. Dr. Sainsbury found an energetic disturbance with my thyroid, without me telling him about it. It was something that I had forgotten about but he found it to be part of the cause of my problems.

The CEDSA (Computerized Electrodermal Stress Analysis) test results showed the migraines, my Raynaud's Phenomenon, female problems, constant metallic taste in mouth, etc., were caused from toxins and nutritional deficiencies in my body. Dr. Sainsbury gave me a plan to balance and heal my body, which included nutritional supplements, herbs and homeopathic remedies to detoxify the mercury, copper, nickel, candida yeast and parasites out that were showing up as the cause of my symptoms. Dr. Sainsbury recommended I have my metal dental fillings removed and replaced with composites.

When I left the exam, I was in tears. For the first time in years, I actually had answers as to what was going on with my body.

Since I've been on Dr. Sainsbury's program and had the silver dental fillings removed, the metallic taste in my mouth has disappeared. Within just a couple of days of taking the supplements the difference I felt was amazing. **The heaviness in my legs was gone, the tingling in my hands and feet was gone, my leg spasms seemed to be gone and I was able to sleep through the night for the first time in years. And no migraines! All this without prescription drug side effects.**

A couple of weeks after seeing Dr. Sainsbury, I had an appointment with my neurologist, who had taken me off the Beta-Serone because the side effects were getting worse. I was getting physically ill after each injection. His suggestion was another type of injection, one that was just recently put back on the market after having been removed because it was causing more damage than helping. Two people died from taking it.

When I refused to take it because of that fact, he was upset with me. I explained to him that I was doing a detox/cleanse program recommended by a naturopathic doctor. He said I was wasting my money and I needed these prescriptions. When I told him how good I was feeling

> *from being on the natural program he shook his head, dropped my chart down, threw his hands in the air and said, "I'm done. There's nothing I can do for you. You'll have to find another doctor." I walked out of that office without a handful of prescriptions and knew I did the right thing.*
>
> *Another benefit from doing the detox and cleansing that I didn't expect was that my hair was coming back. Years ago, my hair had slowly been falling out, and I was told there was nothing that could be done about it, it was just a fact of life. But now, little by little, it's coming back.*
>
> *For the first time in years, I have a doctor who hears what I'm saying and has answers and solutions for me. I feel like I'm living now and not merely existing. I'm not just another prescription.*
>
> *Thank you Dr. Sainsbury*
> *Kim Powell*
> *Newnan, Georgia*
>
>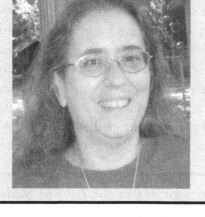

Kim is one of many who was disgusted with her medical doctor's drugs because they didn't work for her and the side effects were devastating. What kind of doctor would get mad enough to throw her chart down and quit when she was feeling so much better? What kind of doctor isn't interested in seeing his patients get well so they don't have to be a slave to expensive toxic drugs? Is he a doctor or a drug-dealing pimp working for the pharmaceutical industry? Kim told me that one of her prescriptions, Beta-Seron injection, was costing her $1700 a month and causing her to be nauseated for the next twenty-four hours!

After performing a CEDSA exam and balancing her energetically with natural nutritional and detoxification formulas, she is healing. Symptoms are fading away as we focus on healing the cause rather then suppressing symptoms with drugs.

When Kim first came to see us we checked her and she had three major issues causing imbalances in her body. These three issues were her thyroid, nervous system and intestinal tract. She is doing ninety percent better, since we have focused on balancing those three areas.

For those who are sick and tired of taking drugs and feeling better for a short time only to crash again and start another vicious yo-yo cycle of more drugs, I invite you to practice what I teach. If it fails to empower you with health, then call me a liar and go back to dulling your God-given senses with man-made chemical drugs. The proof is in the pudding.

> "Do not be angry with me if I tell you the truth."
> Socrates 470-399 B.C.

Most of us did not get in our condition over night and most likely will not heal over night. When the train called disease is going down the tracks at fifty mph, it takes time to bring it to a stop and get it going in the opposite direction towards health. Be patient and consistent. A champion athlete doesn't win the first place trophy by skipping workouts, eating junk food and abusing his body. You get what you pay for. You get what you put in. You reap what you sow. There is no such thing as a magic cure for optimum health.

Doctors will cut out your gallbladder, uterus, tonsils, adenoids and appendix. Common sense ought to tell you that your Creator, All-Knowing God, might have put those things in you for a reason. Just because you are done having babies doesn't mean your uterus needs to go in the trashcan. Wake up to the sad reality that drugs and surgery is a business no different than selling used cars and cell phones. The goal is to make money, not necessarily to do what is best for your health. The more drugs and surgeries, the better business is.

> "When the dollar sign enters the field of health or religion, the sincerity and the love fade away." T.O. McCoye

Radio Signals and Energy

Our solar system is held in place through magnetic polarities. There are magnetic fields that go around the earth from North to South. Just as the earth has north and south magnetic poles, so does every cell in our body.

> "The thought wave is electrical. The energy coming from the eyes is electrical. Muscles work by electrical impulses from the brain. In essence, the human body is an electrical being, and our health, strength and endurance depend upon the energy currents that run through the body."
> C. Samuel West, D.N., N.D. – Author of The Golden Seven Plus One

Whether we understand it or not, we are electrical beings. Every cell functions through very minute electrical currents generated along the cell membrane by the sodium-potassium pump. Our cells have zeta potential, which means they have the ability to retain an electrical charge ranging from 70 to 90 millivolts. When we are sick, the electrical potential goes down. Cancer patients have been known to drop to 15 or lower. Once we lose our electrical potential, the lights go out and it's game over, we die.

In 1994 the Nobel Prize was given to Alfred G. Gillman of the University of Texas Southwestern Medical Center and Martin Rodbell of the National Institute of Environmental Health Sciences for discovering that the cells of the body communicate with each other by sending and receiving "radio" signals.

> **"Signal transduction is the single most important unifying concept in modern day biology and medicine."** Dr. Robert Bell - Head of the Department of Molecular Cancer Biology, Duke University

Have you ever been listening to the radio in your car and drive under a bunch of power lines and get static? Heavy metals and other toxins in the body cause cellular static. When cells do not receive the right signals, they begin to mutate. This is cancer. Make no mistake, cancer isn't a disease, it's a symptom of your cells not receiving the right signals. This is why it is so important to detoxify the body. If the cells can't communicate effectively, then we cannot heal. Any military officer knows that the key to winning a battle is to destroy your enemy's ability to communicate. Without cellular communication there is chaos, which means dis-ease.

Like a military unit caught in battle without a means of communication, it is easy to mistake your own men for the enemy. When cells do not get the right signals in the body, then like confused soldiers, they can begin attacking their own cells. Some examples of this chaos occurring are; ALS (Lou Gerhig's disease), multiple sclerosis, lupus, rheumatoid arthritis and other autoimmune disorders. We almost always see heavy metal poisoning as a culprit interfering with cellular communication lines in these types of illnesses. Where do we get heavy metals? Vaccinations, flu shots, prescription drugs, silver dental fillings, deodorants, beverages in aluminum cans, household cleaners, insecticides and the list goes on. We are surrounded by heavy metals and when they accumulate in your body and interfere with cellular activity, doctors label you with a disease. The name of the disease depends upon where the toxins settle and the manner in which they manifest themselves. So the bottom line to heal and get well is to identify what toxins are where and what does your body need to get rid of them.

> **"All matter is energy."** Albert Einstein 1879-1955

Energy has always been mysterious because you can't see it, but yet it is so powerful. The most powerful things in the universe are unseen. Through the ages, energy has been called many things. Some refer to it as life force or vital force, Christ called it light. The yogis in Eastern India call it prana and the Chinese refer to it as chi. Hippocrates called it "vis medicatrix naturae" (nature's life force). What you call it is not important, however, the reality is, it exists. Many things in our universe are an illusion, not that they aren't real, but that they are much different then what they appear.

> **"Body chemistry is governed by quantum cellular fields."**
> Murray Gell-Mann - Nobel Prize Laureate

We are told that everything in the universe is made up of atoms. Atoms are made up of electrons, protons and neutrons. Science acknowledges that some sort of "energy" is what holds the electron in orbit around the nucleus. The faster those atoms move, the more solid the physical object seems. For example, your desk isn't really solid, but it appears to you as a solid object because the atoms are moving so quickly. The way you see matter is an illusion. Your hands that are holding this book, the chair you are sitting on, the floor and walls around you, all seem so solid, practical and non-mystical. Yet, scientists have found that each of these is made up almost completely of empty space. For example, think of just one of the atoms that is spinning in the period at the end of this sentence. Yes, right there. Think of just one of the millions of atoms in the ink that made that dot. If we were to enlarge the nucleus of that atom to the size of an average orange, the electrons circling around it would be approximately four hundred miles away, with nothing but space in between. No other atoms are in there. And what is the nucleus? It is a universe in itself and is mostly space. Ultimately, we find all of these particles turn out to be no more than energy charges.

> **"Everything is energy. Nothing is solid. Everything vibrates at its own level of reality, and while form appears to be solid, a simple examination under a microscope reveals that that solid object is actually alive with dancing molecules vibrating at a little less than the speed of light and thus appearing to us to be solid."**
> Wayne W. Dyer, Ph.D.

Kirlian Photography

Semoyon Kirlian, a Russian scientist, helped us understand that each of us has an electromagnetic field, sometimes referred to as an aura, surrounding our bodies. Kirlian photography is a way to photograph these energy fields. Through special photographs he demonstrated that disease can be detected in the body's electrical field. Diseased areas of the body will show dark spots while healthy areas of the body will manifest different colors.

It is interesting to note that when Kirlian photography is used with individuals who are missing limbs, the electrical body still protrudes out from where the limb used to be.

> "All living organisms emit an energy field."
> Semoyon D. Kirlian, USSR 1900-1980

If you take a potato and take a picture of it with Kirlian photography you can see a beautiful energy pattern surrounding the living food. Put that living energy food into a microwave and heat it with microwaves for several minutes and then take another picture of it. After it has been radiated, the energy field surrounding the potato has been radically destroyed. It is chaotic, jagged and out of balance.

Harold Burr at Yale University studied energy fields around plants and animals back in the 1940's. He found that we all have this energy field that surrounds us. He taught that an electrical blueprint of the adult body exists at the earliest development, even at the stage of an egg. This electrical blueprint acts as a template that the physical body is destined to follow.

For more scientific research to help you understand energy there are some powerful books available. Two good ones are *The Body Electric* by Robert O. Becker, M.D. and *Vibrational Medicine* by Richard Gerber, M.D. If we are going to heal, it's time we start acknowledging the very energy that allows us to exist.

> "The energy field starts it all."
> Harold Burr, Ph.D. - Yale University

CEDSA (Computerized Electrodermal Stress Analysis)

Dr. Reinhard Voll was a German medical doctor in the late 1940's who was studying Chinese acupuncture meridians. Chinese medicine theory states that at specific locations on the body you have acupuncture points which are sensitive to energy. Just as the blood vessels carry blood through the body, the acupuncture meridians carry energy to every organ and gland. Improper flow of energy through the acupuncture meridians causes energy imbalances in the body that can lead to disease.

Acupuncture points are like lights on a Christmas tree. Each individual light on a Christmas tree is illuminated when electricity flows through the wire. Just as electricity (energy) flows through a wire to bring each light to life so does energy within our body flow through our meridians illuminating our organs and glands with life-force energy. This is what allows us to function and live.

Twenty of these meridians begin or end on the hands and feet. As a result, stress associated with the corresponding organs may be detected by testing indicated acupuncture points. In acupuncture, inserted needles in the skin at these points act as antennas which have the ability to bring energy into the body or release it, thus restoring proper energy balance so healing can occur.

> **"The magnetic electrical research field will come to prove that the human body is an electrical being and our health depends on the energy currents which run through the body."**
>
> George S. White, M.D.

An amazing experiment was done to prove the electrical energy flow in a living body. Chinese scientists attached wires to a person's body and generated enough current to light a small light bulb. We are electrical beings and when the electricity isn't strong enough to light up your organs and glands, you die.

> **"The physician should look for the force and nature of illness at its source. He is not to look to that which can be seen, for we are not called to extinguish the smoke, but the fire itself."**
>
> Theophrastus Paracelsus 1493-1541

Healing Poisoned Medicine

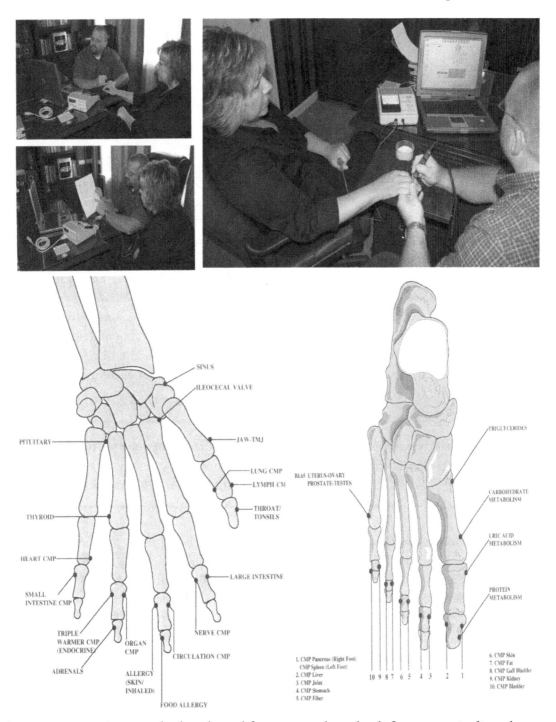

Acupuncture points on the hands and feet are used to check for energetic disturbances within the body. There is no piercing of the skin or electrical impulses felt.

Dr. Voll reasoned that if the Chinese really did have the energy meridians down to a science then you should be able to measure the electrical conductivity of the acupuncture points on the skin using a stylus-shaped electrode made of brass. What Dr. Voll discovered was revolutionary. His experiments proved that you could measure the body's ability to conduct energy. Testing healthy individuals, he found the electrical readings on acupuncture points to measure within a normal range while readings from diseased individuals revealed extreme high or low readings.

The second great discovery made by Dr. Voll was that medicines placed in the energy field of each patient would influence the acupuncture readings. Dr. Voll explains in his own words, *"I diagnosed one colleague as having chronic prostatitis and advised him to take a homeopathic preparation called Echinacea 4x. He replied that he had this medication in his office and went to get it. When he returned with the bottle of Echinacea in his hand, I tested the prostate measurement point again and made the discovery that the point reading, which was up to 90, had decreased to 64, an enormous improvement of the prostate value. I had the colleague put the bottle aside and the previous measurement value returned. After holding the medication in his hand, the measurement value went down to 64 again, and this pattern repeated itself as often as desired."* By using each individual's own unique energy field to test different remedies, we are able to determine which products, (herbs, homeopathics, vitamins etc.,) will bring that individual back into balance. CEDSA eliminates the guessing game as to what products are best for each individual to take as well as finding the correct dosages for each remedy.

> **"Electricity will become as ubiquitous in medical practice as surgery or drugs are; in many instances it will replace them."**
> Dr. Andrew Basett - Columbia-Presbyterian Medical Center

Scientific research has clearly demonstrated that pathways of energy (meridians) within the body can be accurately measured through electronic devices which use an Ohm meter. CEDSA has the ability to identify the cause of specific health problems by identifying which toxins are resonating in the body and which remedies would be best to pull those toxins out. Nutritional deficiencies can be detected as well and thousands of different products in the computer's library can be tested in a matter of minutes to determine which ones will be most effective to bring the body back into balance.

CEDSA is an instrument used to measure energetic stress levels and identify toxic or diseased frequencies resonating in your body. It works by holding a brass bar in one hand which sends three volts of electricity through your body. Of course nothing is felt because the current is so small. Pressing acupuncture points on the hands and feet with a probe allows us to measure energetic stress in the body. There is no piercing of the skin, discomfort or side effects. An Ohm meter is attached to the computer which informs us of the amount of energy resonating in that particular organ, gland or system. The Ohm meter has a scale of 0-100. A 50 reading indicates a good healthy balance. Any reading above 50 indicates inflammation in the area being tested. A low reading (below 50) indicates a chronic, degenerate state. As a result, stress associated with the corresponding organs may be detected by testing indicated points. For example, an inflamed prostate may register at 85 where as a cancerous prostate may measure at a sluggish 15.

> **"If we are beings of energy, then it follows that we can be affected by energy."** Richard Gerber, M.D. - Author of Vibrational Medicine

Conventional medicine uses electrical measurement devices similar to CEDSA. The electrical current of the heart is measured with an EKG, while electrical activity resonating in the brain is measured with an EEG.

Most of us are familiar with X-rays and MRI, but very few actually understand how they work. The electromagnetic energy in the X-ray frequency is concentrated in a specific area of the body and then collected on a photographic plate. The radiation is absorbed by various bodily tissues which create shadows to appear on the plate. From this, we are able to take a picture of the internal body and identify fractures and other health concerns.

MRI (Magnetic Resonance Imaging) occurs when a human or animal is placed in a tunnel surrounded by a strong magnetic field that aligns the nuclei of the body's hydrogen atoms. Then FM radio beams focused on specific desired areas cause a "resonance" of the aligned nuclei. When the radio beams are turned off, energy is emitted and the nuclei return to their normal state. Special sensors measure this energy and send it to a computer which produces three dimensional images of the body. This incredible technology allows us to see inside the body.

Only a fool would choose not to take advantage of such amazing technology when their health was at stake just because they do not understand how it works. How many times do you fly on an airplane but don't have the slightest idea how that hunk of metal actually sails through the sky at 500 miles per hour? How many people do not understand how light bulbs, television, cell phones, batteries, computers etc., work, yet use them everyday?

Computerized Electrodermal Screening works similar to these mainstream medical screening devices (MRI, X-ray, EKG, etc). However, there is an incredible difference. CEDSA can show energetic disturbances in the body before they become visible to the human eye. We can actually fix small problems before they become large problems that are much harder to correct.

> **"Do you remember how electrical currents and 'unseen waves' were laughed at? The knowledge about man is still in its infancy."**
> Albert Einstein

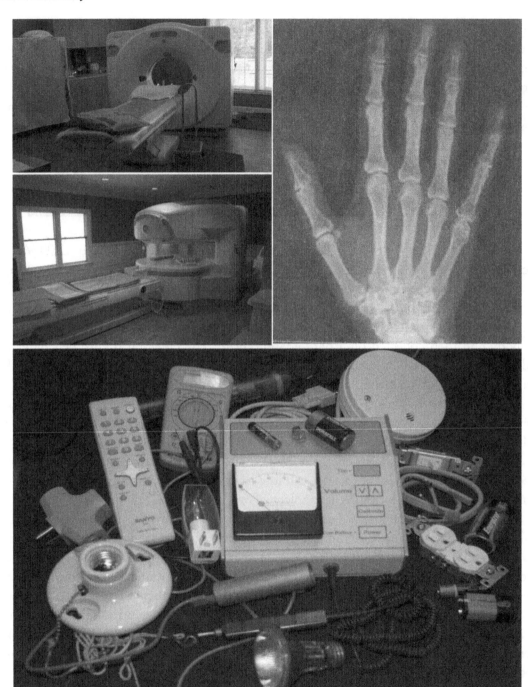

Modern technology allows us to photograph, control and test electricity (energy). Top two pictures - CT scan and MRI machine. Top right picture - An X-ray of a human hand.

> **"Diseases are to be diagnosed and prevented via energy field assessment."**
> George Crile Sr., M.D. - Founder of the Cleveland Clinic 1864-1943

At Harvard medical school a relationship was shown to exist between physical health and energy fields. A cell was found to be held in homeostasis at a certain electromagnetic frequency. When that frequency was altered either positively or negatively, and not returned to equilibrium within seventy-two hours, the cell died. Every health problem is primarily, therefore, an energetic one, which can be detected and influenced prior to physical manifestations of the condition. CEDSA provides us with vital information needed to make wise and informed decisions about our bodily needs and health concerns.

> **"Nothing exists except atoms and empty space; everything else is opinion."** Democritus of Abdera

Physics teaches us that every object on earth has a certain vibrational frequency that can destroy itself completely. Opera singers can shatter wineglasses when high notes are hit with the perfect tone. A plucked string on a guitar can cause another string on a different guitar in the same room to start vibrating. Would it not make sense that every disease resonates at a certain vibrational frequency? CEDSA is an electrical device used for identifying energetic disturbances in the body and which remedies are best for the individual being tested to come back into balance. Balance is the key to health.

> **"Future medicine will be based on controlling energy in the body."**
> William A. Tiller, Ph.D. - Nobel Prize Laureate, Department of Material Sciences and Engineering - Stanford University

CEDSA is on the leading edge of modern medicine. Standard orthodox medicine can only fix what has already happened. They can only cut out a tumor after it has grown. CEDSA has the ability to detect energetic disturbances in the body that favor the growth of a tumor. This is the future of medicine. There will come a time when we'll look back and shake our heads at the fact that for generations we let people get sick before we did anything to help them.

> **"Treating humans without concept of energy is treating dead matter."** Albert Szent-Gyorgyi, M.D. - Hungary (Nobel Prize Laureate 1893-1986)

Benjamin Franklin

Two hundred years ago Benjamin Franklin flew a kite and had an experience with lightning. The electrical energy in lightning had always been around, but no one previously had been able to capture it. When Mr. Franklin did, people said, "Well, Ben, of what possible use is this electricity anyway?"

Life force seems to be a subtle form of electricity that has about the same level of understanding that electricity had two hundred years ago. The possible uses of this life force energy could very well reshape the consciousness of humanity in the next hundred years more deeply than the use of electricity ever will.

> "If we worked on the assumption that what is accepted as true really is true, then there would be little hope for advance."
> Orville Wright – 1st Pilot in History

Have you ever had electrical problems with your car? You get in and it won't start? So you hook jumper cables to your dead car and connect the cables to the battery of a live car. You then turn the key and your car magically starts. Amazing isn't it? Energy travels through those cables and allows the dead to come to life. Energy (electricity) is an amazing thing. Imagine going back in time 500 hundred years and explaining this procedure. You might be hanged for saying such nonsense. We have a tendency to mock and ridicule that which we don't understand.

> "The mind is like a parachute. It must be opened to work."
> James Chappell D.C., N.D., Ph.D.

Energy is something we usually can't hear, see or touch but only a fool would argue that it doesn't exist. How about air? When's the last time you saw the air? When's the last time you grabbed a handful? Confine it and compress it into a rubber tube we call a tire and it will lift a 6,000 pound automobile.

When performing a CEDSA (Computerized Electrodermal Stress Analysis) we always check what is called "The Four Factors." This allows us to pinpoint the cause of the health problem. How do we expect to heal if we don't find the cause?

The Four Factors

> 1. **Organs** – We check the tissue energetically to determine if the organ or gland is resonating at a healthy frequency. A "50 reading" on the meter is considered a normal healthy state. Readings higher then 50 indicate inflammation while readings below 50 are more of a chronic degenerate state.
> 2. **Circulation** – Determines how the circulation is doing to that particular organ or gland. Calcium/arterial plaque build up can restrict blood flow to organs and glands thus starving them of oxygen and nutrients.
> 3. **Nerves** – Every organ and gland needs proper energy flow from the nerves in order to function correctly no different than the wiring in your house that supplies electricity to every light switch and outlet. Testing the nerve point allows us to check for emotional issues, subluxations in the spine impeding nerve function or an imbalance in the sympathetic/parasympathetic nervous system.
> 4. **Lymphatic System** – We always check the lymphatic system to see if the organs and glands are draining wastes sufficiently.

The blood and lymphatic system transports nutrients and also carry waste material out. If you kill cancer in the body but fail to eliminate it from your system, you're still toxic. When the lymphatic system gets sluggish, there is no lubrication. Without lubrication, there is no transportation. When this happens, cells begin drowning in waste materials. Swelling and pain are symptoms of an insufficient lymphatic system.

The following case study is a great example of how people who are sick continue to get sicker and sicker as their doctor prescribes more and more drugs without ever addressing the cause of their illness.

Case Study – June, 2006

In 1989 I started working for the State of Alabama with the Department of Human Resources. My desk was right beside the air conditioning vent and the carpet was always wet. I worked in an office with 80 other women and with them came an enormous array of perfumes, air fresheners, soaps, etc. I soon began having headaches. I went to my medical doctor who tested me and found nothing wrong. He prescribed antidepressant medication? I then went to an Ear, Nose and Throat Doctor who said I needed nose surgery. A couple of years later, that doctor was arrested for fraud. I then went to see an allergist and he put me on allergy pills and nasal spray. I continued to get worse.

Reed T. Sainsbury

I started having serious female problems. I would start hemorrhaging and have a period every two weeks. My doctor put me on serious painkillers that would knock me out for days. He put me on birth control pills, monthly shots and then gave me a hysterectomy.

My health went down hill fast. My joints started to ache to the point that I could hardly walk. I was diagnosed with arthritis. Then I started alternating between cramping with diarrhea, and bloating with constipation. I would throw up almost everyday. The doctor diagnosed me with IBS (Irritable Bowel Syndrome). My blood pressure shot up high, so he put me on blood pressure medication. Then I started getting a metal taste in my mouth right before I would have a reaction of joint pain, stomach pains etc.

By January 2006, my doctor had me on six different medications. I was taking a drug for blood pressure, arthritis, cholesterol, IBS, birth control and anti-depressants. I kept getting worse and worse and gained 35 pounds in three months. I felt so bad that many days I couldn't make it into work.

I did some research and found the only chemical allergy doctor in Alabama up in Gadsden. So I went to have all the allergy tests done. He found me to be allergic to almost everything inside buildings but nothing outside. I was diagnosed with MCS (Multiple Chemical Sensitivity). He told me that I was allergic to my environment and that I would probably be on disability within a year. He said there were people that were better off than me who were already on disability so I needed to get myself prepared. **He said there was no cure and it would only get worse!**

He put me on three different allergy drops (more drugs!) and told me to wear a mask and long sleeves. I had to get rid of all my chemicals in the house, quit wearing makeup and never dye my hair again. I did all this and kept having reactions.

In May my son graduated from high school. I went to the graduation and they had scented candles and flowers. All the chemicals in the air were more than I could handle. After 15 minutes I was so sick that I couldn't see or walk. My husband had to carry me out. I missed my only child's graduation!

I couldn't walk for three days. I went back to the doctor and told him what happened and he looked at me and said, "Well Kay, you've got to stay away from those types of situations." I couldn't believe it! I was 41 years old and I felt like my life was being taken away from me! One day my child would get married. Am I supposed to miss that too?

As I was leaving Gadsden, I was crying and praying for help. I saw a sign that said, "Natural Healing Clinic." I figured that I had nothing left to lose so I pulled in and made an appointment.

A week later, I met my hero, Dr. Reed Sainsbury. This man saved my life! I feel like I've gained 10 years to my life! There are only a few people who have had an impact on my life. Dr. Sainsbury is very high on that list.

When I came in for my appointment I had a reaction from perfume worn by another patient. I couldn't see to fill out the paper work and by the time I went into his office I was crying out of frustration. My hands and ankles hurt. I could hardly think. I was so tired of going to doctors and not getting well. I thought to myself, "This doctor is a quack, I'm wasting my money."

Dr. Sainsbury tested different points on my hands and feet with a probe and the computer would give different readings as to which areas of my body were balanced and out of balance. He found that my liver was very toxic and had an extremely low energy reading. He found that I was allergic to dairy products. He put me on a detoxifying and nutritional program with an emphasis on flushing out my liver. The next thing I knew, I was feeling better.

It's been a year and I'm able to do just about anything now. I'm off all of my prescription medications and feel great. I've started living life again. I've started dancing which was something I thought I'd never be able to do again. I'm even taking some night classes at the local college. It feels so great to be around the living again!

I went back to my old doctor, just one more time, for a physical. He asked me what I was doing because all my lab work came back good. No high blood pressure, no high cholesterol and I have lost 30 pounds. I told him about Dr. Sainsbury and showed him what herbs and other nutritional formulas I was taking. He looked at them and said, "Well, if you believe something works, it will." I told him, "Well – I believed that you and the drugs you kept giving me were going to work too!"

Kay Dement
Montgomery, Alabama

Kay's symptoms were not caused from a deficiency of drugs but that's all her doctors had for her. Are you like Kay, sick and tired of being prescribed more and more toxic drugs without ever finding the cause?

When Kay came into our clinic sick and frustrated, we went right to work to find the cause of her illnesses. Her allergy doctor told her there was no cure for her allergies (Multiple Chemical Sensitivity). Any doctor who claims there is no cure for a disease, does not understand the magnificence of the human body. If your doctor claims that there is no cure for your problem then maybe it's time to find a new doctor?

A toxic liver will many times cause allergies. Kay needed to flush her liver out and when we did her body responded just as it was engineered to do. Once we started cleansing her liver and the nutritional levels were brought back into balance, she got well. She made a liar out of her medical doctor. She is not on disability and she has her life back because we found the cause of her allergies. Are you satisfied playing your doctor's disease maintenance game with toxic drugs or are you ready to heal the cause?

If you want to get better, don't take no for an answer. You deserve to live your life to the fullest. Don't let anyone, including your doctor, tell you to settle. You don't have to settle. There is a way to heal. Use Kay as an example and don't stop until you are dancing again! You can heal and live the life you love. God created your body to heal naturally but it has to have correct nutrition and detoxification tools to work with. In case you haven't realized, diseases are not caused from a deficiency of drugs.

> **"There is a divine current within you that carries healing power."**
> Catherine Ponder - Author of The Healing Secrets of the Ages

Chapter 2
HEALTH CARE OR DISEASE MAINTENANCE?

A large percentage of Americans are tired of the prescription drug game. They want to fix the problem, not just suppress the symptom with drugs. It has been estimated by David Eisenberg at Harvard University that one out of three Americans has used some form of alternative medicine within the last year. Similar statistics reveal that thirty-seven percent of Americans use alternative medicine, and 41.9 percent of households earning over $100,000 per year with post graduate degrees use alternative medicine.

In 1990, according to The New England Journal of Medicine 328:4 (January 28,1993), 246-252, Americans made 425 million office visits to alternative practitioners. The fact that over 13 billion dollars was spent on natural healing, is evidence that Americans are fed up with the symptom suppressing game doctors play as they maintain disease but never address the cause so that true healing can occur. What's even more convincing that Americans are fed up with legalized drug dealers in white coats is the fact that 10.3 billion dollars was spent out of their own pockets because insurance didn't cover it! Wise doctors, who truly are interested in seeing their patients get well, address the cause of disease with natural remedies, diet and exercise and use drugs only as a last resort. Responsible Americans will not tolerate disease maintenance quackery. Drugless solutions to their illnesses are sought out and employed because their health is worth it.

America's Disease Maintenance System

> "Perhaps the words health care gives us the illusion that medicine is about health. Modern medicine is not a purveyor of health care but of disease-care." Carolyn Dean, M.D., N.D.

Americans spend over 500 billion dollars on drugs each year! That's a staggering number. Most medical doctors treat symptoms. They wait until something breaks down before anything is done. Then they cut, burn, radiate or poison it with drugs or chemotherapy. They treat symptoms. They fail to correct the cause of disease and rarely are there ever any preventative measures taken. They simply prescribe drugs to maintain disease symptoms. There is no correcting the cause so the body can heal with nutritional and detoxification therapies.

> "The intrusion of money into science means 'medicine' will never arrive at what truly works, unless they can patent it for maximum profits!" Joel Wallach, D.V.M., N.D.

In case you haven't put two and two together yet, this country has a health care system or better put "disease maintenance system," that is controlled and influenced by the almighty dollar sign. And if you don't believe it, try taking something natural, let's say an herb and start advertising that it can cure a certain medical condition. It won't be long before you come to understand that the AMA, FDA and pharmaceutical industry have a monopoly on maintaining disease in this country and have patents on the words diagnose, treat, cure or prevent disease. Any competition claiming to cure disease from a non-patented drug will find you in violation of their law. That is how powerful and protective of their monopoly they are. If they feel it a threat to their multi-billion dollar empire that has been built through their hard work and clever business tactics, then action will be taken to squash all competition.

The fact that they can shut down competition (anything natural besides patented, expensive and toxic drugs to be used by medical doctors to treat disease) is their fear-based attempt to maintain disease through prescription drugs with no intention of ever healing the cause. Who cares what is prescribed as long as it works right? If a group of doctors claim they can cure arthritis by using a combination of herbs, vitamins, minerals and enzymes and they are having a ninety percent success rate in doing it, then shouldn't insurance companies be in favor of it? Of course they should. However, they are not. Why? You have to see the whole picture to understand how the puzzle pieces line up. We'll address that corrupt, rotten sack of fecal matter later.

> "A free society, if it is to remain free, cannot permit itself to be dominated by one strain of thought." William J. Baroody, Sr.

Doctors who are truly committed to helping their patients heal recommend natural remedies that cleanse and nourish the cells, unlike drugs that add more toxins to the body and cause cellular acidosis, thus providing the body with the terrain that favors even more disease. These doctors have their hands tied in this country. They must prescribe drugs or else the "big boys" put the kibosh on those who step out of line. When doctors decide to stop poisoning their patients with toxic drug therapies, then the noose is cinched and they either "play by the rules," stop working with insurance companies, leave town, or give up their license. I personally know several good medical doctors who have been bullied around and persecuted to the point of giving up their license or leaving the country. It is a sad reality that you would hope would never happen in the great land of the free and home of the brave. How free are we?

> "None are more hopelessly enslaved than those who falsely believe they are free!" Johann Wolfgang von Goethe 1749-1832

If you visit some of the alternative cancer clinics in Mexico, you'll see how many doctors from the U.S. have left the great "home of the free," because they are not free to treat their patients using natural remedies that don't have toxic side affects like drugs do. Health care practitioners are not free to do what really allows people to heal themselves of disease. There is simply too much money involved in dealing drugs and maintaining disease by suppressing symptoms.

> "Unless we put medical freedom into the constitution, the time will come when medicine will organize into an underground dictatorship...To restrict the art of healing to one class of men and deny equal privileges to others will constitute the Bastille of medical science. All such laws are un-American and despotic and have no place in a republic... The constitution of this republic should make special privilege for medical freedom as well as religious freedom."
> Benjamin Rush, M.D. - Signer of the Declaration of Independence and personal physician to George Washington

Eliminating Competition

William F. Koch, M.D., was a famous professor at the University of Michigan, Detroit College of Medicine who had great success in curing cancer, especially leukemia. He had a forty-six percent success rate curing advanced cases of cancer and averaged a seventy-two percent success rate curing patients not yet in a terminal stage of cancer. He was using a formula he called "Glyoxylide," a nontoxic, oxidative catalyst which has the capacity to reverse neoplasms and viral parasitism. It works by restoring oxygen to non-oxygenating cells. The FDA and pharmaceutical industry found out about his formula and decided it was an infringement upon their multibillion-dollar cancer monopoly. He was arrested and put on trial. He had over 4,000 other doctors using this cure also. Two of those doctors came to the trial to testify in Dr. Koch's behalf. Both of them were mysteriously murdered. One was hit by a car and the other poisoned.

The cancer industry does not like competition. When something other than radiation and chemotherapy becomes a threat to their multibillion-dollar monopoly, they eliminate the competition. Dr. Koch won the court case but in the process was nearly assassinated thirteen times. He realized that he would soon be dead if he didn't flee the good ol' USA, land of the free (as long as you don't cure people of disease and take business away from the drug lords).

Dr. Koch found refuge in South America and continued helping sick cancer patients heal. In Brazil he was offered the highest position in the Brazilian medical services. Shortly after accepting that position, he was mysteriously murdered.

Those who don't want cures finally won and the Glyoxylide formula was lost. This was a blatant attack on freedom and health. Where were all the protesters? Of course, since the same group of people who had Dr. Koch murdered control the media, no mention was ever made about it. You hear the news they want you to hear.

A Cure for Cancer – Outlawed in the USA

> "The opposite of fact is falsehood, but the opposite of one profound truth may very well be another profound truth."
> Niels Bohr – Nobel Prize Winner (Physicist 1885-1962)

American medical inventor Raymond Royal Rife, created the Rife Frequency Generator-a device that transmits specific electronic signals to destroy cancer and other pathogens. How does it work? Every cancer, bacteria and virus resonates at a specific frequency. When a pathogen's specific frequency is matched with an electronically transmitted frequency, it causes the cancer cell or pathogen to explode from an excess of energy.

Rife found that by using his Frequency Generator on people who were infected with different bacteria like osteomyelitis (recurrent bone infection), viruses and other chronic infections, he could cure them just like he had with cancer. These pathogens could be destroyed when tuning in to the right frequency just as an opera singer shatters a wine glass by producing its resonate note.

In the 1940's, some people were getting excited about healing cancer using this technology. Milbank Johnson, M.D., wanted to know if the Rife Frequency Generator was a hoax or if it actually worked. He and his Medical Research Committee at the University of Southern California conducted the first and only study on it for a possible cancer treatment device.

Dr. Milbank took sixteen patients with terminal or "incurable" cancer and for the next three months treated them with the Rife Frequency Generator daily for three-minute durations. After three months of treatment, fourteen of the sixteen terminal cancer patients were declared clinically cured and in good health by a staff consisting of five medical doctors and Alvin Ford, M.D., group pathologist. Strangely enough, the cancer industry dismissed the research done by Dr. Milbank Johnson and the FDA outlawed the Rife Frequency Generator. No further research has been done on this technology that could very possibly help us heal cancer.

So why did research stop and why don't we use this nontoxic cure for cancer in the USA? The answer is simple. If you don't want a cure then you don't find one.

Uncovering a medical rat's nest we have found that authorities under the direction of Morris Fishbein, a highly influential editor of JAMA (the Journal of the American Medical Association) attempted to control the Rife technology by purchasing ownership. After being declined, Fishbein made it his mission to destroy Rife's cancer cure technology. It was no accident that a special laboratory built to study Rife's technology was mysteriously burned down after Fishbein's offer was refused. Rife was harassed and even taken to court on phony trumped-up charges and Fishbein himself was eventually convicted of racketeering charges.

So instead of using nontoxic, safe and effective cancer treatments in this country we cling to the kill, kill, kill approach with toxic chemotherapy. Why? Because the average cancer patient spends $175,000 for chemotherapy treatments. Treating cancer with chemotherapy is a money-making business. Curing cancer with energy frequencies doesn't meet the pharmaceutical industry's financial goals.

The Rife Frequency Generator technology is still used today in other countries where the FDA can't bully people around because it works. As a matter of fact, Geronimo Rubio, M.D., and medical director of American Metabolic Institute in La Mesa, Mexico uses the Rife technology and other nontoxic natural healing modalities in his clinic. He has an eighty percent success rate in reversing stage I and II cancers. For more information go online to http://www.amihealth.com.

> "The American public has no idea how politics secretly control the practice of medicine." James P. Carter, M.D. – Tulane University, Author of Racketeering in Medicine The Suppression of Alternatives

Americans Have the Most Expensive Health Care, But Not the Best

We in the U.S. are ranked seventeenth in life expectancy. Japan and Sweden are ranked number one and number two. It is interesting to note that their health care costs are fifty percent to seventy-five percent less than the U.S. Why is that? Japan and Sweden focus on prevention rather than disease maintenance.

> "There is only one thing more powerful than all the armies of the world, that is an idea whose time has come." Victor Hugo

A tremendous amount of money is generated through sickness and disease. Cancer alone is the second largest revenue producing business in the world next to the petroleum industry. By being sick and using drugs, you support the "disease maintenance" business. If America was suddenly to adopt the 10,000 year old system of traditional Chinese medicine and only pay the doctor when you were well and stop paying him when you became sick, doctors would learn real fast about safe, effective, natural healing or else go out of business.

Americans have the wealthiest, highest priced, most technologically advanced health care system in the world, yet we rank seventeenth in longevity and nineteenth in healthfulness. We spend over two trillion dollars on health care and our doctors write over three billion prescriptions each year. If we have the best, why aren't we number one? Perhaps we don't have the best health care system available? Maybe we aren't being told the truth about health and medicine? Could our search for health possibly be headed in the wrong direction?

> "America's health care system is second only to Japan, Canada, Sweden, Great Britain ... well, all of Europe. But you can thank your lucky stars we don't live in Paraguay!" Homer Simpson

What's going on in this country that is keeping us from being healthy? It doesn't make sense. It's about as ridiculous as a Ferrari getting beat by a Ford Pinto in a drag race. Something just doesn't add up. A century ago one in thirty-three people were diagnosed with cancer. Experts are now reporting that one in three Americans will develop cancer at some point in their lives and two thirds of these patients will die within five years. What is wrong? Do other countries have more intelligent doctors than us? Do they eat healthier or know health secrets that we "smart and educated" Americans don't? We have the most expensive health care system in the world, but not the best. Do you suppose money has an influence in our capitalistic society where prescription drugs are used extensively for every symptom you can say, write and imagine?

Would you be concerned if the nutritional formulas naturopaths recommended people take to get well sent over 700,000 people per year to the emergency room due to adverse reactions? That would be absolutely ridiculous now wouldn't it? An article in the Journal of the American Medical Association (JAMA 2006; 296 (15):1858-1866) reports that 700,000 people visit the emergency room every year due to adverse drug reactions. The fire alarm has been pulled for us to wake up.

In the South when tornadoes are a possibility, sirens go off to warn people to take cover and seek safe shelter. When your doctor prescribes a new drug you may be wise to look at the warning sirens that have been sounded in the Physicians Desk Reference (PDR) about possible adverse side effects. In order to list them all, it takes approximately 3500 pages!

You can call me conservative, but when it comes to my health, I don't like to gamble. I believe we Americans deserve medicine that doesn't harm and kill in the process of attempting to achieve health. Is not the fact that drugs have adverse side effects evidence enough that they are poisons and should only be used in emergency situations?

> "There is no such thing as a safe, harmless drug. All drugs, including common aspirin, are potentially dangerous."
>
> Paavo Airola, Ph.D., N.D.

In a disturbing article written by Barbara Starfield, M.D., MPH, professor at Johns Hopkins School of Public Health, in the Journal of the American Medical Association (JAMA) – vol. 284. No. 4 483-5 – July 26, 2000, the research reveals that our mainstream medical system kills 225,000 Americans per year. Considering that this figure does not include adverse side effects from drugs, only death figures, this is a shocking, red-flag-waving wake up call that something is terribly wrong with our lousy attempt to get people well in this country.

JAMA Journal of the American Medical Association) vol. 284 #4

Incidents Per Year
- **12,000 - Unnecessary Surgeries**
- **7,000 – Medication Errors in Hospitals**
- **20,000 – Other Errors in Hospitals**
- **80,000 – Nosocomial Infections in Hospitals**
- **106,000 – Adverse Effects of Medications**

Our way of practicing, but never getting medicine right, in this country is killing us. American medical doctors write an average of ten prescriptions per person every year in this country and it's slaughtering us. In 1991 Harvard University, school of Public Health study reported that 1.3 million injuries and 198,000 deaths occur in American hospitals each year as a result of "iatrogenic" or doctor caused problems and adverse reactions. Go online to **http://www.iatrogenic.or/** for more information. Dr. Sydney Wolfe (director of the Ralph Nader-founded watchdog group, Public Citizen Health Research Group, Washington, D.C.) in a 1993 news release stated that, *"300,000 Americans are killed each year in hospitals alone as a result of medical negligence."* In 2001 the California Sun newspaper stated that, *"Allopathic doctors kill more people than guns and traffic accidents."*

Carolyn Dean, M.D., and Gary Null, Ph.D., in Death by Medicine, Journal of Orthomolecular Medicine, 2005, report that 783,936 iatrogenic deaths occurred in America in 2005. This is catastrophic, outrageous and totally unacceptable. When the prescriptions that are supposed to help you get well end up backfiring and killing people, then it's time for change. It's time for a safer solution.

> **"When the number one killer in a society is the healthcare system, then, that system must take responsibility for its shortcomings. It's a failed system in need of immediate attention."**
> Carolyn Dean, M.D., N.D.

The New England Journal of Medicine says that adverse drug reactions occur in one out of every four individuals who visit their family medical doctor. (April 17, 2003 volume 348:1556-1564 number 16) Even more shocking is that USA Today states that adverse drug reactions are the fourth leading cause of hospital admissions. They estimate that 2.2 million Americans are so severely injured from doctor-prescribed drugs that they are either hospitalized for an extended period of time or permanently disabled. What a vicious cycle to get mixed up in! Go to the hospital to get well and the medicine they give you backfires and makes you worse. If you're a betting man, you might be better off playing the odds and just stay home and deal with your illness rather than play Russian roulette with their poisonous drugs that have a good chance of killing you or making you sicker than you already are. It's time to wake up, start thinking things through and take responsibility!

> "If you choose to go to a hospital, go into hospitals with your eyes wide open. Medical care, like so many other things, is problematic; it's not a sure thing. Patients must understand hospitals are hazardous and medical care is a dangerous enterprise – you must be willing to put a considerable amount of energy into self-protection."
> Lowell Levin, M.D. - Yale School of Medicine

Would you put your trust in an institution that accidentally killed 225,000 people every year? If Delta airlines killed 225,000 people each year from airplane accidents, would you risk flying with them? I certainly wouldn't let my children or loved ones take the risk. It's just not worth it. Unfortunately, most brainwashed Americans fall for it, hook, line, and sinker. They fall right into the trap like a desperate, non-thinking, stupid mouse who is pinned down by a metal hinge with its' greedy snoot on a piece of cheese. It got the cheese but now the metal hinge on the trap is suffocating the life right out of it. The mouse never saw it coming.

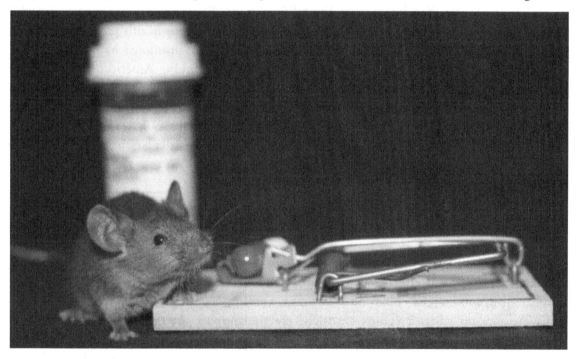

Are we Americans any different than greedy mice who fail to understand that if we mess with the cheese on the metal trap it, will release the spring and trap us down on the wooden block, suffocating the life out of us? Do we not see the consequences of our choices? Do we not care about tomorrow as long as we feel good today? Make no mistake about it, suppressing symptoms with toxic drugs and never addressing the cause of illness is going to have a price to be paid. The illusion created by a quick fix drug that the problem has been fixed is similar to the metal hinge crushing the mouse's neck. The metal hinge was never a threat to the hungry mouse until it snapped across its fuzzy neck when he took the bait. The man-made chemical drugs we take may at the time help us feel better, but the acidic terrain, clogged lymphatic system and toxic liver residue left behind may very well prove to be the metal hinge we never see coming that puts us six feet under.

> **"Basically you die earlier and spend more time disabled if you're an American rather than a member of most other advanced countries."**
> Christopher Murray, M.D., Ph.D. - World Health Organization

We are lulled into a hypnotic trance to follow doctor's orders to "take meds." These good-health fairy tales at the pop of a pill are seductively given to us every day in doctor's offices as well as the media. You know what I'm talking about. You can't watch TV at night with out seeing clever ads promoting drugs as the magic answer to your health problems, without changing diet, exercise and lifestyle. These laughable myths are promoted by pharmaceutical drug companies whose business relies upon obedient, nonthinking Americans (doctors and patients) who care more about the ball game on TV then their own health. One can't help chuckling when they start naming all the possible side effects which in some cases are worse then the symptom you are taking the drug for in the first place. What a joke! What kind of person would risk ruining their liver or kidneys with a particular drug to lower their cholesterol?

> **"There are some remedies worse than the disease."** Pubilius Syrus

As I sit here this evening I hear ads on TV by law firms inviting people who have taken Vioxx and suffered side effects to file a claim against Merck & Company. Ten minutes later another drug commercial comes on with some exciting new news for depressed males who don't measure up when it counts and need erectile support. At the end of this nice little spiel they report possible side effects. My favorite part of the whole commercial is when they say, "If erection lasts for over four hours consult your physician." My wife and I no longer bother going to the movies for a good comedy, we just watch the drug commercials at home and laugh up a storm. I can't help imagining the poor desperate man taking this drug and the problems he'd face at work in the office with his four-hour erection side effect. Cups of coffee being knocked over on desks and what not as he uncomfortably and embarrassingly promenades through the office slouched over like an old man trying in a feeble attempt to hide his drug induced problem. The poor fella could probably get his doctor to sign a note excusing him from work due to his unfortunate condition. What a joke!

Am I the only one who finds drug ads like this so ridiculously stupid that it becomes hilarious? It's kind of like stupid movies such as, *Dumb and Dumber* and *The Naked Gun*, that are filled with such absurdity and nonsense that it magically becomes hilarious. The only difference between stupid, funny movies and drug ads is that people know movies are just movies and not real life, whereas, despite the drug ads being ridiculously funny, Americans still continue to follow doctors orders and take the poisonous chemicals that have adverse side effects that may be worse then the original reason for taking the drug. And even more ridiculous is that they go back for more and more from the same doctor. At least mice who experience the force of a trap and somehow manage to get out are smart enough not to mess with it again despite a delicious piece of cheese tempting a hungry belly.

When are we going to wake up and get the joke that pharmaceutical drugs do not promote health. It's not funny anymore, 225,000 people are being killed each year and who knows how many are being harmed and are suffering from adverse side effects! It's time for change and you have a choice. What are you choosing? Knowledge is power. And with the knowledge of what things cause disease and which things promote health, you can begin to heal disease. You no longer have to be a poor victim, a helpless guinea pig for the doctor's latest drug experiments with the surprise side effects.

QUESTION:	Why are prescription drugs being advertised on TV?
ANSWER:	They want you to tell your doctor what you need.
COMMENT:	Too bad your doctor wasted all that time and money on medical school.

If medical doctors prescribed the right drug for each patient to be healthy, then why advertise prescription drugs? After years of medical school wouldn't you think your doctor would know what you need without some slick pharmaceutical advertisement persuading Americans to, "ask your doctor if drug X is right for you." If patients can learn about a new arthritis drug from a commercial on TV and then go ask their doctor for a prescription for it, then where is the expertise in that?

When someone comes in our clinic we perform a Computerized Electrodermal Stress Analysis to identify what nutritional deficiencies and toxins are causing their symptoms. We check each organ, gland and system to find out which areas of the body are most compromised. We only recommend each individual taking what their body needs to be balanced.

We have people bring in their bags of supplements all the time and ninety-five percent of the stuff they are taking they don't need for balance. Why? Because if it was working, they wouldn't be in our office with symptoms seeking our help.

> "The cause of most disease is in the poisonous drugs physicians superstitiously give in order to effect a cure."
> Charles E. Page, M.D.

The news media is highly censored. When you consider the pharmaceutical companies spend over five billion dollars every year on advertising alone, then you can bet the only reports you hear about in the mainstream media are the ones they want you to hear.

Our sick care industry only offers drugs and surgery for health. There is no nutritional or detoxification programs in mainstream medicine employed for people to truly heal. And the fact that the FDA has made it a law that, "Only a drug can cure, prevent and treat disease," is evidence enough of a conspiracy to maintain disease by suppressing symptoms and never address the cause so healing occurs. This is what Dr. Benjamin Rush warned us about. Americans will never be healthy and free as long as we are addicted to chemical drugs to make us function in life, legal or illegal.

> "During 1991 it is estimated that approximately five billion dollars was spent by the pharmaceutical industry on advertising alone to encourage us all to use these chemical agents in spite of the massive amounts of medical documentation and governmental investigation indicating the serious and very dangerous side effects they possess, in addition to their devastating addictive potential." George Berkley
> (Harvard University associated review - Nieman Reports)

The National Center for Health Statistics (vol. 54 number 19) revealed the leading causes of death in the USA for 2004. It is interesting how they conveniently left out prescription drugs as a major cause of death. The third leading cause of death, medical drugs, was added by the author.

LEADING CAUSE OF DEATH IN USA (2004)	
1. Heart Disease	654,092
2. Cancer	550,270
3. Medical Drugs	225,000

4. Stroke	150,147
5. Chronic Lower Respiratory	123,884
6. Accidents (Unintentional injuries)	108,694
7. Diabetes	72,815
8. Alzheimer's Disease	65,829
9. Influenza / Pneumonia	61,472
10. Nephritis (Kidney Disease)	42,7562

The most shocking fact in medical history is that the leading cause of death in the U.S. is heart disease, cancer and **PRESCRIPTION DRUGS. Prescription drugs are the third leading cause of death in the United States of America.** Can you believe that doctor-prescribed drugs kill more people than car accidents, AIDS, and street drugs combined?

> "The conventional approach of treating specific symptoms with specific drugs or remedies, without taking into consideration the patient's total condition of health and correcting the underlying causes of his ill health, is as unscientific as it is ineffective."
>
> Paavo Airola, Ph.D., N.D.

If the medicine you choose to take that is prescribed by your medical doctor is supposed to help you get well, but in actuality ends up killing 225,000 people every year who trust it and it tops the chart as the third leading cause of death, then something is terribly wrong. Anyone with an ounce of common sense would realize drugs are poisons and that they should be used with extreme caution and mainly in emergency situations. Occasionally, there may be a rare exception, when Mother Nature's remedies fail to produce the desired results and a drug may be needed, but that should be the great exception and certainly not the rule.

> "Only 15% of all medical procedures are scientifically validated."
> David Eddy, M.D., Ph.D. - Health Policy Research & Education – Duke University

Case Study – Aug, 2004

I was 16 years of age and had yet to begin my period. Out of concern, my mother insisted that I see a gynecologist. Upon my arrival to the doctor's office, I explained my situation and without question or hesitation, the doctor wrote me a prescription for birth control pills. Although I was somewhat concerned about taking the pills, the gynecologist insisted that my problem was "normal" and that the pills would be the solution. So, I started the pills and started having a period. I went to the gynecologist annually and was written another birth control prescription at every visit.

Four years later, and still on the pills, I began to get concerned for my health. My concern was not so much for my immediate health but, rather, for my future health. As I got older I realized that being on the birth control pills year after year could not be good for the future of my body. After bringing my concern to the attention of my gynecologist, she said I could try coming off the pills and I would, perhaps, be able to have a period without the aid of the pills. I did as she said and came off the pills. I did not, however, have a period. At the age of 20, after being off the pill and without a period for several months, I decided I had better begin taking the pills again.

Approximately one year later, I became aware of Dr. Sainsbury and his naturopathic approach to health. I went in for an appointment and he performed a CEDSA test on me. He explained in detail, the natural products he was giving me were to balance and support my endocrine system. After discontinuing the use of my birth control pills and using the natural products from Dr. Sainsbury, I began having a period. Once I finished Dr. Sainsbury's program, I continued to have my period. I am now over a year out of the program, I am on no herbs, pills or products of any sort, and I continue to have my period (like clockwork) every month.

I can not say enough about Dr. Sainsbury and the way that he has helped teach me the way my body is designed to work. The products he gave me helped my body heal itself, rather than simply concealing the problem with prescription medication. I highly recommend Dr. Sainsbury to anyone. I am a living example of the fact that it works!

Lauren Grier
Rainbow City, Alabama

Horse Urine for Health?

The hormone replacement drug, Prempro, made from pregnant mare's urine is a combination of estrogen and progestin that is reported by JAMA to develop Alzheimer's at twice the rate of those taking a placebo. (JAMA 2003;289:2651-2662) The Framingham Heart Study published in the 1985 New England Journal of Medicine showed that women who had taken estrogen were fifty percent more likely to develop heart disease. Evidence keeps stacking higher when JAMA 283(4):485-491, 2000 produced a study revealing that a woman increases her risk of breast cancer by eight percent for each year that she takes combined hormone replacement therapy. The National Institutes of Health have warned how Prempro increases a woman's risk of breast cancer, heart disease, and stroke.

Stanford University's pioneer in cell biology and former professor at the University of Wisconsin's School of Medicine, Bruce Lipton, Ph.D., explains how doctors prescribe synthetic estrogen that does not focus the drug's effects on the intended target tissues. He explains, *"The drug also impacts and disturbs the estrogen receptors of the heart, the blood vessels and the nervous system. Synthetic hormone replacement therapy has been shown to have disturbing side effects that result in cardiovascular disease and neural dysfunctions such as strokes."* He points out why iatrogenic (doctor caused) illness is a leading cause of death in this country, as we foolishly take drugs to suppress symptoms with no regards as to what the long term consequences may be.

> **"Given that hormone replacement therapy is known to be associated with serious increases in breast cancer, and may pose other risks as well, this trend is disturbing. Why aren't doctors making available the natural, plant-derived forms of estrogen and progesterone, substances that are known to have fewer side effects than their laboratory-produced analogs? The answer reflects the economics of medicine: Since the natural substances are not patentable, there is no incentive for drug companies to study their benefits, and so the vast majority of M.D.s, who get their information about drugs from the drug companies, don't even know about them."** Candace B. Pert, Ph.D. - Research Professor – Department of Physiology and Biophysics at Georgetown University Medical Center & Author of Molecules of Emotion

Dr. Otto Sartorius, Director of the Cancer Control Clinic warns, *"Estrogen (and its derivatives) is the fodder on which cancer grows."*

Some years ago, a book written by Dr. Robert Wilson, entitled, *Feminine Forever* was used as a marketing strategy to promote the use Hormone Replacement Therapy as a cure-all for depressed, unattractive, menopausal women. Dr. Wilson and his wife Thelma, who was a registered nurse, taught that menopausal symptoms were caused from a woman's ovaries not producing estrogen. Menopause is a natural change of life when a woman stops menstruating. However, Dr. Wilson and the pharmaceutical empire would have us believe it is a disease that must be treated with HRT. Entangled in this web of lies was the false theory that cancer, osteoporosis and other dreaded diseases were the result of a lack of estrogen. These scare tactics resulted in massive numbers of women beginning HRT.

Time has an interesting way of proving our ignorance. The truth about hormone replacement therapy began to surface and the Wilson's teachings began to crumble underneath their own feet. Dr. Wilson's wife, Thelma, who was on HRT, ironically developed breast cancer herself.

It turns out that Dr. Wilson was paid big bucks by Wyeth Drug Company to market his hormone replacement book. When it was all said and done, Dr. Wilson had received 1.3 million dollars from drug companies for his book encouraging HRT. After the pharmaceutical industry got what they wanted from Dr. Wilson, he was hung out to dry. His own son, Ron, tells how his dad was sued by several drug firms and eventually turned to drugs and alcohol. In 1981 Dr. Wilson committed suicide.

> "...much of what is called 'scientific evidence' is really disease mongering designed to sell more drugs." John Abramson, M.D. – Clinical Instructor at Harvard Medical School and author of Overdosed America The Broken Promise Of American Medicine

In the meantime, many women continue their hormone replacement therapy and gain weight as if they were pregnant, all the while ignorantly increasing their chances of cancer, Alzheimer's, strokes, blood clots and cardiovascular disease because a doctor told them to take HRT.

Why not just give the body what it needs to be balanced so that we don't have to fight the symptoms? Oh yes, I almost forgot, if you can't put a patent on something and sell it for $180 a bottle then why bother? The goal is to make money, not heal. Think about it. If medical doctors and pharmaceutical companies focused on things that actually healed you, then they both would be out of work. And the purpose for work is to make money, not diminish the possibilities.

When we feed the endocrine system with nutritional support so that the glands can work like they were designed to, symptoms clear up naturally. Many women are deficient in essential fatty acids which affects the hormones. Evening primrose oil helps balance out hormonal issues naturally. It is great for circulation, falling hair, dry skin and loaded with antioxidants. Doesn't that sound like a healthier choice compared to an unnatural drug that has unwanted side effects? Another big culprit causing female problems can be low magnesium and zinc levels. A few natural super-foods that help balance the endocrine system are; kelp, yarrow, dong quai, wild yam (natural progesterone cream), suma and maca. A CEDSA (Computerized Electrodermal Stress Analysis) will identify which remedies are best for your body chemistry to be balanced and symptom-free.

> "Doctors are always warning their patients about the dangers of consulting 'medical quacks' or resorting to 'unscientific, unproven remedies.' Meanwhile, they have made a living dispensing therapy from their own bag of unproven, unscientific, and often worthless 'cures'." Robert Mendelsohn, M.D.

The following case study is a great example of what happens when we give a woman's body what it needs nutritionally so the endocrine system can balance the hormone levels naturally without a bunch of toxic drugs.

Case Study – May, 2007

In March of 2007, my health began to deteriorate. My hair began to fall out and I started having miserable hot flashes around the clock every hour or two even while sleeping which made it extremely hard to rest well. I would wake up at 2:15 A.M. every night and it would take hours for me to get back to sleep.

When I first came to Dr. Sainsbury I had not had a menstrual cycle in over three months. Prior to my appointment with Dr. Sainsbury, I went in to see my gynecologist to check my hormone levels to see if I was experiencing menopause. The lab work came back completely normal with no signs of menopause.

My beautician, Ava Berry, told me about Reed Sainsbury, a naturopathic doctor who could help with these types of problems. I was somewhat reluctant to try this holistic health care, but decided to give it a shot since my regular doctor had no solution for my problems.

My first visit with Dr. Sainsbury was on May 10, 2007. After a CEDSA exam we found that I had several issues. He recommended a few herbal and nutritional formulas (including borage oil, Lunazon & Sumacazon) to bring my body back into balance. I began my nutritional program that same day and have not had one hot flash since!!! It worked that quickly for me. I started having my period again and since being on this program have had one each month. I began sleeping all night within a week, I do not wake up at 2:15 A.M. any more like I used to. I feel so much better and more rested during the day now. My hair not only stopped falling out but is so shiny and healthy looking now. Not only did the problems that I went in for improved but my joints that used to ache are better. My skin is no longer dry, it feels like I have lotion on even when I do not. My fingernails do not split and crack anymore, in fact, I have to trim them and I have never had to do this before! Constipation is no longer a problem either.

I had previously had a bone density test in 2004 which showed that I had Osteopenia. My GYN doctor prescribed calcium for me but I didn't take it because it caused constipation. In August I went in for my gynecological visit and another bone density test. When my bone density test came back this year (Aug, 2007) it showed improvement. My doctor was very impressed because he said hardly anyone my age shows improvement. He wanted to know what I had been doing that caused such remarkable improvement. I told him about the Liga-Plus formula and some other natural formulas for bones and joints that Dr. Sainsbury put me on.

After being on Dr. Sainsbury's seven week program I went back in for another CEDSA evaluation. Every point that was out of balance at my first appointment checked balanced, near perfect. I am so grateful for the opportunity to have met Dr. Sainsbury and heal my body naturally. Not only do I feel better physically and have more energy but I feel better mentally as well. I feel that my life is in balance. I am on a maintenance schedule now, but if I ever have a feeling of being 'out of balance' again, I know where to go. Thank you Dr. Sainsbury and Karen for your help and kindness.

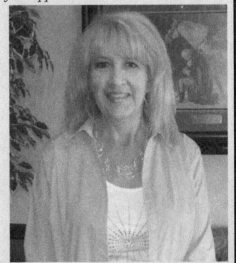

Leigh Reynolds
Hokes Bluff, Alabama

Dr. Semmelweis - Killed for Teaching the Truth

Back in the 1800's, before man developed the microscope to see the "unseen microscopic world of germs," there lived a doctor named Ignaz Semmelweis. He believed that infection was caused primarily from decaying particles of flesh carried on the hands of the physicians who failed to disinfect their hands after working with cadavers and then touched live patients. He discovered that just soap and water would not kill bacteria that was causing childbed fever. Dr. Semmelweis insisted that physicians (obstetricians) in his section wash their hands with his special formula he developed, a chlorinated lime solution to disinfect their hands after working on a cadaver and then moving to a pelvic exam on live patients. As a result of this, the mortality rate in his section dropped from 18.3 percent to almost zero.

What great news right? Simply wash your hands with this special lime solution that kills germs and save lives. What did the medical profession do to show their appreciation for such progress in saving lives? They mocked and ridiculed Dr. Semmelweis for such foolish nonsense. He was cast out and labeled a lunatic.

Although Dr. Semmelweis could not prove his theory true because microscopes had not been invented yet and despite the fact that mortality rates dropped considerably when physicians washed their hands in his special chlorinated lime solution, mainstream medicine rejected him for "going against the grain." He was hauled off and put in a Viennese insane asylum where he was tortured and beaten. On August 13, 1865, forty-seven year old Dr. Semmelweis died from internal injuries sustained from the guards at the asylum and no one at the asylum was held accountable for the abuse that cost him his life.

> **"Each progressive spirit is opposed by a thousand mediocre minds appointed to guard the past."** Maurice Maeterlinck

Most of his colleagues in medicine and even his own wife and children did not attend his funeral. They killed this doctor because he stood up for what he believed in and even had the success record to prove it, but doctors didn't want to hear the truth. How many ignorant and arrogant doctors today do not want to hear the truth?

It has been said that science and medicine progresses funeral by funeral and of course with the invention of the microscope we can see why one must disinfect their hands after working with cadavers and then working on live patients. Today, Dr. Semmelweis is honored as a medical pioneer and a hospital bears his name. They even turned his childhood home into a museum of medical history. I guess this is their feeble attempt to apologize for rejecting the truth out of ignorance and pride. This story is tragic. But my purpose for writing this book is to sound another alarm of tragedy that is occurring right now out of pride, arrogance and greed. Just as Dr. Semmelweis was ignored and ridiculed, so is natural healing spit upon and made fun of by the pharmaceutical empire and many medical doctors. People being healed of cancer, arthritis, diabetes, multiple sclerosis etc., by using natural nontoxic remedies is seldom given media attention and honor for its accomplishments. Instead, we are brainwashed into believing we must bow down and and worship the engraven image of prescription medication to "be healthy."

> **"There is a principle which is a bar against all information, which is a proof against all argument, and which cannot fail to keep a man in everlasting ignorance. That principle is condemnation before investigation."** Herbert Spencer 1820-1903

Murder by Prescription

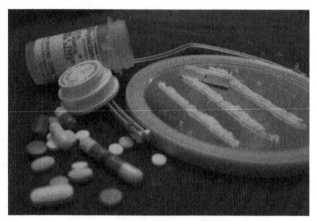

Medical science is constantly changing with time. What is the definition of science anyway? At what point do we really "know" how things are?

Before 1976 all medical books stated that the "thymus gland atrophies at puberty," implying that the body no longer needs it. When the 1980's came along our medical scientists said, "Uh, we made a mistake, that thing called a thymus gland, well it turns out that it is actually the boss of your immune system."

> **"There is nothing so powerful as truth, and often nothing so strange."** Daniel Webster 1782-1852

Fifty years ago medical doctors prescribed PCP, also known as "Angel Dust" and LSD. It was once believed to be safe and beneficial, otherwise our wonderful FDA and AMA surely wouldn't have let it go on the market now would they?

What about heroin, the first synthetic version of opium that was portrayed to be non-addictive cough medicine by the Bayer Company? It too, was just a matter of time and experience before it was discovered to be addictive and a bad news drug. The streets are full of this addictive junk brought to us by medical science at one time used for sick people.

> "We are prone to thinking of drug abuse in terms of the male population and illicit drugs such as heroin, cocaine, and marijuana. It may surprise you to learn that a greater problem exists with millions of women dependent on legal prescription drugs."
> Robert Mendelsohn, M.D.

In 1982, Eli Lilly invented an arthritis drug called **Oraflex**. He sent his drug reps out to convince medical doctors to start dishing the wonder pill out to the masses. This little terrorist in sheep's clothing caused kidney and liver failure. Approximately four months later, seventy-four people were killed from the once thought of safe drug. The FDA finally said enough is enough and the poison was removed from the market. Those poor seventy-four people were guinea pigs for the pharmaceutical company's latest attempt in creating another magic miracle pill that proved worthy of the trash can, not the human body.

In 2000, **Lotronex**, a drug used for treating irritable bowel syndrome was yanked from the market by the FDA after people were dying from taking it. Some had to have their colons removed after this chemical did cellular damage beyond surgical repair.

Reports identifying **Redux**, a diet pill, was the main suspect in killing 123 people. Obviously this outrage forced the FDA to ban it in September of 1997. Heart valve damage and pulmonary hypertension was detected in patients using the drug.

To demonstrate how much power drug companies have, an advisory committee even voted against letting the drug go on the market in the beginning. Obviously money talks and the advisory committee was ignored like a four-year-old child crying for candy before dinner. With dollar signs dancing in their heads, the drug went public. Unfortunately, the advisory committee had good reason to advise against the drug going on the market. It turns out they were right after all. Oops, I guess they owe an apology to those 123 innocent people they killed with their chemical death pill.

Posicor, a blood pressure medication found its way onto the doctor's prescription list. It is shocking to know that warnings from FDA specialists about adverse affects of the drug causing abnormal heart rhythm were ignored prior to Posicor going on the market. Data from the congestive heart failure trials were presented to the FDA Advisory Committee that showed more people treated with Posicor died than taking a placebo. The potential to make big bucks off this drug muscled its way through the warnings and it was finally approved to go public.

The results killed more than 200 people before it was finally taken from the market in 1998. Hoffman-LaRoche Inc., the manufacturer of Posicor, assured everyone that the drug had been proven safe, well tolerated and effective for use. They lied, 200 people were killed from taking the garbage.

Painkiller drugs harm the liver, cause constipation and do a lot of unseen damage at the cellular level. **Duract** proved to be no exception, despite FDA medical officer's warnings when it somehow slipped through the cracks and was being recommended by doctors who, (I hope had no idea) what this killing-drug was capable of doing. The drug was a suspect in sixty-eight deaths.

Diabetes is a favorite disease to treat with drugs for mainstream medicine. Dr. John Gueriguian of the FDA recommended not allowing **Rezulin** to be put on the market because it showed no significant advantage over other diabetic drugs and it caused inflammation of the liver. When a few key executives complained to high up FDA officials, Dr. Gueriguain was mysteriously removed from the approval process for this drug and it was allowed to go public in 1997. After 1.8 billion dollars of this liver-destroying trash sold, over 400 cases of liver failure and 391 deaths linked to the use of Rezulin they took it off the market in 2004. Dr. Janet McGill told the Los Angeles Times that Warner-Lambert pharmaceutical company, "clearly places profits before the lives of patients with diabetes." It was also reported by the Los Angeles Times that no fewer than twelve of the twenty-two researchers overseeing the diabetes study were receiving fees and grants from Warner-Lambert. Obviously, researchers that are paid by a drug company will have a tendency to make that company's product look good. Money motivates. For more corruption-exposing scandals performed by those dearly trusted researchers, read David Willman's article from the Los Angeles Times, December 7, 2003, "Stealth Merger: Drug Companies and Government Medical Research." The bottom line is that hundreds of thousands of dollars are paid by drug companies to research experts. It gets their products on the market regardless of how unsafe they are.

Propulsid was a drug used to kill heartburn symptoms. It not only got rid of the heartburn, it also killed the heart rhythm, which caused 302 innocent people to die. They finally took this killer away in July, 2000. Too bad they didn't spend more time researching this assassin and less time and money marketing it before it took the lives of innocent Americans who just wanted to get rid of heart burn when they laid down to sleep at nights.

Pondimin was a drug taken for weight loss, however it did more then destroy fat. It destroyed the heart valve and caused blood pressure to shoot up like fireworks on the 4th of July. In 1997 they finally decided to remove this destroyer from the market.

Allergies are a nuisance for many people. Instead of identifying the cause for the irritation and correcting it, the pharmaceutical industry manufactured **Seldane**. It stifled allergies all right, however, it also stifles the liver. When you shutdown your liver you die. In 1997 they realized that this liver damaging drug was too dangerous, so they took it off the market. What kind of insane ridiculousness is it to take something for allergies and end up destroying your liver so you die of liver failure? Wouldn't you rather live and just deal with sneezing and itchy eyes?

> **"Arrogant ignorance has followed science and medicine throughout history."** James P. Carter, M.D. – Professor of Nutrition - Tulane University

One evening I picked up the newspaper. On the fifth page of The Gadsden Times, September 29, 2002 it read, "Food and Drug Administration Recalls BAYCOL – A popular cholesterol-lowering drug." The recall notice informed that the FDA pulled **Baycol** from the market because it has been linked to at least forty deaths. It then went on to explain how the drug is linked to destroying muscle tissue which causes severe pain and eventually kidney failure and death.

Now doesn't that make sense, lower your cholesterol with this drug and ruin your kidneys, muscles and possibly die, but at least your cholesterol levels will measure right up to snuff on your doctor's chart. Come on folks, it's time to wake up. It's almost embarrassing to me that we Americans are so ignorant and foolishly desperate that we take harmful drugs in an attempt to achieve optimum health. Is any one thinking out there? Or are we already addicted, caught in the trap, pinned down by the metal hinge and just following blindly in a foggy drug-induced haze trying to make it through each day like hypnotized zombies?

> **"Ralph, what did you do (in school) today? Think or believe?**
> (Ralph Nader's father)

Are we thinking or just merely believing in what they want us to believe in? I hate to shatter the bubble you've been living in, but your health doesn't matter to them. What matters is the hundreds of thousands of dollars you will pay to take their toxic drug poisons for the rest of your life that never heals disease. And, as you take the poisons, adverse reactions will ensure you need more drugs to combat adverse side effects.

Eli Lilly, the founder of Prozac, who makes over $100 million every month off Prozac sales alone is a businessman who knows how to generate residual income. Despite over 20,000 Prozac related suicides since 1987 according to the FDA's own analysis, the drug remains on the market. (James D. Hagarty - Suicidal and violent behavior associated with the use of fluoxetine) Go online to www.hsph.harvard.edu/Organizations/DDIL/prozac.html for more details.

> **"A drug without toxic side effects is no drug at all."**
> Eli Lilly – Founder of Prozac

Vioxx and **Celebrex** are popular arthritis drugs that have also been linked to kidney problems and an increased risk in heart attacks. As a matter of fact, the FDA showed that people taking Vioxx increased their risk of heart attack by nearly 400 percent! Get rid of your arthritis pain and die of a heart attack. Who in their right mind would take this risk? The truth of the matter is when you start researching the possible side effects from different drugs, the wise person is scared into using an alternative, natural and safe approach. It's time to turn off the TV, do some homework and find a safe solution to your health problems.

According to an ad by an attorney in the Gadsden Times 2004, Vioxx, a Cox-II inhibitor, was estimated by the FDA to have caused 27,785 heart attacks and sudden cardiac deaths. The Associated Press launched a whistle-blowing article by FDA scientist, Dr. David Graham on January 3, 2005. Dr. Graham informs that the number of Americans who died or were seriously injured by Vioxx is 139,000, not the original low 28,000 outdated estimate. In September of 2004 the FDA finally pulled this poison from the market.

Hismanal, Raxar and Raplon are a few more killers that at one time were on the loose but have now been caught and removed from the market. To hammer a couple more nails in the drug coffin, these prescriptions were deemed safe at one time until these ticking time bombs exploded and doctors were given orders to stop prescribing the poisonous trash to their patients. What drugs do you take now that will be recalled in the future because they harm and kill, even though the FDA has claimed that they are safe?

> "More men die of their medicines than their diseases." Moliere

When the FDA approves a drug, it is supposed to be fully convinced that the drug is both effective and safe. Obviously, the FDA is failing miserably in their so-called attempt to keep us Americans safe from harmful drugs and foods. Perhaps a little money is nonchalantly slipped under the table here and there to make sure certain concoctions pass "the test" and make it to the market. Go to www.drugvictims.com for more medical mayhem.

> "If all the medicine in the world were thrown into the sea, it would be bad for the fish and good for humanity."
> O.W. Holmes - Professor Of Medicine, Harvard University

Vioxx – A Killer Drug

It is interesting to note that most drugs are not removed from the market until they have reached a high enough financial status to be worth the manufacture's efforts. For example, Merck spent 160.8 million dollars advertising Vioxx! So how much money did Vioxx make before it was pulled in September of 2004? Medical doctors began prescribing the heart-attack causing trash in 1999 and during their five years of prescribing Vioxx to their trusting patients it was a 2.5 billion-dollar seller! No wonder drug companies can afford to pay out millions to people who file law suits when loved ones are killed from the dangerous poisons that are supposed to help you feel better, but unfortunately cause heart attacks, strokes and death.

Why is it that doctors who prescribe these poisons not held accountable? Since our doctors have good malpractice insurance, and we trust them to always do their best regardless of how toxic the drugs are that they use, they become exempt.

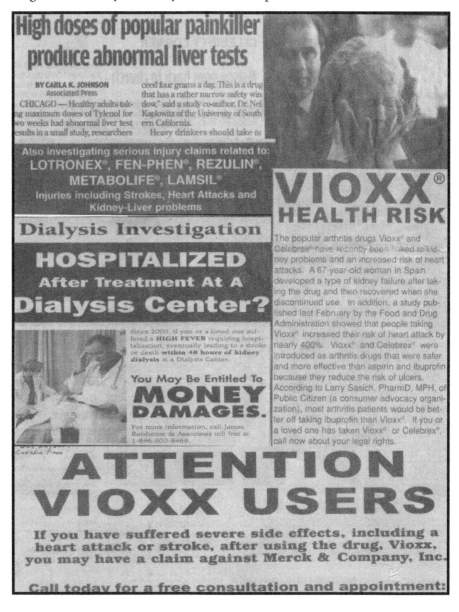

A disturbing event took place after the FDA came out with the recall notice for Baycol. Wouldn't you expect doctors to contact all their patients who they had prescribed Baycol to? Did this happen? No! When someone comes in our clinic with a list of prescriptions their doctor has them on, we always ask, "Did your doctor inform you of the possible adverse side effects of these drugs? Are you aware that the FDA has recalled this drug?" We are still waiting for a yes; unfortunately, it's always a disappointing "no."

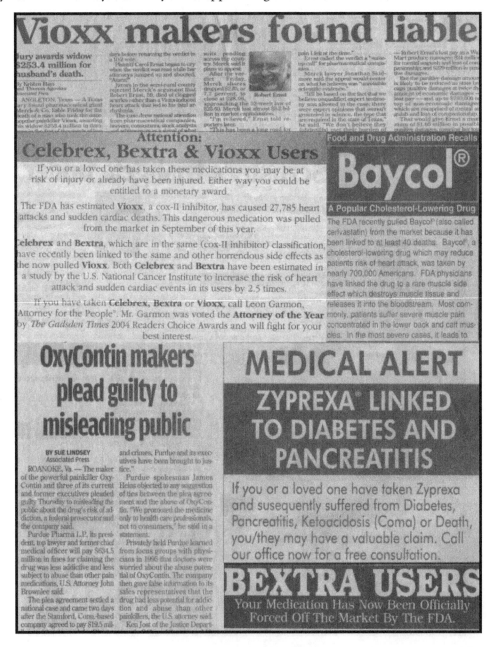

> "We are made in the image of God…popping a pill every time we are mentally or physically out of tune is not the answer. Drugs and surgery are powerful tools, when they are not overused, but the notion of simple drug fixes is fundamentally flawed. Every time a drug is introduced into the body to correct function A, it inevitably throws off function B, C or D." Bruce Lipton, Ph.D.

One of my clients went in for a shoulder operation. The doctors had him on a combination of drugs and when they gave him anesthesia before his operation his body could not handle it. The chemicals exploded in him like an eighth grade science experiment and when he came out of the operation it was as if he had had a stoke. When he woke up his speech was slurred, he was dizzy and his muscles were extremely weak. His doctor assured him that the anesthesia would soon wear off and that he would be back to normal. After days, weeks and months of no improvement they began running tests to find out what was wrong. He was later diagnosed with Lou Gerhig's disease and was told in a nice way to prepare to die, he had 18 months left.

It reminds me of an experiment I once saw with a two-liter bottle of Diet Coke and the candy called Mentos. Open up the Diet Coke and drop as many Mentos in as possible and the Diet Coke begins shooting uncontrollably in the air. I suspect the combination of drugs did something similar to this man's nervous system. What did his doctor have to say? "Oops, sorry."

When he contacted an attorney about the doctor/drug caused condition, the attorney did some investigation and informed him that it's very expensive to pursue these types of cases and rarely do they ever win. He was encouraged to drop it.

I guess that's what malpractice insurance is all about. It's the ticket to keep prescribing harmful drugs, but when these killers show their real face and finally harm enough people, the FDA takes the murderers off the market and the doctor throws up his hands and points his finger to escape responsibility and says, "Well, the FDA is the one who told me it was safe to prescribe."

Disease is really two words, DIS-EASE. Something is not at ease, it's out of balance and harmony. The solution is to identify what is causing it to be out of balance and correct that cause, thus eliminating the dis-ease. Usually, it is out of balance because of a nutrient deficiency and toxins built up. When you take a drug and your body attempts to break it down, you are left with an acidic, toxic, poisonous residue for your liver and kidneys to deal with.

> "As a young medical student, and even as a young doctor, I naively believed that the army of detail men who were on the road representing drug manufacturers were there to help me save lives. It didn't take me long to realize that this wasn't the primary motive of pharmaceutical manufacturers. They're out to make money and to make everyone think their products will save lives.
>
> ...I watched detail men march in my office,...Of course, they knew and I knew that many of these drugs were dangerous, untested on humans, and possibly ineffective for the purpose for which they were to be prescribed. As I got to know them better, many of them confessed that what they were doing made them sick."
>
> Robert Mendelsohn, M.D.

According to JAMA, May 1, 2002 (287:2215-2220) a group of Harvard University professors warn physicians not to prescribe new drugs because their safety has not been proven, despite FDA approval. To support their warning they point out that adverse drug reactions from FDA approved drugs are the leading cause of death in America!

> "There isn't a single medication on the market that couldn't be replaced by a botanical remedy." James Duke, Ph.D. – Ethnobotanist, Author of The Green Pharmacy

Terrorists Among Us

When used as prescribed, prescription drugs kill more people than car crashes, AIDS, street drugs and terrorism combined. The mass murders committed by prescription drugs every year that claims the lives of 225,000 people in this country alone is a terrorist attack that Americans need to wake up to. It's time to wake up and identify the enemy within our own gates before we grab our guns and run off to other countries declaring war and seeking vengeance and justice.

Synthetic drugs and the doctors who prescribe these harmful chemicals are murdering innocent people everyday and no one protests! These attacks are brutal because these "doctor-prescribed" remedies are supposed to heal. Unfortunately, they often harm and sometimes kill. They are the big bad wolves disguised as dear grandmother.

> "How modern medicine has come to be the number-one killer in North America is as incredible as it is horrifying. Doctors certainly don't think of themselves as killers, but as long as they promote toxic drugs and don't learn non-toxic options, they are pulling the trigger on helpless patients." Carolyn Dean, M.D., N.D.

When great white sharks begin attacking people in a particular body of water off the coast of Florida, they close the beach. After hundreds of thousands of people being attacked and killed by the pharmaceutical industry you'd think we'd wake up to the insanity and close the beach where these deadly toxic medications are coming from, right? Come on, we do it with shark attacks, drunk driving, three-wheelers, lead based-paints and any other thing proven to harm and kill. We don't even give motorists the opportunity to choose whether or not to wear a seatbelt, the law says "you have to." We use common sense for things that have proven to hurt and kill people in the past by banning them or inflicting heavy penalties upon those who refuse to listen. So why don't we do something about the deadly prescription medications? Why is it with drugs we choose to put our heads in the sand? The answer is found in your King James Bible.

> "For the love of money is the root of all evil..." 1 Timothy 6:10

Americans Demand Justice

When two jet planes deliberately crashed in to the World Trade Center towers on September 11, 2001 killing some 3,000 innocent Americans we clenched our fists, declared war on terrorism and came out fighting. The country jumped to its feet like Rocky Balboa battling for the world heavy weight boxing championship. Our founding fathers in America were fighters and that independent spirit has been passed down to us. On the radio we heard songs like Toby Keith's, *The Angry American*, which has been renamed, *Courtesy of the red, white, and blue*. The song's message is very clear. It warns terrorists that since you sucker-punched us from the back and picked a fight, the Statue of Liberty started shaking her fists. It carries on, "Justice will be served and the battle will rage, this big dog will fight when you rattle his cage, and you'll be sorry that you messed with the U.S. of A. 'Cause we'll put a boot in your ass. It's the American way." Fighting songs like this, kindled with revenge, echoed throughout the land.

We sent military troops and billions of dollars over seas and declared war, but when 225,000 Americans are killed each year according to JAMA from doctor prescribed drugs, nobody even blinks an eye. We accept it like a bunch of whipped dogs running with our tails tucked between our legs, afraid to ask questions and make someone responsible when a loved one is killed.

Are we intimidated by the schoolyard bully and afraid to retaliate? Do we want to put our head under the covers and hope the boogieman goes away? As Jack Nicholson plays colonel Jessop in the movie *A Few Good Men* he replies to Tom Cruise who plays a young questioning attorney, *"You don't want the truth because you can't handle the truth."* Some people are afraid of the truth because it hurts, not to mention how scary it can be, so they remain silent and do nothing, hoping the horror will magically disappear and they'll soon wake up and the nightmare will be over. By putting your head under the covers and pretending nothing is wrong, you support the insanity and corruption. Which corner are you in and whom do you fight for? Who do you serve? Who do you worship? Your actions speak louder than what you are saying. A wise man once stated, *"All that is required for evil to triumph is for good men to do nothing."*

> **"This collection of serial killers with reckless disregard for human life, extinguishes the hopes and lives of over 100,000 Americans every year. In the past decade they have been responsible for over one million innocent deaths, yet not only have they not faced justice, they have enriched themselves with profits that would make Bill Gates envious. These parasitic killers come not from some cave in Afghanistan, but from plush office suites…"** Jay R. Cavanaugh, Ph.D. - California State Board of Pharmacy (talking about prescription drug manufactures) DrugWar.com

Many years ago a Galilean witnessed corruption in the temple. Instead of turning the other cheek he made himself a whip, a scourge of chords (a weapon) and went into the temple and overturned the moneychanger's (bankers) tables and drove them out by force. Jesus Christ took a stand for truth and put an end to corruption in the temple. What are you choosing to do? Cowards always take the easy path. Judas Iscariot felt life wasn't worth living any longer after he chose the easy path. Then to deal with his conscience, he found a sturdy rope and a tree and did his business according to what he felt would justify his betrayal.

> **"Disease cannot live in a body spiritually and physically clean and well nourished."** LaDean Griffin - Author of Is Any Sick Among You?

Most people know deep down within that prescription drugs are not a wise investment for health. They openly admit it time after time. Divine intelligence within gives us this intuition, but most of the time it is told to, "Shut up!" because we are slaves to our flesh. We eat and drink what tastes good and not what our cells need. Many are addicted to alcohol, tobacco, sugar, coffee, painkillers, over-eating, laziness and anything else you crave because it makes you feel good at the moment, with no regard as to how we will feel later. Later may be the next day when we have a headache or the next ten years when we have cancer.

> **"No man is free who is not master of himself."** Epictetus

Almost every one knows that fruits and vegetables are healthy foods. But how many of us use them as the staple of our diet? Meats, breads, sugars, pastas, soda drinks, processed and artificial foods are the staple of most diets and the results are obvious as we stuff our faces with these acidifying junk foods that produce dis-ease.

Most Americans can name you all the diseases they have been diagnosed with by their doctor. It never ceases to amaze me that most consider themselves healthy despite being on three or four prescription drugs for different symptoms they have. "Oh, I'm healthy because my blood pressure, cholesterol, headaches, and depression are all maintained with my drugs," is a common response. Healthy people do not need drugs. If you take a drug to suppress a symptom then something is out of balance in your body. Something is dis-eased.

In our clinic we focus on balancing the body naturally and pulling the toxins out. By supplementing the organs, glands and systems with the nutritional formulas they require for balance and optimum health we find that people no longer need many of their drugs. Likewise, after we fix the problem, they no longer need the herbs either. However, a wise person practices preventative medicine by doing a few things to maintain good health, especially when the food we eat is depleted of minerals and other vital nutrients.

> "You need to be aware that modern medicine is biased, largely unscientific, extremely dangerous, and ignorant of therapies that really can improve your health with virtually no risk." Julian Whitaker, M.D. - Founder of Whitaker Wellness Institute & The Whitaker Health Freedom Foundation

The Truth Hurts

It would be nice if this book was a fictitious drama packed figment of my imagination and after reading it you say, "Boy that was a scary book," just like you do after watching a disturbing movie like *The Shining* where Jack Nicholson turns against his family and hunts them down. But because it is just a made up movie and didn't really happen we all come back to our happy little perfect reality here in the good ol' USA, where everyone has the best of intentions.

The sad, scary and startling fact that 225,000 deaths each year from medical negligence comes from JAMA (Journal of American Medical Association) is our wake up call to a failed system. These facts demand our attention and scream for you to wake up, no different than the good people of Asia who were caught off guard by the merciless tsunami that destroyed their communities and killed thousands. Different news reporters might tell different stories and statistical figures, but the facts are thousands of good people lost their lives. Only an ignorant fool would argue against the mass destruction of the 2004 Asian tsunami.

And now in 2005, Hurricane Katrina plowed into New Orleans and demolished the city and killed thousands. Fierce hurricanes are killers and so are doctor-prescribed drugs that are used to suppress symptoms, without ever addressing the cause of illness.

It's time to look at facts and logically think things through so you can start making informed decisions about your health and stop following blindly like a Black Angus steer to the slaughter house. His life will provide a few steaks and hamburgers for you and your friends to wolf-down when you get together for your next barbeque.

> "My People are destroyed for lack of knowledge." Hosea 4:6

Knowledge is power and as you turn the pages you will be empowered with information to heal. To be completely honest, the power to heal is already within you. Your Creator engineered your cells to be self-healing. All we need to do is to give the cells some tools to cleanse, nourish and regulate. Herbs and homeopathic detoxifiers are the tools we use to do that.

Some trusting Americans are so brainwashed about health that they can no longer think for themselves. We need to understand that no drug has ever cured anything. In fact, the only real difference between what we label a drug versus a poison is dosages and intent. Understand that drugs cannot build new tissue. Only food can do that. In case you didn't know, herbs are food. Herbs are loaded with nutrition; including minerals, vitamins, amino acids, fatty acids and enzymes.

If we want to be healthy, it is crucial that we understand the simple fact that the human body runs on nutrients, not drugs. Like a gallon of gasoline that has the potential to thrust a 3,000 pound automobile six miles into the air when extracted in the right form, so do herbs. When combined with organic, whole living foods and homeopathic remedies, healing miracles become possible. These living plant life forms contain the vibratory energy frequencies that are the tools for cells to heal. Packed with antioxidants these plants cleanse and nourish the body so it can heal itself of dis-ease. This scientific fact is deliberately withheld from young medical students for financial purposes orchestrated by the almighty billion-dollar pharmaceutical/oil industry that was started back in the 1800's by John D. Rockefeller, Sr. and I.G. Farben. There will be more on that later.

The Paradox of Modern Medicine

> "If modern medicine really cares about the patients it treats, it shouldn't continue to use questionable drugs and procedures until there is proof that they do kill people; it should be refusing to use them until there is proof that they don't."
>
> Robert Mendelsohn, M.D.

It's time to incorporate the, "JUST SAY NO TO DRUGS," campaign, they are too risky. When it comes to your health, you deserve something that is (1) SAFE and (2) EFFECTIVE.

The facts are; drugs are (1) DANGEROUS and (2) many times INEFFECTIVE with adverse side effects and (3) sometimes FATAL. It's your choice. It's your health. It's your life. You are responsible for you, not the man in the white coat that some bow down and worship. Wake up to the sad fact that the first thing a smart doctor does is buy malpractice insurance. Why? He knows the drugs he will be prescribing for you and your loved ones to take are dangerous, risky, will have adverse side effects and may prove fatal. His medicines cause harm and kill, but you are supposed to trust him right? Is this not a ridiculous paradox and obvious attempt for drug manufactures to make billions off of the ignorance of Americans?

> **"Every educated physician knows that most diseases are not appreciably helped by medicine."**
> Richard C. Cabot, M.D. - Massachusetts General Hospital

Pharmaceutical companies send their drug reps out to indoctrinate our medical doctors about their magical powers. Medical doctors relying upon what the pharmaceutical rep has told him then begins writing prescriptions like a thief writing bad checks in the night and you and your loved ones trust him with your lives. You crack your heels and salute when he tells you what to take to cover up your symptoms. Open your eyes to the business of disease maintenance.

> **"89% of doctors rely on drug company salesmen for their information."** The Australian Doctor 1989

I guess we can't blame the doctors. They only know what the pharmaceutical rep tells them about the drug. They weren't involved in the manufacturing of the drug so how would they know the possible disastrous side effects the little colored pills? They don't have a clue about the drugs they are told to prescribe, they just follow orders like any other successful company. They go through the different levels of command in order to market and sell a product for gain. If this were not true then why would doctors have prescribed all the drugs mentioned previously that have killed and harmed so many good trusting Americans? And why would drug companies need to advertise on TV and tell you to, "ask your doctor about it." Shouldn't your doctor be smart enough to prescribe what your body needs to heal?

> **"When 250 million people believe in a bad idea, it's still a bad idea."** Terry A. Rondberg, D.C.

It really doesn't make any difference which drugs the FDA approve and which ones they ban. The bottom line is, all drugs are toxic and will eventually begin to manifest their toxic side effects with use. Some may be visible and other symptoms may be hidden internally in the confines of the cells, only to come out in the form of arthritis, tumors or cancer later on. Remember, you reap what you sow.

> "Our figures show approximately four and one half million hospital admissions annually due to the adverse reactions to drugs. Further, the average hospital patient has as much as thirty percent chance, depending how long he is in, of doubling his stay due to adverse drug reactions." Milton Silverman, M.D. - Professor of Pharmacology, University of California

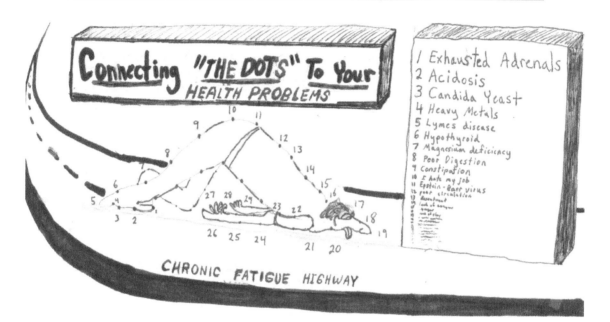

Most people never connect the dots of their drug-taking puzzle. Young children who are diagnosed with asthma get on inhalers and take drugs to help them breathe. After years of drug abuse, routine vaccinations and high sugar/white flour consumption, the pancreas cannot keep up with the body's insulin demand. The drugs burn the adrenal glands out like a flashlight that was left on all night at scout camp. Finally the body retaliates and the poor child is diagnosed with diabetes. Now the doctor displays his dis-ease maintenance plan and instructs the parent how to give insulin shots. No adrenal, liver and pancreas support is ever mentioned or prescribed. Why? Those are the organs and glands that malfunction when the blood sugar is unstable. The cause is never corrected in mainstream medicine because if it were, perhaps the body would no longer need expensive medication and routine checkups to maintain the diseased state for years to come.

> "The person who takes medicine must recover twice, once from the disease and once from the medicine." William Osler, M.D.

Are the experts protecting our health, or are we guinea pigs for the clever pharmaceutical chemists who make billions off their inventions in a lab while they addict the majority of our country to drugs? It's just a matter of time before these drugs harm, cripple and kill enough people before our so-called protective agencies (FDA) remove the foreign man-made synthetic chemical poisons from the market. But for every drug removed, there are hundreds more waiting in line for their turn to gleam in the spotlight on the doctor's list to be dished out to the masses. Have you ever wondered where all those free samples come from?

> "The people in charge (FDA officials) don't say 'Should we approve this drug?' They say 'Hey, how can we get this drug approved?'"
> Michael Elashoff (Ex-FDA Biostatistician)

The following story is a lady who has never even stepped foot in our clinic but through phone consultations I knew right off the bat what she needed in order to heal. And yes you are correct, the seventeen prescription drugs doctors had her on were killing her.

Case Study – November, 2003

In 1990, I was in a terrible car accident. I attended physical therapy three times a week for four months. I ended up needing TMJ surgery, the left side of my face was totally misplaced and the right side destroyed. It had to be totally rebuilt. After eating everything out of a straw – I recovered (or so I thought). I had to exercise for months to learn to open my mouth again.

Over the following years my health and well-being slowly went down hill. By 1995 I thought I was going crazy and becoming a complete hypochondriac! I was becoming sicker and sicker by the week. My co-workers, bosses, doctors and even my family thought I had just become lazy. I looked perfectly normal – I even ended up having a 3-year career as a professional model-well into my 40's!

Things got worse and I could no longer pretend, I was so tired, no energy. My Edema, Raynaud's (numbness), vertigo (loss of balance, ringing in ears), rapid-irregular heartbeat, skin rashes, headaches, lack of memory, acid reflux, stomach aches, inward trembling, hot flashes, night sweats and depression was unbearable. I started falling down, everything was spinning, each time I fell, I hit my head. I had aches and pains all over.

Eventually I lost my hearing (loud ringing in my ears was all I could hear), sight (only vague images), speech (thick tongue). My only comment in my memory was "what was I saying?"

I could no longer walk (I crawled), smell or taste food. My sense of touch was long gone. I was dying…

Eventually doctors diagnosed me with "Endolymphatic Hydrops/Meniere's disease" with some undiagnosed neurological disorder.

We (my husband and I – by now I was a crumbled ball of vomit) searching for a cure – he was told there was no cure – eventually all of my organs would just give up and die. He wasn't ready to let me go – I wasn't ready to go!!!

My daughter, Jennifer's college advisor, Joe Shinkle, told her about Dr. Sainsbury, a friend in Alabama who is a naturopath. My husband was reluctant, so many doctors, so little hope – NO CURES!

Dr. Sainsbury said he could help – but my husband had to commit to making sure I took all of my herbal/nutritional supplements, (I wasn't able to do anything on my own). My husband agreed! This was December 2002. I was taking 17 prescription medications at the time.

I improved by the week! It is now November, 2003 less than one year later. I am healthy, happy, strong, and full of energy! I am alive!!! I am off all my medication except for one.

Dr. Sainsbury saved my life!!! How do you ever thank someone for such a gift? In July of 2003 I was finally able to speak to Dr. Sainsbury myself…what does one say – the words truly do not exist!

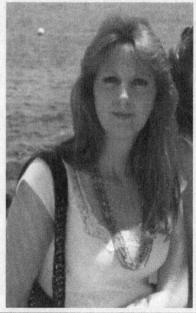

I will continue to keep his phone number by my side for the rest of my natural, healthy life! I have referred so many people. They are all so amazed at my recovery!

P.S. I have never even met Dr. Sainsbury. He had me fill out a clinical appraisal form and fax it back and then we would do phone consultations and he would send me the nutritional formulas I indicated I needed. There is no way to thank him.

Very sincerely, forever grateful,

Farrell Pelletier
Keizer, Oregon

How did we help Farrell to heal? The first time I talked to her and she explained her symptoms to me I knew her lymphatic system was not draining toxins which will cause many symptoms like Meniere's disease. Drugs shut down the lymphatic system. We put her on a program to drain the lymphatic system, balance her immune system, drain the liver, spleen and kidneys. While supporting her body to dump toxic drug residue, we also gave her nutritional support (wheat grass, alfalfa, barley, spirulina and other alkalizing greens to get nutrition into the cells. We supported her endocrine system and built her depleted adrenal glands back up along with increasing her circulation.

As we opened up her body's elimination channels and focused on getting toxins to drain out so that cells were no longer drowning in toxic waste materials, swelling and pain subsided. By nourishing her body with cell foods, healing occurred. It's really quite simple when you understand that all dis-ease is caused by **1. Malnutrition and 2. Toxins**. Focus on giving the cells what they need and stop playing the symptom-chasing game and healing occurs.

> **"A doctor's main focus should always be to get people off drugs and onto dietary supplements."** Carolyn Dean, M.D., N.D.

Every dis-ease can be healed if the cause/stressors are removed and the body is properly nourished. This book is dedicated to those friends who suffered and died because our medical system failed to address the cause of dis-ease. I am fed up with people coming in and saying, "My doctor doesn't know why I have such and such dis-ease so he prescribed these (toxic drugs) for me to try out to see if the symptoms will magically disappear."

We are long over due here in America for a change. It is time to stop playing the insane symptom suppressing drug game and start finding the cause of dis-ease and providing the body with what it needs to heal.

Hippocratic or Hypocritical?

> "The oath of Hippocrates requires that I administer no poisons to my patients even if I am requested to do so. The ancient teacher also advised his students that the first law of healing was, 'Above all, don't make things worse.' In a report from the World Health Organization, we are advised that one of every four people who die in hospitals is killed by the drugs he or she is prescribed. It is believed that this is the result of the physicians being unfamiliar with the dangers of the new drugs, which they freely prescribe. The 'pill for every ill' approach to disease has backfired. We are killing as many people or more with the "cure" as does the unchecked disease." Dr. Irving Stone 1903-1989

Last time I heard, medical doctors still take what is known as the Hippocratic Oath and promise to, (primum non nocere) *"First do no harm."* Hippocrates, the father of medicine, would be turning over in his grave if he knew that medical doctors swear an oath on his name to not administer anything harmful and then turn around and prescribe toxic drugs that have adverse reactions and kill 225,000 Americans every year!

Hippocrates was an herbalist and nutritionist. He believed in your food being your medicine and the fact that our toxic drug-prescribing doctors swear an oath on his name in order to become "legalized drug dealers," is the biggest joke in the world.

> "Drug companies freely offer this 'education' so they can persuade doctors to 'push' their products. It is evident that the massive quantities of drugs prescribed in this country violate the Hippocratic Oath taken by all doctors to 'First do no harm.' We have been programmed by pharmaceutical corporations to become a nation of prescription drug-popping junkies with tragic results. We need to step back and incorporate the discoveries of quantum physics into biomedicine so that we can create a new, safer system of medicine that is attuned to the laws of Nature." Bruce Lipton, Ph.D.

This book is an answer to Dr. Lipton's cry to create a new, safer system of medicine that is attuned to the laws of nature. It is absolutely shocking and outrageous to know that the third leading cause of death in the USA is the medicine doctors give that is supposed to make you well. It's about as ridiculous as an atheist who doesn't believe in God standing up in court and putting his hand on the Holy Bible and swearing to tell the truth, the whole truth and nothing but the truth, so help him God. He might as well lay his hand on a Playboy magazine, because God and the Bible means nothing to him or the moral principles found within its pages. He can swear to tell the truth all day long as many times as you want him to but it doesn't make a bit of difference if he's in court, church or a whore house because if you don't believe in God then there is no law and if there is no law then everything is legal. Why tell the truth or even attempt to do good unto your neighbor when you believe there is no Creator?

I don't understand how 225,000 innocent people (Moms, Dads, children and friends) killed every year because of the toxic effects from man-made chemical drugs is "doing no harm?" Is not this a ridiculous paradox? Is the whole nation so drugged up that we can't even logically think for a minute and put a stop to this medical genocide? Just one person killed a year would be harm, wouldn't it? Could you imagine the media attention and punishments inflicted if a naturopath, chiropractor, herbalist or homeopath killed patients with their treatments and procedures? It is a given, common knowledge, that we don't live forever and some sick people are going to die, but they shouldn't die from the medication that is supposed to help them be well, right?

Americans being killed each year due to medical negligence screams at us to wake up, we obviously aren't using effective and safe medicine. Ironically, doctors and their drugs do a lot of harm regardless of the oath that they take to practice medicine. Why even take the oath if all your remedies are poisons that have adverse side effects and kill some people?

> **"Those who have lived the longest seem to be those remote from medical practice."** Ruth Wegg, M.D. - University of Southern California

Heroes in the Emergency Room

In this country we have some great doctors, no doubt about it. Our emergency room physicians are brilliant geniuses when it comes to emergency situations and deserve the utmost respect. Let's give credit where credit is due. Do not be mistaken, there is a time and place for modern medicine. They save lives and help millions of people in emergency situations.

Car accidents bring mangled crushed bodies into emergency rooms on stretchers. Skilled doctors work fast and effectively to give each individual the very best. Their knowledge and skills alleviate pain and suffering and save many lives. In some instances surgery is absolutely necessary to save lives.

If it's a kidney or heart transplant then the body's T cells will recognize the organ as an illegal alien, and begin attacking it because it does not have the proper identification to be in the body. Your cells are highly intelligent and almost every cell has a protein molecule (MHC) like a flag on a ship to indicate what army he represents, so his immune system will know whether he is friend of foe.

Doctors administer a drug called cyclosporine which suppresses the body's immune system from rejecting the life-saving organ so we can live. What a wonderful blessing to have in emergency situations. These surgeons who are skilled enough to successfully achieve such a feat and use drugs to allow a successful transplant are truly awesome. The drug companies that have managed to manufacture drugs like cyclosporine to help save lives deserve to be applauded as well. In emergency situations is when drugs can be wonderful lifesavers. This is where prescription drugs are needed and should be used.

The problem comes when our non-emergency room physicians begin and continue to hand out toxic, cell-harming drugs for dis-ease maintenance year after year as the poor patient gets sicker and sicker. Doctors who never focus on addressing the cause of dis-ease with nutrition and detoxification routes are doing their patients a great disservice.

> "What hope is there for medical science to ever become a true science when the entire structure of medical knowledge is built around the idea that there is an entity called disease which can be expelled when the right drug is found?" John H. Tilden, M.D.

One of my seventy-two year old female clients reported to me that her doctor admitted that her diabetes medication has caused cirrhosis of the liver and has now sent her home to die with six months left to live. What an honest doctor should say is, "If you continue to take the toxic drugs I give you and follow my disease maintenance plan, you will die in six months." If your doctor gives you a death sentence or tells you there is no cure for your illness, then obviously you don't have the right doctor. Perhaps there is a chance to live following a different program that doesn't destroy your liver with toxic drugs and who knows what else.

> "I am dying with the help of too many physicians."
> Alexander the Great 356–323 B.C.

Could you imagine taking your car to a mechanic who says, "Sorry Lester, but we can't fix your Dodge Dart, you'll just have to learn to live with this problem and the best we can do is to keep this metal rod shoved in the carburetor. You'll have to adjust it every time you want to accelerate and decelerate but other than that you can still drive." No one in their right mind would buy in to that hunk of baloney. They would take the car to someone who could fix the problem.

Insanity

> **"Insanity is doing the same thing over and over and expecting a different result."** Rudyard Kipling

Are we insane when we continue to take our arthritis drugs that damage our liver and kidneys and eat away the lining in our stomach, causing ulcers and many other imbalances that we aren't even aware of and still suffer from arthritis pain? If it's not working why are we still doing it? Even if it is working and it magically suppresses our symptoms, do we not care about our long-term health? Are we so naive to believe that we can take man-made chemical drugs and escape pay-back day? It's time to wake up and use the round thing that God put on the top of your shoulders. Yes, I know it is a beautiful hat rack, but it does have other functions too.

The Cancer Industry

> **"It is my position that the truly healthy body and mind rarely need chemical drugs. Within each of our own bodies exists a far more powerful and efficient weapon with which to combat disease than any drug could possibly provide: the human immune system."**
> Jau-Fei Chen, Ph.D. Author of Nutritional Immunology

The hospitals are full of sick and dying people. Cancer is like a snowball rolling downhill, picking up more speed with each revolution second by second. In fact, every sixty-three seconds some American dies of cancer. By the time you finish reading this page someone else will have just died of cancer. Every day 1,350 people die of cancer here in the great USA. That's over 500,000 a year. Thirty years ago cancer wasn't so popular, but lately it has come in to style like bell-bottom jeans did in the 1970's disco era. A century ago, one in thirty-three people had cancer. Today more than one in three have cancer and it continues to increase each year.

Larry Dossey, M.D., former chief of staff of Medical City Dallas Hospital sounds the alarm for us to wake up. America's health care system is long overdue for a change.

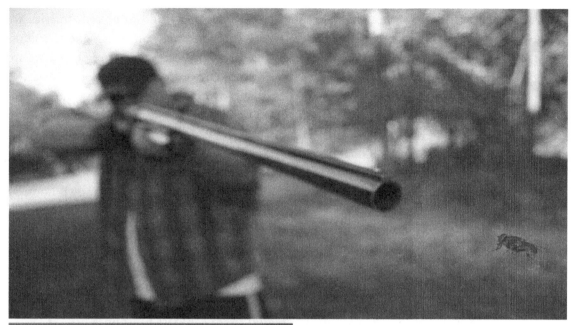

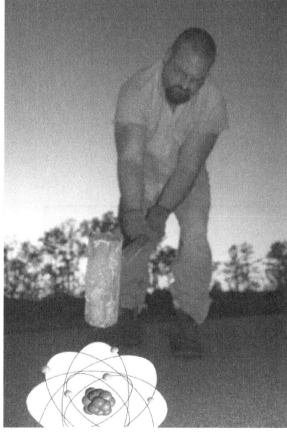

"One does not kill flies with shotguns nor manipulate electrons with hammers; and neither will many human maladies be 'fixable' with our current shotguns and hammers, our drugs and surgical procedures."
—*Larry Dossey, M.D.*

President Richard Nixon declared war on cancer back in 1971 and promised America we would have a cure within five years. He lied. After $200 billion spent on research, one-trillion spent on therapy and seven million casualties, we are losing the war. As a matter of fact, we are being slaughtered and throwing away money like a drunken compulsive gambler in Vegas.

Clifton Leaf, Executive Editor of Fortune magazine wrote an article, "Losing the War on Cancer," March, 2004. Hundreds of millions of dollars are being wasted by drug companies in pre-clinical models of human cancer. Leaf points out that just because a drug can shrink a tumor doesn't improve a person's chances of survival. What difference does it make if we can shrink tumors but the patient dies?

We are looking for a cure in the wrong place. The cure is found within your own body by having a balanced immune system. No man-made chemical drug will ever cure cancer, AIDS, a cold virus or any other dis-ease. Stop believing in that fictitious fairy tale dream that the pharmaceutical industry wants you to put your faith and money into.

> **"The significant problems we face cannot be solved at the same level of thinking we were at when we created them."** Albert Einstein

The only way to be healthy is by allowing your own immune system to work how it was designed to work. You can't, cut, burn, kill, drug and radiate your way to good health. Am I starting to sound like a raving lunatic? Good, because so did our founding forefathers when they declared war and won our freedom July 4, 1776. People thought Benjamin Franklin was crazy when he tried to tell everyone about electricity and they did the same with Thomas Edison when he talked about doing away with candles and using light bulbs. In fact every great invention or discovery you benefit from was probably laughed and scoffed at when it was first brought up.

> **"If everyone is thinking alike, then no one is thinking."**
> Benjamin Franklin 1706-1790

Modern medicine likes to ridicule any theory using natural remedies to build and balance your immune system because there's no money to be made at it. Some like to make fun of things that are beyond their money-driven, drug-indoctrinated mind's comprehension. They poke fun at things they don't understand out of ignorance and pride. And of course when the check they draw each week depends upon them not understanding something then that becomes the leash that leads them to research and study only topics that line up with that source of money.

> "Were it not for this immensely lucrative "malignancy market", the medical profession would have abolished slash-burn-and-poison (surgery, radiation, and chemotherapy) treatment long ago because the records of success simply aren't there. But the profits are, and these are too alluring for those in the cancer industry to turn down." Burton Goldberg Author of An Alternative Medicine Definitive Guide to Cancer

Don't hold your breath waiting for that same pharmaceutical gang who has wasted billions of dollars in the name of "cancer cure research," only to have cancer statistics still on the rise, to come up with a cure for you. Live your life to the fullest with no regrets so that when that day comes for you to fly on out of here you go in style and class leaving behind good memories. Remember, we all have the ability to make a difference if we choose.

Healing Cancer

> "Each one of us produces several hundred thousand cancer cells every day of our lives. Whether we develop clinical cancer or not depends upon the ability of our immune systems to destroy these cancer cells. That's because cancer thrives in the presence of a deficient immune system." Douglas Brodie, M.D.

When former chief orthopedic surgeon of San Francisco General Hospital, Lorraine Day, M.D., was diagnosed with cancer she had to make a decision about how to treat herself. Did she choose chemotherapy or radiation? No. Why not? She explains in her own words, *"Cancer doesn't scare me anymore. I had it...and got well by natural, simple therapies that you seldom hear about. I refused mutilating surgery, radiation and chemotherapy because studies in the medical literature and common sense told me that you shouldn't destroy your immune system while you are trying to get well."*

To order her videos on how she healed herself of cancer call 1-800-556-4846 or go online at www.drday.com. Any one with cancer who feels they need a medical doctor to tell them what to do and how to do it would be wise to watch her videos. They are simple, easy to understand and powerful.

> "Everyone should know that the 'war on cancer' is largely a fraud, and that the National Cancer Society and the American Cancer Society are derelict in their duties to the people who support them."
> Linus Pauling (Two-time Nobel Laureate)

Discussing cancer, Robert Atkins, M.D. informed, *"There is not one, but many cures for cancer available. But they are all being systematically suppressed."* The Lancet medical journal reported a study which compared chemotherapy and no treatment at all. The conclusion was that no treatment proved a significantly better policy for patients' survival and for quality of life.

> "My doctor gave me six months to live, but when I couldn't pay the bill he gave me six months more." Walter Matthau

James Hawver, N.M.D., owner of Standard Enzyme Company teaches that cancer patients always have four main issues:

(1) Poor circulation – arterial plaque build up/calcium plaquing etc.
(2) Acidosis – The body's pH is very acidic.
(3) Miasms – Inherited genetic weaknesses.
(4) Emotional issues – something eating them up inside.

> **The Nobel Prize was awarded in 1936 to Dr. Otto Warburg for discovering the cause of cancer. Do you know what causes cancer? Oxygen deprivation & Acidosis (Acidic pH).**

Tumors thrive in an oxygen deprived environment. Oxygen gets to cells via the blood. If your circulation is compromised in a certain area of the body, then most likely there will be low oxygen levels as well which sets the stage for cancer.

As mentioned earlier, an acidic body provides the environment to favor cancer growth. Cancer loves acidosis. Everything you eat either feeds cancer or fights against it. Sugar feeds cancer as well as weakening the immune system.

Cancer is no different than any other living form of life. Take for example tomatoes. What allows tomatoes to grow? Good soil, air, water and sunlight. Remove any one of those vital elements and tomatoes won't grow. Change the terrain in your body and stop feeding cancer sugar and starches and you'll starve it to death. Many people have cured themselves of cancer by changing their diet to only living foods with an emphasis on wheat grass juice, barley greens and sprouted grains. The Ann Wigmore foundation is a healing center that has helped thousands of sick people overcome all types of so-called incurable diseases by focusing on raw, organic, whole living foods.

> "My studies have proved conclusively that untreated cancer victims actually live up to four times longer than treated individuals... Beyond a shadow of a doubt, radical surgery on cancer patients does more harm than good." Dr. Hardin Jones - University of California

What a slap in the face to cancer treatment here in America! Dr. Jones, from the University of California is basically saying you'd be better off not going to a medical doctor for cancer treatment. The treatment is worse than the disease! Need anything else be said about our sick-care industry in this country? Obviously, there are exceptions to the rule and every case is different, but for the amount of our tax dollars that has been wasted by our government on cancer, it is an absolute travesty.

WHAT DO YOU THINK OF THE WAR ON CANCER?

- "...Largely a fraud." Linus Pauling, Ph.D., twice Nobel laureate
- "...a qualified failure." John Bailar, M.D., Ph.D., former editor of the Journal of the National Cancer Institute
- "A medical Vietnam." Donald Kennedy, former President of Stanford University
- "A bunch of sh_t." James Watson, Ph.D., Nobel laureate, co-discoverer of the DNA code

I grew up with Ada, Angela and Jeff. After high school, tragedy struck. They were diagnosed with cancer and died shortly after being diagnosed and treated by conventional medicine. How many people do you know who have died from cancer?

In naturopathy we believe there is a cause for the cancer. If a doctor fails to identify the cause and remove it, then the person's chance to heal and live is drastically reduced. Poisoning the body with chemotherapy is as ridiculous as spraying Round-Up weed-killer all over your lawn to get rid of dandelions. Of course you'll kill the dandelions, but you'll kill the grass too! Just as we don't want to kill the grass in order to get rid of dandelions, we don't want to harm your immune system with poison in an attempt to kill cancer, like chemotherapy does. Let's think before we begin poisoning the body with drugs.

> "If you rush to take it (a new drug), do so with the full knowledge that you are being a guinea pig. The longer a drug is on the market, the more will be known about the side effects."
>
> Robert Mendelsohn, M.D.

Poison for Health?

Chemotherapy, a descendent of chemical weapons and biological warfare developed during World War II came on to the cancer seen in the 1950's. Mustard gas is a poison. Chemotherapy is a poison. We have many poisons to kill. Does it make sense to poison ourselves in order to kill cancer cells? I don't think our Creator intended for us to poison our bodies in an attempt to be healthy. The problem with Chemotherapy is that it does not have intelligence to govern it. There are no captains and generals directing the troops on what to attack and what to leave alone. It goes into the body and attacks and kills everything; healthy cells along with cancer cells. This kamikaze approach to health is detrimental to trillions of delicate healthy cells. It's a chaotic assault which many times leads to death because it destroys the immune system beyond repair. Let's take a common sense look at this.

If you want to clean your garage, you have a few options.
1. Go in and hand sort through all your stuff and throw away everything you don't want and keep the good stuff organized in boxes. **Or**
2. Throw a hand grenade in your garage and run for cover. Yes, the grenade will clean it out, but it will not distinguish between the good stuff and bad stuff.

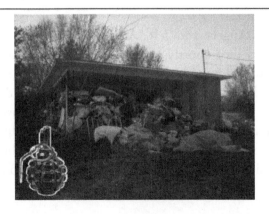

If we would quit trying to poison our cells with toxic drugs and shift our focus to strengthening our immune system so that it can do its job, then we would eliminate ninety percent of our problems.

> **"The greatest part of all chronic disease is created by the suppression of acute disease by drug poisoning."** Henry Lindlahr, M.D

Cats: Created by God to Kill Mice

Growing up on a farm in Moses Lake, Washington, I learned that farmers could keep mice outbreaks under control by having healthy cats around. Cats are created with an instinct to hunt and kill mice. Now if you happen to love mice then you might hate cats because they hunt, kill and eat the little creepy crawlers. It's part of their diet just as humans inherit an instinct to eat fruits and vegetables. Get rid of your cats and you'll have mice everywhere as long as there is something for them to eat.

Suppose your body is like a farm in operation. Mice are like diseases (viruses, fungals, bacteria, cancer etc.) that are looking for a place to live. Cats are like your white blood cells or your immune system. When functioning normally, they roam around hunting those foreign invaders in your body just as cats do mice on the farm.

We had a six-toed gray mother cat that was an excellent mouse hunter. Trotting up the ditch bank with a fat mouse in her mouth was a common sight for us to see. She did a great job keeping the mice population down.

You have a choice. How do you want to get rid of mice? You could put poison out that will kill mice, the family pet, and any toddler that happens upon it. Or you could keep your cats healthy so they can go out and do what they have been created to do–kill mice. They are your immunity to mice infestation. Just as cats know how to kill mice, your immune system knows how to kill cancer, viruses, bacteria and fungals. Let's quit poisoning everything to death. The kill, kill, kill, approach to health is not working. It's time to shift our focus to strengthening what God has given us so that we can live at our fullest potential. Working with Mother Nature instead of against her most always results in peace, prosperity and health.

Reed T. Sainsbury

Without Herbs We Would Die

An herb is defined as a medicinal plant. Weeds are simply plants that we haven't found medicinal purposes for yet. Through a process called photosynthesis, plants (herbs) combine sunlight, carbon dioxide and water to release oxygen that we humans breathe. So, the next time you hear someone say, "I don't believe in herbs," tell them to stop breathing for a minute because they are using the oxygen produced by herbs. As an old friend from back home used to say…

> **"Don't open your mouth and reveal your ignorance."**
> Lester Klingemann 1916-2004

Did you know that through mathematical calculations and other scientific formulas, bumblebees should not be able to fly? It's physically impossible. Scientists admit that the fact bees can fly defies our current level of scientific understanding. Obviously, in man's limited capacity in the field of science we don't know everything because bumblebees fly regardless of what science says. Jesus Christ walking on water and resurrecting three days after they killed him doesn't seem to fit into their scientific formulas either. Keep in mind that what you hold on to as the "truth" may be completely absurd in fifty years.

> **"Never try to teach a hog to sing. It frustrates you and aggravates the hog. In other words, don't throw your pearls before swine."**
> Author Unknown

Chapter 3
HEALING THE CAUSE OF DIS-EASE

The Lymphatic System and Cellular Activity

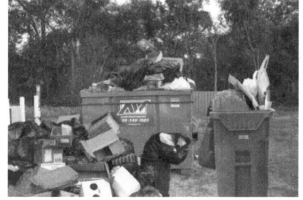

Mainstream medicine has a tendency to ignore your lymphatic system with its 2 ¼ million miles of lymphatic ducts and 650 lymph nodes (garbage dumpsters), because they do not have drugs to clean and drain it. As a matter of fact drugs clog the lymphatic system up and when cells can't get rid of waste material dis-ease thrives. Every solid structure in the body is bathed in lymph. The average human has approximately twelve quarts of lymph in the body.

Lymphatic drainage is a crucial therapy for optimum health. Every one of the 100 trillion living cells in your body produces waste material and, without the lymphatic system draining properly, then waste material builds up similar to garbage cans and dumpsters after a month of not being emptied. When this garbage is not picked up, we attract infection into the body. Swelling and pain are warning signs that our lymph nodes (garbage dumpsters) need to be emptied. The lymph nodes are the garbage cans in the body. When they are full they swell. That is why sometimes when you have a cold the lymph nodes under the cheekbones swell. They are fighting infection, cleansing excess mucous and toxins out.

Swollen lymph nodes are warning signs for us to empty our trashcans. When we ignore these signs and suppress them with diuretics and pain killers, then we can literally drown from our own metabolic wastes. A sluggish lymphatic system will almost always leave the immune system depleted and susceptible to infections. Remember that Dr. Carrel proved how important it is to keep waste materials cleaned out when he kept a chicken heart alive for twenty nine years. It died when someone failed to remove the wastes.

The Lymphatic System

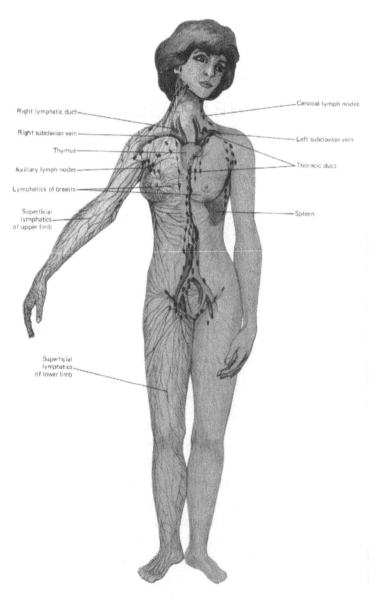

A fish aquarium in my office teaches us how important circulation is to life. There is a filtering system that circulates the water to keep it clean. When that filter gets clogged to the point that the water stops circulating, what happens? The water turns a dark murky color and fish die because of the disease-producing environment of stagnant water.

The fish are alive and living creatures excrete waste and fecal matter. Just as circulation is essential in having a clean aquarium, so is circulation in your body also essential. This is especially important for the lymphatic system, which drains toxins and fights infection. Your lymphatic system and immune system work like a pitcher and a catcher on a baseball team. They both need each other to work effectively.

A swamp is dead water because it has no outlet and when water is stagnant, disease thrives. It provides the perfect breeding grounds for mosquitoes and all kinds of infection. Similar to a disease infested swamp, so is our body stagnant and asking for disease when the lymphatic system is not draining toxins sufficiently. Edema (swelling) is a warning sign that lymph channels are blocked.

The Dead Sea receives thousands of gallons of fresh water every day yet it continues to remain dead. Fish can't live in it. Why? In order for life to exist it must receive and give. If water comes in, it must go out. And if it doesn't let anything out, the cycle of life is disrupted, circulation is hindered and dis-ease sets in.

The lymphatic system draining improperly can be compared to the sewer system in your house being clogged up. First of all, what is required for your sewer system to drain? **WATER,** is required to drain wastes. You can't wash the dishes, your clothes or anything else without water. Water is a cleaner and you can't flush the toilet to get rid of wastes without it. In the same sense, a great number of people have insufficient drainage due to dehydration. They simply do not have enough water in their bodies to clean and drain wastes. Constipation and headaches are two common symptoms when our water reserves are low. If you take your body weight and divide it by two that is how many ounces of water the average human should drink per day (a person weighing 150 pounds needs seventy-five ounces of water per day). Secondly, the lymphatic system doesn't have a pump like the circulatory system has. The blood moves through veins and arteries by a pump that we call the heart. The lymphatic system requires bodily movement in order for wastes to be flushed out. That brings us to our next health secret, **EXERCISE**.

> **"If the lymphatic system stops circulating for just 24 hours, death will occur."** Arthur C. Guyton, M.D. - Text Book of Medical Physiology

Wise doctors understand that the lymphatic system is part of your highly skilled military defense that we call the immune system. Our immune system is similar to a military operation. Tonsils in our throat are like guards at a gate that protects us from any incoming harmful pathogens. The adenoids are used to guard against any toxins that you may breathe in through your nose. The appendix acts as an overflow valve for the large intestine and also guards against foreign invaders that may come in through food.

> **"Longevity and beauty are not in your genes; they are in your lymph."** Paul Chhabra's great grandmother who lived to be 111.

A sluggish lymphatic system plays a key role in maintaining your disease. Our mainstream medical system is right up to snuff when it comes to ignoring the lymphatic system. With a sluggish lymphatic system you'll be a perfect routine customer for their drugs, surgeries and eventually the high dividend payer, "cancer." Cancer is the jackpot that pays. They'll have you right where they want you to bleed you of your life savings as they ignore the cause of your illness and continue to poison your body with expensive drugs and mutilate you through surgery as body parts are removed.

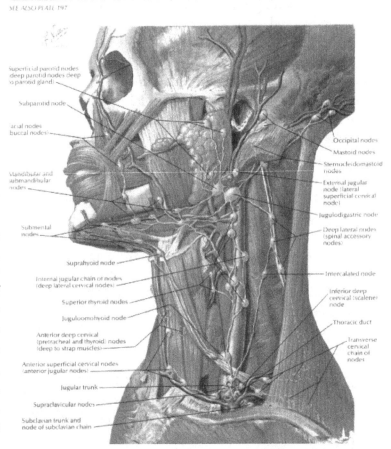

Lymph Vessels and Nodes of Oral and Pharyngeal Regions

*Notice how many lymph nodes are in the neck and under the cheek bone. It is common for the nodes to swell when you have a cold or fighting infection.

> **"Man does not die, he kills himself."** Seneca

Rebounding (Lymphasizing)

We are born with a natural instinct to bounce. Children naturally love to jump on the bed, pogo sticks, trampolines and anything else that acts as a spring. Drive by a school and watch how many kids are jumping rope and other bouncing exercises on recess. When small babies cry what do we do? Bounce them of course, because the bouncing motion pumps the lymphatic system which soothes inflammation and makes us feel better. As we grow older some of us stop bouncing for some reason or another and dis-ease prevails. We would be healthier if we all had a label on our foreheads like salad dressing that said, "SHAKE WELL BEFORE USING."

A rebounder is a small mini-trampoline that enables you to use it almost anywhere. By bouncing up and down you activate the lymph flow as much as ten to thirty fold. The up and down motion while rebounding activates the one-way lymph valves to their maximum. For more information go to www.healthbounce.com or www.immunesystem.org.

> **"Rebounding is by far the most efficient, the most effective form of exercise yet devised by man."** Albert Carter - The National Institute of Reboundology and Health

The heart starts beating before you are born and continues to beat until you die. But it only pumps blood. It does not pump lymph fluid. You have three times as much lymph fluid in your body as you do blood. Lymph fluid surrounds the tissue cells of the body. When the cells of the body need nutrients, they have to get it from the lymph fluid. When they excrete metabolic waste, it goes into the lymph. Like a fish aquarium or any other body of water, the more circulation your lymph fluid receives, the healthier you are going to be. The problem is that we have never taken this mystifying system seriously. For example, we are able to hear the heart, measure the beat, and monitor the pressure of the blood. But, because the lymphatic system just quietly goes about its job, not making waves, we don't study it. In fact, we have done just the opposite.

Because we don't understand the lymphatic system's importance, we have tried to get rid of it. We started forty years ago by removing tonsils and the adenoids from healthy children. These are two of the drainage organs of the lymphatic system. We have no love for the appendix either, another lymphatic drainage organ. Removal is in order most of the time a surgeon gets close to one. Lymph veins are stripped from the arms during a mastectomy.

How many women do you know who have had lymph nodes removed? In actuality when your lymph nodes swell that means they are working. They swell because they are fighting infection. Do you get sore and swell when you workout with weights for the first time in five months? That doesn't mean we should cut your legs and arms off because they are sore and swollen, does it?

> "The name of a dis-ease depends upon where the poisons settle."
> Bernard Jensen D.C., N.D., Ph.D.

Suppose you live in a city where every week a deliberate fire is started by arson. So the city mayor sends out an order to crack down on crime so arsonists can be caught. Let's suppose these guys are sneaky and very difficult to catch. After two more months, twelve more businesses have been burned down. The mayor throws his hands up in the air and says, "I don't know what to do." In a rage of desperation he sends out an order to destroy the fire stations.

Does this sound ridiculous? Why in the world would you want to destroy the fire stations? They are where the fire fighters come from who put the fires out! But since every time there is a fire (swelling) the mayor (doctor) sees firemen (swollen lymph nodes) they assume that fires are caused by firemen. They are the ones fighting to save the businesses and stop the fires (infection).

A similar situation occurs in your body when doctors detect swollen tonsils or lymph nodes. They first crack down on crime, or infection with f. After months of antibiotics failing to get rid of the inflammation, the doctor throws his hands in the air just like the mayor and says, "We're going to have to do surgery and remove your tonsils, lymph nodes etc." Why would you remove lymph nodes, tonsils, adenoids, etc., that are swollen because of the fact that they are fighting infection? Doctors are destroying the fire stations that are fighting infection in your body out of desperation. The reason they are swollen is the same reason your legs swell after jogging five miles. They are working, only a fool would cut his legs off because they are swollen after a grueling workout.

> "Some people study all their lives, and at their death they have learned everything except to think." Domergue

Healing Poisoned Medicine

Rebounding a few minutes every morning to pump the lymphatic system and strengthen every cell in the body is energizing and invigorating. It is a great time to meditate and focus on goals by speaking them into existence through the power of the spoken word. It can be used as a time to create what you want in life so your mind has a blueprint. It's one of the most powerful ways to start the day.

The human body functions through electricity produced by the sodium-potassium pump of each cell. Some of the new flashlights on the market do not take batteries. In order to make them shine, you simply shake them. By shaking them, enough energy is generated to illuminate the bulb. Rebounding is an effective way to generate a tremendous amount of electrical energy so your light can shine. When you are electrically charged and your light is shining then you are empowered to reach your goals and bless the world with your talents. Living powerfully means that you make a difference in every situation.

> **"Every cell generates an electrical field. It is an actual electrical generator."** C. Samuel West, D.N., N.D.

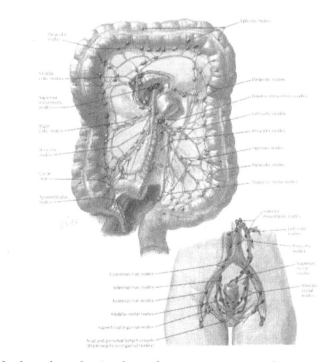

Lymph Vessels and Nodes of Large Intestine

Notice all the lymph nodes (garbage dumpsters) surrounding the colon. Can you imagine how filthy they are if one does not have 2-3 bowel movements per day?

The solution for swelling and infection is to drink plenty of water, rebound to pump the lymphatic system (or some type of exercise) and take herbs and homeopathic remedies to boost up the immune system. Cutting part of your lymphatic/immune system out when it swells and throwing it in the trash every time there is inflammation is insulting to the intelligent self-healing person that God created.

Some may argue, "My tonsils stay inflamed and infected all the time!" The question is what are you eating to feed the infection? Does your diet include dairy products, white flour, sugar and chemicals in processed foods? Stop putting garbage into your temple and start eating fresh fruits, vegetables and whole grains. Let your food become your medicine taught Hippocrates. Start taking some immune boosting herbs that cleanse the bloodstream and expel mucous. A few minutes of CEDSA testing can identify food and inhalant sensitivities that can be contributing to inflammation.

Some great herbs to heal infection and swollen tonsils, lymph nodes etc., are; echinacea, elderberry, cat's claw, astragalus, goldenseal, garlic and myrrh. CEDSA testing identifies which herbs are best for your body's chemistry.

Make sure your bowels are moving at least two or three times per day. Trust God, your body will heal when you nourish it with mild foods and herbs. It knows how to get well. It just needs the right tools to heal.

Finding the Cause of Dis-ease

> **"We doctors are taught in our medical training that virtually 80 percent of diseases have no known cause. We are not taught to treat the underlying cause of the disease, we are only taught to treat the symptoms. This does not get a person well."** Lorraine Day, M.D. - Former Chief Orthopedic Surgeon, San Francisco Hospital

Cancer, lupus, fibromyalgia, chronic fatigue syndrome and a host of other new diseases are emerging everyday and doctors are prescribing drugs that have disastrous side effects and simply don't work. How many people do you know who have been cured of cancer, arthritis, diabetes etc., by taking prescription drugs? Like an honest medical doctor I spoke with recently told me, "There's not much we can do when someone has fibromyalgia." Of course they can't do much because they don't know what's causing it. Medical doctors do not look for the cause most of the time. If you don't know what's causing a disease how are you going to cure it? Even if they do find the cause, their prescription drugs, do not heal, they only mask symptoms by stimulating or shutting down which creates major imbalances in the body and pushes the toxins deeper into the tissue only to manifest later on in a different form, fashion or location.

Take shingles for example. The chickenpox virus suppressed with drugs or vaccines is not allowed to run its course and so the immune system never fully terminates the virus and becomes immune to it. It lays dormant in the body for twenty-five years. Then the immune system becomes weak from poor eating habits and prescription drug use. On top of that some very stressful emotional experiences beat you up pretty good. In this weakened state, when the body is out of balance, the virus can now show its face. Suddenly, you begin to experience this chickenpox virus now evolved into shingles ripping through you like a raging tornado causing extremely sensitive blisters and pain.

You and your doctor never connect the dots but many tumors, cancer etc., are caused from years of prescription drug abuse suppressing your symptoms and now the piper must be paid. You reap what you sow. Just because a drug magically makes your symptoms disappear like the great magician (David Copperfield does animals in cages and girls in sparkling clothes), it does not mean that you have fixed the problem. As a matter of fact, you are creating the terrain that will favor major disease in the future. This is not health; it is disease maintenance and it is one of the world's largest money making businesses. It is nothing more then a neat magic trick, an illusion created by a clever scientist's drug to make your current symptoms disappear so you think the problem has been solved. It would be nice if good health was achieved that easily.

It is time for us to wake up and begin to understand the fundamentals of health. First of all, disease is not caused by bacteria or viruses that attack poor innocent people. It is time for us to stop playing the poor-me victim game. Everything you choose to eat and drink either promotes health or weakens your body, thus leaving you vulnerable to bacteria, viruses and dis-ease. Mainstream medicine plays this game well. They have most Americans believing that bacteria, germs and viruses are out there and if you happen to come in contact with them you will inevitably become sick. But that's okay, because your medical doctor can become your personal savior by giving you an antibiotic to kill the germs or inject you with the flu shot and other germ-killing agents to "cure" you.

> **"Antibiotic resistance comes mainly because of inappropriate or improper use of antibiotics by physicians. Some 150 million prescriptions are written annually in this country. And 60% of them–that translates to 90 million prescriptions–are for antibiotics. Of those, 50 million are absolutely unnecessary or inappropriate."**
> Dr. Philip Tierno - Director of Clinical Microbiology and Diagnostic Immunology, New York University Medical Center

Most diseases are not caused by germs, bacteria and viruses but an imbalance in the immune system that causes a weakened resistance created by our own health-destroying living and eating habits. If we want to truly heal and be healthy, we must stop being poor victims and start taking responsibility for our health and dis-ease. A wise teacher once told me, *"If you want to watch your flowers grow, treat the roots, not the leaves. If you want to heal disease, treat the cause, not the symptoms."*

If the body has the power to inflame a joint or grow a tumor, then it has the power to remove it. Remember, if it has been created, then it can be uncreated. You have that power. Take responsibility and be the cause, not the effect. YOU are the source! Be a creator not a reactor and start living the life you choose, the one you love. You can heal but you have to give up being a poor victim and start taking responsibility.

> **"Who looks outside, dreams; who looks inside, awakes."**
> Carl Gustav Jung

Mother Nature's Food Chain

Understand that Mother Nature has a food chain. When a rabbit is killed on the road vultures gather around for dinner. Flies come and lay eggs and maggots emerge. We always have been and always will be exposed to every kind of germ science can identify under a microscope. Bacteria, viruses, molds, funguses, parasites and any other type of microbe/pathogen we can think of will always be in our midst, despite how clean we think we are. They are in your house, car, work, water, food and air. There is no way to escape these microbes. As long as you live on planet earth you will come in contact with millions of these "germs."

If you want to get rid of flies in your house what do you do? Oh sure, you can buy poisonous fly spray and poison them to death and harm yourself in the process. You can spend all day swatting them against the wall with a fly swatter, but more flies will eventually come back in time. They'll come back because the cause is still there and you are only chasing symptoms. What's the cause? Probably a dirty trashcan, food left out or maybe a dirty bathroom with something for flies to eat. The environment either attracts or repels different life to it.

Clean your house and get rid of the fly attracting food and you cure it. If there's nothing there for the scavenger flies to eat or lay eggs in, they leave. They cannot survive in a clean environment. It's Mother Nature's way of cleaning house. It keeps the world turning and promoting life. If something needs cleaning up, she sends ants, maggots, flies, vulture's etc., to clean up the mess, and they do a great job, don't they? Just leave a piece of candy out and watch the ants devour it within a few hours. Watch the vultures feast on a dead carcass next to the road whose slow moving feet proved fatal. What is trash to one is a meal to another. Mother Nature has things figured out. We would be wise to work with her instead of against her. Be calm, relaxed and harmonized with the universe. Stop resisting what God has created. Cleanse your temple within and give up the need to worry about the evils outside.

> "Why would a patient swallow a poison because he is ill, or take that which would make a well man sick." L. F. Kebler, M.D.

If Americans want to be healthy, then we have to apply health-building habits. You reap what you sow. If you never take the trash out, you'll attract bugs of all sorts, mice, and rodents that carry diseases. Why? Because God created a life cycle that works this way. Every living thing eats something. Everything has a purpose. If you plant carrots in the garden, you won't harvest tomatoes. Put a low octane fuel in your car, never change the oil, air filter, spark plugs etc., and it will run sluggish. Eat a lot of processed, dead food packed with sugar, white flour, nitrates, chemical dyes, artificial color etc., and you'll catch colds, coughs and every virus that comes your way.

Every time you eat sugar it has a paralyzing effect on your immune system. A candy bar and coke suppresses the immune system for up to six hours. Did you ever wonder why you get sick if you eat a lot of candy? How many kids get sick right after Halloween? Cold and flu season always accompanies the holidays because we fire an assault on our immune system with all the Thanksgiving and Christmas goodies. The consumption of large amounts of sugar leaves us wide open to illness.

So what is the solution to being healthy? Ingest antibiotics every week to kill bacteria? Of course not, because new ones will come your way as fast as you kill the first. If we want to heal dis-ease and get rid of infections, then we have to change our body's terrain so that it no longer favors the growth of infection and illness.

Do you know people who start on one antibiotic and it seems that every four months they are sick again? That's because they did nothing to change the terrain that has allowed the bacteria to exist in the first place. The solution is to break the food chain cycle. Stop poisoning your body so the critters have something to feed on. Clean up the dead rabbit on the road and the vultures and flies won't come around, because there is nothing to feed on. Cleanse the body of undigested proteins, mucous, built up fecal matter etc., and these microbes will have nothing to eat. You see, these microbes only proliferate in an unclean body where there is much garbage to feed on, like vultures do flattened opossums on the side of the road.

Just as a full garbage can will attract ants, flies, maggots, cockroaches, mice etc., so does an unclean body. Put a clean trash can out and if there is nothing for our little friends to eat, they do not come and stay like they do when you see a heaped up trashcan with watermelon rinds, ice cream cartons and other garbage with food particles for something to eat.

The survival of every human, animal, insect, fish, plant, bird, virus, bacteria, fungus, mold, germ, microbe, etc., what ever you can identify big and small that is alive only continues living if it's environment allows it. You will never see polar bears living naturally in the Sahara desert nor alligators at the North Pole, because these animals cannot survive in those environments. We humans would all be dead without oxygen from plants. Water and food are next in line but everything either lives or dies depending upon its environment. We become diseased when our internal terrain favors disease. Reverse that condition and we begin to heal.

> "DNA does not control biology and the nucleus itself is not the brain of the cell. Just like you and me, cells are shaped by where they live. In other words, it's the environment, stupid."
> Bruce Lipton, Ph.D.

Germs are very seldom the cause of disease. In most cases, they are the result of disease. When your body's pH (fluid in and around your cells) is acidic, then your immune system will be weak and there is usually lots of undigested protein and other trash backed up in the lymphatic and blood system. This sets the stage for infection and illness. You are preparing the terrain (garden) to attract and grow a fine crop of infection by eating and drinking acidifying foods. You might want to know that all drugs are very acidic and actually contribute to an acidic terrain that favors dis-ease. On the other hand, herbs are alkaline. Doctors who understand how the body heals will recommend remedies that counteract cellular acidosis, not drugs that cause it. Healthy people have a pH (saliva) of about 6.8. We'll focus more on pH later.

Healthy people around the world who eat only wholesome organic foods and beverages rarely get sick. Some people can honestly say they haven't had one cold, the flu or a headache in the last ten years. How can this happen when they are around sick, coughing, sneezing people just the same as you and I? The secret is; healthy people don't get sick. If your immune system is balanced, you have nothing to fear.

> "Disease symptoms are an effort of the body to eliminate waste, mucus, and toxemia. This system assists Nature in the most perfect and natural way. Not the disease but the body is to be healed; it must be cleansed, freed from waste and foreign matter, from mucus and toxemia accumulated since childhood." Professor Arnold Ehret

Own Your Dis-ease and Be Healed

Every cold I have ever had in my life is because I earned it. Illness is a result of broken natural laws. It was created by my body to get rid of excessive mucous and other garbage created from eating and drinking acidifying, unhealthy foods. Too much white sugar and white flour laden junk foods create illness. Anything that Mother Nature doesn't produce naturally is usually a junk food that compromises the body.

Negative thoughts and fear-based emotions add stress that can lead to an imbalance in your immune system as well. Have you ever had an argument or some negative emotional battle and the next day woken up sick?

> **"We, ourselves, choose the time of illness, the kind of illness, the course of illness, and its gravity."** Dr. Arnold A. Hutschnecker

One of the first steps to healing is to take full responsibility for your illness and own it. Empowerment comes from taking ownership of your very situation and realizing that we create our experiences. God gives us our free agency to experience whatever we choose.

Every illness I have ever had is because I created it. Understand that if I have the power to create something, then I also have the power to uncreate it. I am no longer a victim of circumstances. This is called living powerfully. This is being one with source.

> **"Everything you see has its roots in the unseen world. The forms may change, yet the essence remains the same. Every wonderful sight will vanish; every sweet word will fade, but do not be disheartened. The source they come from is eternal, growing, branching out, giving new life and new joy. Why do you weep? The source is within you. And this whole world is springing up from it."** Jelauddin Rumi

If you have a disease like cancer and you believe and feel you are a poor innocent victim, then you will never be completely healed. Oh sure, surgery and radiation might get rid of it for the time being, but nothing has been done to pull the roots out that nourished it to grow in the first place; therefore you are not truly healed. Many times those roots are negative mental/emotional patterns that cause you to self-destruct (subconscious way of committing suicide). Without changing your destructive thought patterns, that same illness will be recreated perhaps in a different form or part of the body. In the meantime, your doctor has performed another magic trick to make the cancer look like it is gone, but if he is honest, he will admit it is impossible to get 100 percent of the cancer cells. They'll be back again someday soon, just like Frosty the Snowman sings every winter when the temperature readings get high enough to melt snow. When that cancer does come back, it will come with a vengeance. Oncologists see this quite often.

Stop giving away all your power to the cancer. You have given something else more power then yourself when you do this. If you want to heal, then you need to start by taking ownership of the cancer. Be the source of it. Be the creator of it. By owning it, you can do what you want with it. Instead of it controlling you, you control it. This belief in your mind is crucial in order to heal and overcome disease. This is empowerment. If you are the source of it, meaning you created it, and then you also have the power to destroy it and create something different.

> "I can do all things through Christ which strengtheneth me."
> Philippians 4:13

Sick people have lots of faith. They have a tremendous amount of faith in the wrong thing. What do you worry about and fear? Whatever you allow your mind to dwell upon is where your faith is. In the Bible there is a story about Job. By focusing on what he didn't want, he was plagued with boils. The very thing that he feared came upon him. What you dwell upon creates your reality. Focus on what you want, not what you don't want. What you dwell upon is what you give your attention to and this will eventually manifest itself in your life. What you feed grows. Your life is a reflection of your innermost thoughts and beliefs.

> "Reality is that which, when you stop believing in it, doesn't go away." Philip K. Dick

Understand that all the prayers in the world cannot heal you when you continue to give your attention to ill health. Focus on what you want. See and feel yourself completely healed. Give your attention to health, not disease. Put those energetic vibrations of health in your mind so they can physically manifest themselves in time.

De-Nile is not just a river in Egypt. Accept full responsibility for your condition. If this makes sense to you and you believe it, then congratulations because you just took your first step to creating a healing environment to get well. You no longer have to feel sorry for yourself and be a poor victim while your doctor maintains your disease with his magic drugs. You no longer have to sit around hoping and praying that they'll create the perfect drug to cure you someday.

> "What lies behind us and what lies before us are small matters to what lies within us." Ralph Waldo Emerson

Take ownership of your situation. If it is cancer, then own it. If it's a bad relationship, then own it so that you have the power to create something different, because what you previously created isn't working out. Like an artist painting a masterpiece, your life is whatever you choose to create. What you choose to create is who you are BE-ING. If you don't like that, then try creating something different.

Weight Loss Without Trying

> "I know what Victoria's Secret is. The secret is that nobody over thirty can fit into their stuff!" Gary R. Oberg, M.D.

Twenty-five year old Rhonda came into our clinic after her chiropractic physician sent her to the emergency room because he suspected she was having a heart attack. In the emergency room, all the tests came back normal so they sent Rhonda home with painkillers, despite her pounding heart that felt like it was going to explode. She was also experiencing tightness in her throat, fatigue, nausea, high blood pressure and severe panic attacks. She came in our clinic and complained that she felt like she was having a nervous breakdown and was so jittery she couldn't even drive her car. Her mother had to bring her in and keep her hands on her, trying to calm her as she sat in our office.

We did a CEDSA (Computerized Electrodermal Stress Analysis) exam on Rhonda to find out what was causing her to be so far out of balance to produce these symptoms. We obviously knew that her symptoms were not caused from a deficiency of painkillers so why take a remedy that wasn't going to address the cause? Within fifteen minutes of testing, we found a major imbalance in her gallbladder, spleen and thyroid. Further testing revealed her nervous system was causing these organs and glands to be compromised.

Checking her body for nutritional deficiencies, we detected her magnesium and potassium levels to be extremely depleted. We immediately opened up a bottle of magnesium and potassium and had her take three capsules. Within ten minutes the nervous, panicky, jittery feeling decreased dramatically. She was calm and relaxed and felt ninety percent better. "Wow! That is powerful stuff, can it really work that fast," she asked. Why didn't the emergency room doctors check her magnesium levels?

She left our clinic with some nutritional remedies for the deficiencies that showed up and also some herbal formulas to flush out her gallbladder and spleen. Some kelp and thyroid support was given as well as circulation support.

Six weeks later Rhonda came back a new person. Her nervous system was stable, her energy levels were up and she had lost twenty pounds without even changing her diet. She felt great and appeared to be healthy.

When we balance the nervous system and thyroid which controls body temperature, metabolism and weight gain in the body, then overweight people let go of excess pounds. Why? Because we fire-up the furnace that burns calories. It's hard to lose weight when you have a sluggish metabolism due to hypothyroidism, even if you only eat one meal a day and exercise.

Balancing the endocrine system, especially the thyroid, is a key to losing weight. Unfortunately, most medical doctors do blood work to check the thyroid which is many times inaccurate. Emotions, diet, stress, exercise and menstrual cycles can all influence the blood chemistries which may or may not give us accurate thyroid readings. We recommend the Barnes Basal Temperature Test: a mercury thermometer check of your temperature. Keep the thermometer on your nightstand next to the bed so you don't have to get up. Obviously, if you get up and move around your body temperature goes up. We want an accurate reading, so first thing in the morning put the thermometer in your armpit and go back to bed for ten minutes and then check your temperature. Record your readings for several weeks. Normal temperature should be 97.8-98.2 degrees Fahrenheit. If your morning temperature consistently registers less than 97.8 degrees, then you most likely have a sluggish thyroid. If the readings are higher than 98.2, you probably have a hyperthyroid.

After approximately fifty years of research, Dr. Broda Barnes, M.D., Ph.D., claims that no less then forty percent of the adults in the U.S. suffer from hypothyroidism (low thyroid). How many of the following symptoms do you experience?

> "Without thyroid, there can be no complexity of thought, no learning, no education, no habit formation, no responsive energy for situations as well as no physical unfolding of faculty and function. No reproduction of kind with no sign of puberty at expected age and no exhibition of sex tendencies thereafter." Louis Berman, M.D. - World Renowned Endocrinologist

Signs of Hypothyroidism

Weakness	Dry skin	Lethargy	Slow speech
Swelling	Cold hands/feet	Diminished sweat	Thick tongue
Coarse hair	Pale skin	Constipation	Weight gain
Hair falls out	Breathing (hard)	Swollen feet	Hoarseness
Loss of appetite	PMS	Nervousness	Heart palpitations
Brittle nails	Slow movement	Failing memory	Emotional instability
Depression	Headaches	Sleepiness	Goiter (Enlarged neck)
Ringing in ears	Acne	Irritable	Mental dullness
Numbness	Low energy	Low sex drive	High cholesterol

High Cholesterol or Sluggish Thyroid?

> "There are doubtless a great many people who are mildly deficient in thyroid hormone and would be benefited by taking it orally but are not ill enough to see a physician."
> Dr. Roger J. Williams - Discoverer of Pantothenic Acid

Why would a sluggish thyroid cause high cholesterol? Have you ever tried to spread cold butter from the refrigerator on toast? It spreads a lot easier if it has been sitting out at room temperature all day doesn't it? After you fry fatty hamburger meat and let the pan sit and cool down, a thick white solid lard covers the pan. After hot fat cools, it turns to a solid. If your body temperature is low, it has a tougher time breaking down and metabolizing fats similar to a hot or cold frying pan. When your body temperature is normal, the body can move the fats through a whole lot easier. If the body temperature is low, then fats build up in arteries and cause blockages. Thyroid hormones control blood fat and cholesterol levels. So if you have high cholesterol, a low thyroid could be a factor.

An enlarged thyroid gland, (where the individual's neck swells) is called a goiter. Why does it swell? All of your blood (about five quarts) circulates through the thyroid every hour to take hormones to your cells. Every one of your 100 trillion cells requires thyroid hormones to catalyze metabolism, similar to your car's engine needing spark plugs to ignite the fuel to excel the car into motion. When the thyroid is not getting enough iodine, it swells in an attempt to capture more iodine from the blood. We don't need a drug to shrink the thyroid so we have to be on synthetic hormone support for the rest of our lives. What we need is to give the thyroid nutritional support, like kelp which is high in iodine. Taking kelp is the most effective way to get iodine levels up. Magnesium, vitamin A, B2 (riboflavin) and amino acids may also be needed to balance the thyroid. Natural desiccated thyroid supplement (Armour) may be beneficial. By supporting the thyroid nutritionally, we solve many health problems.

It has been proven that after removing the thyroid from test animals, arteriosclerosis develops. Dr. Kocher of Switzerland found that after performing surgery to remove thyroids (thyroidectomy) from individuals with goiters, they developed arteriosclerosis just like the test animals (Journal of Clinical Endocrinology & Metabolism June 2003, 88(6): 2438-2444). Austrian pathologists have also concluded that thyroidectomy contributes to hardening of the arteries.

> "Hidden in the throats of unsuspecting millions is the reason for many-if not most-heart attacks: a subnormal thyroid gland."
> Stephen E. Langer, M.D.

By addressing the cause of dis-ease and not just suppressing symptoms with drugs, we can bring the body back into balance with natural remedies. When we do this, symptoms disappear. This is called health and it is earned by giving your body the nutrition it cries out for by sending warning signals most Americans view as annoying symptoms. Listen to your body, it is trying to get your attention so you will make a change for a reason. You don't ignore the red flashing light on your dash when it starts to blink do you? How much more important to you is your health than your car? Stop ignoring the warning signals and fix the problem before you end up in the emergency room wishing you would have taken better care of yourself.

> **"Those who fail to take time to be healthy will ultimately have to take the time to be sick."** James Chappell D.C., N.D., Ph.D.

It is important to know that many drugs (sulfa and antidiabetic) interfere with the formation of thyroid hormones by blocking iodine uptake. Prednisone and estrogen (for women on birth control or hormone replacement therapy) according to Stephen Langer, M.D., should be used very cautiously because these drugs indirectly worsen already subnormal thyroid function. He also warns that cough medicines, lithium and aspirin can also contribute to hypothyroidism. Gee, look at all the medicines Americans take and it is easy to understand why so many have sluggish thyroids that lead to obesity, depression, fatigue and cold hands and feet.

> **"Cellular health depends upon three factors, a steady supply of nutrients, oxygen, and thyroid hormones."**
> Broda O. Barnes, M.D., Ph.D.

Losing Weight and Keeping It Off

How many overweight people do you know who drink diet sodas? The key to weight loss is not artificial sweeteners. Artificial sweeteners actually cause you to crave carbohydrates and gain weight according to diabetic specialist, Dr. H.J. Roberts.

The key to weight loss is to make sure your endocrine system is balanced. Even if you only eat one small meal a day, you will not lose weight if your endocrine system is out of balance. The biggest culprit with obesity is a sluggish thyroid gland. The thyroid regulates metabolism and body temperature. So, by turning the oven thermostat up, we can burn and metabolize our foods. Kelp and raw thyroid extract can make a world of difference in weight loss if the thyroid is sluggish.

The adrenal glands and pituitary need to be balanced as well for the whole fat burning process to work. It's kind of like a football team. You will not win very many games with just a quarterback, receiver and one lineman functioning. However, if you get all eleven players on the field to each do his job and work as a team, you'll have success. The same holds true for all of your glands. They work as a team and each of them requires nutrition to function and do their specific job in order for you to be healthy.

Toxins, especially heavy metals and pesticides, can accumulate in the body and interfere with glandular functions. The thyroid has a tendency to be a magnet to metals. If heavy metals in your body are interfering with glandular functions, then you probably won't have much success until you detox them out. A CEDSA exam is an effective way to scan your body for heavy metals.

> "A friend of mine confused her Valium with her birth control pills. She had fourteen kids, but she doesn't really care."
> Gary R. Oberg, M.D.

It may surprise you to know that the average glass of store bought milk contains over 100 different antibiotics. All those antibiotics and steroid growth hormones fed to animals are stored in their tissues. We eat the meat from animals and drink the milk and are bombarded with concentrated forms of these toxins which effect our health. How many people eat very little and can't lose weight? Perhaps eating foods that contain these stimulant growth hormones prevent us from losing weight?

Some people believe that if they drink water they will feel bloated and gain weight. This is absolutely false. Dehydration is one of the biggest inhibitors of weight loss. When people are dehydrated they retain fluids. The body's cells are intelligent like camels crossing a desert. They know how to conserve water when they haven't received enough in the past. As a result, your cells prepare for future droughts by holding onto fluids because in the past, you have made them wait until you experience thirst to get a drink. If you wait until you are thirsty to drink, you are way too late. First thing in the morning upon arising drink sixteen ounces of purified room temperature water. This will tell your cells from the start of the day that you won't be crossing the desert today and they can use the abundance of water to clean, bathe and flush out toxins. The colon will be hydrated and your bowels will move. Healthy people have a bowel movement every morning. Remember, just as a toilet requires plenty of water to flush wastes out, so do the cells in your body. Drink water so they can release toxic waste materials.

If you have ever let a really dirty casserole dish sit out over night and the next morning tried to scrub clean the baked on, dried out crust, then you can understand just how important water is to weight loss. Let's look at the casserole dish as your body and all of the muck on it as the excess weight that you would like to cleanse out of your body. Everyone knows there is a big difference between the amount of effort it takes to scrub clean a casserole dish that has been soaking overnight versus one that has sat out and dried into a crusty mess. Our body works similar to this. With the proper amount of water intake, it is significantly easier to cleanse excess weight than it is to try and lose weight without proper "soaking" of our cells.

As mentioned previously, drink at least half of your body weight in ounces of water a day. Of course, if you are roofing a house in Alabama in August and it is 100 degrees out with high humidity, you will need more water than the secretary sitting at her desk in an air-conditioned office. Use good judgement.

Another culprit for not being able to lose weight is constipation. The bowels need to empty out two or three times a day. If you eat a meal, the wastes need to be expelled instead of clumped up in your intestinal tract adding to your waistline and sluggishness.

A key to getting the pounds to come off is not starving or depriving yourself of food. If you skip meals then your metabolism goes into slow gear to conserve fuel and energy. Eating smaller meals (five or six a day) keeps your metabolism burning calories. Always eat breakfast. Start the day off by cranking up your furnace with something to burn. Some Americans will skip breakfast or lunch but eat a large dinner and go to bed full. This will cause you to gain weight. Instead, eat your biggest meals at the beginning of your day and do not eat after 6 P.M. Your meals need to be healthy foods with a large percentage being vegetables. As a matter of fact, if all you eat are healthy foods, fruits and vegetables, you will lose weight. The roadblocks people hit are when they eat the fruits and vegetables and then snack on crackers, cookies, chips etc. That's when the spare tire begins to inflate.

You eat what's in your house. Having healthy snack foods like raw almonds are good. If you have a food pantry filled with Pop-Tarts, Pringles, Twinkies and ice cream in the freezer, you are setting yourself up for failure. Get rid of the junk food! If it's Friday night and you have done well on your diet all week long, then maybe it's time to reward yourself with a good dinner and dessert. Remember, all things in moderation.

Taking digestive enzymes with your meals to help break down your foods can be extremely helpful with weight loss and energy. Taking a couple of teaspoons of apple cider vinegar before each meal can help with indigestion, acidosis and balance your metabolism so you don't gain weight. It tones the digestive system.

Exercise is very beneficial to kick the metabolism up. The key is to consume less calories than you burn. Rebounding is very beneficial as well as a fast walk. Jogging can help, but it's hard on the joints. Find an exercise that works for you. Cleaning house like you do an aerobic workout can be great exercise as well as the other obvious benefit. Be creative. Find a way to get what you need done in a day and a cardiovascular workout too. An hour a day is good. Some may have to work their way up to this. Be smart and do what you can handle.

Doing some emotional release work can help you break through barriers that have prevented you from losing weight in the past. Most people who are overweight eat to fill a void. There may be a traumatic experience from the past causing you to subconsciously eat to be overweight. Why do you subconsciously gravitate to overeating? Do you get to be right about something on a subconscious level? Does it make you feel safe or comfortable to carry a spare tire?

Stevia – Mother Nature's Sugar Substitute

> "Stevia has virtually no calories. It dissolves easily in water and mixes well with all other sweeteners. I use it myself in a delicious home made ice cream that is extremely low in carbohydrates."
> Robert C. Atkins, M.D. – Founder of the Atkins Diet (1930-2003)

Most Americans consume too much sugar, which causes weight gain and blood sugar disorders. Stevia is an herb from Paraguay that is 200-300 times sweeter than sugar with no calories. This makes it an excellent 100 percent, all natural sugar/artificial sweetener substitute. A couple of drops will sweeten anything you desire. Research has shown that Stevia helps regulate the pancreas and stabilize blood sugar levels. Naturally, it is highly recommended for diabetics, those who have blood sugar problems and those who need a healthy sugar substitute.

> "Stevia is not only non-toxic, but has several traditional medicinal uses. A digestive aid and also has been topically applied to help wound healing. Recent clinical studies have shown it can increase glucose tolerance and decrease blood sugar levels. Of the two sweeteners (Aspartame and Stevia), Stevia wins hands down."
> Julian Whitaker, M.D.

Some companies like Wisdom Naturals are taking Sweet Leaf Stevia and offering different flavored blends that are delicious. The English Toffee is a popular favorite, but they also offer blends such as Milk Chocolate, Lemon Drop, Vanilla Creme, Cinnamon and many more.

Nutrition and Detoxification

> "Great spirits have always encountered violent opposition from mediocre minds." Albert Einstein

If you fail to periodically employ cleansing your liver, kidneys, spleen and intestinal tract, then no doubt your doctor can and will chop and cut on you faster then Hirito Takaushi can slice your steak and shrimp on a Saturday night at the Japanese restaurant. If doctors would learn how to cleanse organs and systems instead of cutting them out, then perhaps you could avoid expensive surgical procedures and might feel and be healthier.

Most Americans do what their doctor says because their insurance covers it. Is that a responsible way to treat your temple that God has given you? It is a sad fact that what insurance will cover is what persuades many health decisions for people in this country. Some people's health isn't worth $200 and others are delighted, when after a few months of being on intense nutritional/herbal program, their cancer is completely gone for a few hundred dollars compared to over $100,000 spent on chemotherapy hand grenades thrown in the body that kill (good and bad) cells. You have a choice when it comes to health; man-made poisonous chemicals or divine intelligent healing plants.

When your $800 Kirby vacuum cleaner stops working the way you want it to clean, do you start cutting parts off of it? Or do you change the belt, filter bag, and clean all the lint and thread build-up out of the suction chamber? Of course you clean it because you know it requires periodic cleaning and maintenance in order to function properly and last many years. Unfortunately, your medical doctor hasn't been trained to cleanse and service your body to prevent dis-ease. He has never taken a herbology class on cleansing the liver and gallbladder of stones. Most have never studied how to cleanse the colon or any other safe, effective and nontoxic herbal cleansing procedure. The fact that most of the world outside the U.S.A. uses homeopathy is evidence that in this country we use what pays the most, not what heals. Just because homeopathy was never mentioned in medical school and therefore is laughed and scoffed at by most medical doctors does not prove it to be ineffective.

If mainstream medicine was really interested in preventing colon cancer and gallbladder surgeries, then doctors would begin prescribing yearly cleanses and colonics. The Rockefeller/I.G. Farben conglomerate made sure that the instruction manual to cleanse and service your body was dropped like a bad girlfriend at the turn of the century by most medical universities for financial/business purposes.

The fact that drug-chemicals do not cleanse your cells, they actually add toxicity to the body, is evidence of a clever drug conspiracy whose purpose is to create income through maintaining your disease. By keeping people sick and dependent upon drugs, business is at an all time high for doctors and pharmaceutical companies. If you get well, their source of income diminishes.

> "A junkie is a junkie, whether he or she is using legal or illegal drugs. ...Other than the fact that your drug supply was doctor-prescribed, your situation hardly differs from that of the ordinary street addict." Robert Mendelsohn, M.D.

Skin Lesions Healed

Puss and blood oozed out of huge open lesions on fifty-eight year old Fran's legs. Her legs looked as if wild animals had attacked her. Never in my life had I seen legs that looked that bad. It scared me just to look at them, not to mention the fowl smelling stench that came from the open sores. She came in for an appointment because all of her previous medical doctors had failed to help her. She informed me that she had been to six different medical doctors and tried every type of cream and salve available. They put her on a ton of antibiotics, round after round, but to no avail. She had been suffering for thirteen years and no doctor had been able to help her. Common sense finally forced her to try something different than what her medical doctor's drugs were failing to achieve. She came in to our clinic to see if a "naturopathic doctor" using natural remedies could help her. Like many of our clients, she had no other options and didn't really believe in what we did, but was willing to give it a shot.

The medical mystery case as to why she couldn't get well was in full swing and I was determined to crack the case and find the cause of her skin lesions. I did some CEDSA testing and found out that her skin lesions were not caused from a deficiency of antibiotics, cortisone creams or any other man-made drug. It's a good thing doctors can't cut your skin off and throw it in the trash like they can a gallbladder or uterus because if they could, I'm sure it would have already been done.

Her test revealed to us that she had chemical and heavy metal poisoning. I asked Fran about her history and found out that she use to work in a chemical manufacturing facility. Her liver was completely toxic and her spleen was running over with toxins like a clogged up toilet. The cause had nothing to do with the skin. Due to her liver, spleen and lymphatic system being backed up and unable to process and drain the garbage, her body was excreting the toxins through her skin. When the internal filters (liver, spleen and kidneys) of the body become clogged, instead of shutting down and dying, our body will save its life by pushing the toxins out through the skin. What an amazing creation the Lord has designed!

Chasing the symptoms by rubbing salves and creams on the sores was not getting to the cause and therefore wasn't helping her get well. When your liver and spleen are toxic, we develop boils, acne, skin rashes etc., as the body attempts to excrete the toxins.

Suppressing rashes and skin problems can actually make the problem worse. It interferes with what the intelligence in your body is doing. Trying to stop the toxins from coming out through the skin is equivalent to you stuffing a sock in your mouth when vomiting. When food poisoning, flu viruses, etc., are present in the body, the intelligence within automatically creates nausea. This diminishes the appetite so more food is not eaten to complicate matters in a sick body. The doctor within then causes the person to vomit and the toxins are expelled. In an effort to keep us alive and healthy, the body tries to get rid of poisons and we fight what our body's own wisdom/intelligence is doing by trying to push the toxins back in! Only a foolish doctor would stuff a sock in your mouth if you were vomiting, but it's not much different when you suppress what the body is naturally trying to get rid of through the skin or any other part of the body.

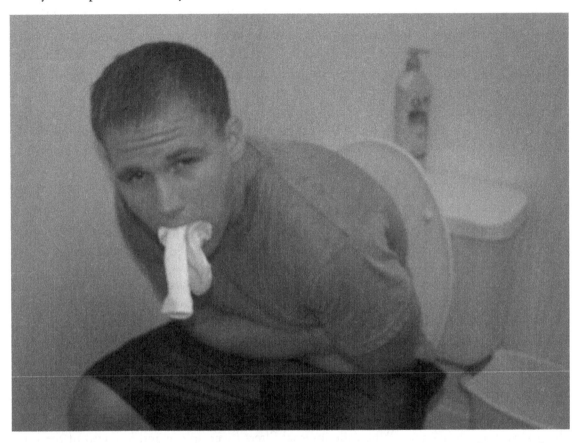

Our skin is capable of eliminating three pints of poison a day. Anything we do to suppress the body from detoxifying is counterproductive. It is believed that if we were to inject those three pints of poison back into the blood stream, we would die in three days of blood poisoning.

When it comes to health, always remember if you step on a cat's tail, it's the other end that yells. Just because the problem manifests itself on the skin doesn't necessarily mean that's what needs the attention. Always look for the cause and work to eliminate it and then the symptoms will usually fizzle out like a 300-pound out of shape slob in a tough-man competition after two rounds.

> **"The problem is not where the pain is."** Dr. Burt Espy

Your Spleen - The Septic Tank of Your Body

Your spleen can be compared to the septic tank at your house. When the septic tank gets full and will no longer drain, then the sewer begins backing up. If you try to flush the toilet and there is no where for the wastes to go, then it begins overflowing. No one wants to live in a house with toilets that won't flush caused from a malfunctioning septic tank. Removing the wastes is essential to a clean house just as it is in your body. When your spleen gets clogged or backed up, then the toxins come out through the skin similar to the toilet overflowing onto the floor. Without proper sewer drainage your house and body stinks. Fran's liver and spleen were swamped with toxins, unable to drain. As a result, they were backed up leaking out through her skin in an effort to save her life.

We put her on a homeopathic lymphatic drainer as well as a heavy metal/chemical detox formula, and a herbal liver and spleen cleanse. Within three weeks the sores on her legs were completely healed. When we address the cause and find the herbs, homeopathics and other nutritional formulas that resonate well with that individual's body chemistry, then healing occurs. The doctor within can do the job quickly and efficiently when we provide the tools to cleanse and nourish at the cellular level.

> "Medical practice has neither philosophy nor common sense to recommend it. In sickness the body is already loaded with impurities. By taking drug-medicines more impurities are added, thereby the case is further embarrassed and harder to cure."
> Elmer Lee, M.D. - Former Vice President, Academy of Medicine

It's also important to find the correct dosage for the individual with a CEDSA exam. Obviously a 400-pound man will need a larger dosage of herbs then a 120-pound woman. With CEDSA, we eliminate the guesswork as to how much to give of each remedy. Very sick people might need 300 drops three times a day of a particular herbal drainer whereas others might only require twenty drops once a day for balance. Everyone is different. In our clinic, we work with individuals and what their body chemistry needs to be balanced, healthy and symptom free.

The body is an amazing healer when you focus on eliminating the cause and quit worrying and focusing on symptoms. Fran's skin sores were only a symptom of a clogged liver, spleen and lymphatic system. Her doctors in the past didn't understand cellular detoxification and failed to support what the body was attempting to do in order to heal her skin problems.

The intelligent doctor within each of us knows exactly what to do each and every time. Medical doctors prescribing a drug to interfere with what your body's doctor within is doing creates a major conflict. Oh sure, you may feel better temporarily, but understand, no medical doctor is smarter than the intelligence that governs your body. Remember the power that created the body, heals the body. No other doctor or outside force can heal you. Healing comes from within. Don't think for one second that your doctor is smarter than the DNA intelligence encoded in every one of your cells. If it had the power, wisdom, intelligence and energy to create you in mother's womb, then it certainly knows what to do to heal you. But in order to heal, the cells need oxygen, nutrition, water and the detoxification channels opened.

> **"It's supposed to be a secret, but I'll tell you anyway. We doctors do nothing. We only help and encourage the doctor within."**
> Albert Schweitzer, M.D. - Nobel Laureate 1940

Don't Ignore Your Body's Warning Signs

If your medical doctor is failing to check your liver, spleen, kidneys and lymphatic system to make sure they are filtering and draining sufficiently so toxins don't back up and come through the skin, then you might want to consider finding a new doctor. Be bold and fire him or her if they fail to focus on prevention. A doctor who understands the importance of proper drainage from your 100 trillion living cells could save your life.

Our Creator gave us a way to deal with sickness and to detoxify. A fever allows us to sweat toxins out. Diarrhea, vomiting, sneezing and coughing are other safety features we come equipped with to expel toxins from inside. Anything done to suppress what the body does naturally is inviting disease to visit us tomorrow.

Edema (swelling) and pain are warning signs from your body crying out for help. Mainstream medicine teaches us to ignore those vital warning signals by suppressing them with painkillers, diuretics and anti-inflammatories. The surgeon for the King of England understood this healing secret long ago and informed the world of this wisdom when he stated,

> **"There is but one disease and that is deficient drainage."**
> Sir Arbuthnot Lane, M.D. - Surgeon for the King of England

Choosing to ignore the warning signals in your body is no different than you putting duct tape over an annoying red-flashing oil light in your car. The wise automobile manufactures put the oil warning light there to prevent disaster when the oil level gets dangerously low in your car. When I was younger, my older brother failed to heed the warning sign in our Buick. He kept driving and burned the engine up, needless to say Dad wasn't necessarily dancing a German Polka jig and sashaying across the living room humming "Oh what a beautiful morning…"

Like the warning lights on the dash of your car, The Creator engineered your body with warning signals as well. Headaches, swelling, pain, heartburn, diarrhea, hunger, thirst, lightheadedness, fatigue etc., are some of those signs you come equipped with. Most of us address the hunger and fatigue signals by eating and sleeping, but suppress the other signals with drugs.

> **"Most diseases are the result of medication which has been prescribed to relieve and take away a beneficial and warning symptom on the part of Nature."** Elbert Hubbard

Let's analyze lightheadedness, one of the ingenious warning signs your custom designed body has. Lightheadedness, which can result in fainting, is the body's way of making you lay flat so blood can flow effortlessly to the brain without fighting against gravity. As you collapse and lay flat, the blood can carry the needed sugar or oxygen to the brain that you weren't getting, probably caused by sluggish adrenal glands from the over consumption of sugar or coffee also known as hypoglycemia. Within a few minutes, the nutrients flow in to the brain and you feel fine again and you stand back up and go on your merry way.

If you choose to ignore the warning signs that your body sends out long enough, then it will shut down in an effort to solve the problem. Taking time out to address the cause of dis-ease is an investment in the quality of your life. Suppressing your symptoms with toxic drugs is a quick fix that invites trouble into the body later on. We live in a quick-fix, ignore-the-cause society. Suppressing all of our little symptoms with drugs here and there has a price to be paid. The symptoms we suppress today with drugs create the cancer and other diseases of tomorrow.

In his book, *The Biology of belief*, cell biologist Bruce Lipton, Ph.D., from Stanford University's School of Medicine, relates a story to illustrate how ridiculous it is to suppress symptoms with drugs.

"Our drug mania reminds me of a job at an auto dealership I held while in graduate school. At 4:30 on a Friday afternoon, an irate woman came into the shop. Her car's "service engine light" was flashing, even though her car had already been repaired for that same problem several times. At 4:30 on a Friday afternoon, who wants to work on a balky problem and deal with a furious customer? Everyone was quiet, except for one mechanic who said: "I'll take care of it."' He drove the car back into the bay, got in behind the dashboard, removed the bulb from the signal light and threw it away. Then he opened a can of soda and lit a cigarette. After suitable time, during which the customer thought he was actually fixing the car, the mechanic returned and told the woman her car was ready. Thrilled to see that the warning light had stopped flashing, she happily drove off into the sunset. Though the cause of the problem was still present, the symptom was gone.

Similarly, pharmaceutical drugs suppress the body's symptoms, but, most never address the cause of the problem." For more information go to www.brucelipton.com

> **"An ounce of prevention is worth a pound of cure."**
> Benjamin Franklin

Americans have foolishly been taught by a money-oriented medical system to "cut the wires" so we can go on our merry way with life and not be annoyed with warning lights and symptoms. Like a businessman once told me as he swallowed his painkillers, "I don't have time for this nagging headache and this little pill does the trick." There's no doubt that drugs do a wonderful job at keeping the signals suppressed, however we run the risk of burning up the engine. When he's laying ten toes up in a hospital bed because he just had a heart attack or he has colon cancer, then he'll all of a sudden, abracadabra magically have time. When your health fails, you have all the time in the world to lay in bed and mope around sick because you can't work or play. Don't wait until you are flat on your back in a hospital bed lying ten-toes up to start focusing on health. By then, you have one foot in the grave and the other one on a banana peel. Your health is your wealth. Wake up and be responsible for your life and your health! Now is the time to start a healing environment for your body.

> **"Drugs never cure disease. They merely hush the voice of nature's protest, and pull down the danger signals she erects along the pathway of transgression. Any poison taken into the system has to be reckoned with later on even though it palliates present symptoms. Pain may disappear, but the patient is left in a worse condition, though unconscious of it at the time."**
> Daniel H. Kress, M.D.

Diarrhea

Diarrhea is another way the body attempts to get rid of toxins, taking a drug to stop diarrhea is interfering with the wisdom of your body's healing efforts. Almost everyone at one time or another in life experiences diarrhea. Running to the toilet every hour to sit down and experience straight liquid coming out as if someone turned on the faucet gets old real fast when you are not feeling well. Keeping the body nourished so you do not dehydrate is very important, but at the same time allowing the toxins or infection to come out of the bowels so that the portal vein that wraps around the intestinal tract quits absorbing toxic infectious waste is a key to healing.

> "In the 50 years I've spent helping people to overcome illness, disability and disease, it has become crystal clear that poor bowel management lies at the root of most people's health problems."
> Bernard Jensen D.C., N.D., Ph.D.

Fever

When your military-like immune system identifies invaders like bacteria or viruses in the body, it automatically heats up. White blood cells come onto the scene like police and firefighters do at a car accident. This is nature's way of bringing toxins and impurities to the surface to be eliminated. It is your innate intelligence's way of saving your life. It isn't something to fear but to be thankful for because the body is healing. A fever occurs when other channels of elimination are not removing waste material fast enough..

> "Give me the chance to create fever and I will cure any disease."
> Parmenides (2,000 years ago)

What do we do as soon as our child gets a fever? We run to the medicine cabinet and grab our Tylenol to reduce the fever. This interferes with the health restoring power of the body and the illness is supressed internally. The body's intelligence is not given a chance to raise the temperature high enough which increases white blood cells so that they move extremely quickly into troubled areas and take care of problems. It has just been shoved in the corner so we can deal with it later on in a different form.

Drugs suppress the body's toxin releasing activities. If we want to truly heal and get well, we must allow toxins to surface and be released. Your body knows how to heat up and create a fever to burn out the toxins. Anything done to reduce the temperature such as drugs or sponging is counterproductive. When we interfere with this intelligent, safe and natural means of getting well by suppressing the symptoms with drugs, we are asking for problems later on in life. Wisdom beckons us to stop interfering with what God engineered the human body to do in an effort to be healthy. You can rest assured that He knew what He was doing when He created you.

> "Natural forces within us are the true healers."
> Hippocrates - Father of Modern Medicine, 460-370 B.C.

How high can a fever get before it becomes dangerous? Every parent would be wise to read Dr. Mendelsohn's book, *How To Raise A Healthy Child In Spite Of Your Doctor*. He states that fevers below 105 degrees do not pose any lasting threat to ones health. *"Every doctor learns in medical school that for every degree of rise in temperature the rate of travel of the disease-fighting leukocytes in the blood stream is doubled. This process is known as leucotaxis,"* informs Dr. Mendelsohn. For example, if you have a 104 degree fever, the ability of your white blood cells to move and fight infection is increased sixty-four times compared to normal body temperature of ninety-eight degrees. It makes no sense for a doctor to slow or interfere with the mechanism that is trying to get the person well by burning out the infection.

Many doctors have shown that the body produces a fever to prevent infection from spreading to other areas. Experiments performed by G.W. Duff and S.K. Durum have demonstrated that at two degrees centigrade of fever, T-cells and antibodies rapidly increased by 2,000 percent above their normal number at regular body temperature. If fever increases our ability to fight diseases, then possibly a low body temperature (which may be caused from hypothyroidism) makes us more susceptible to infections?

> **"The Intelligence within you is the same Intelligence that created this entire planet."** Louise L. Hay - Author of You Can Heal Your Life

Colds

We do not catch colds. The common cold is a good thing. It is your body's natural way of cleaning house. We get rid of toxic garbage, which produces symptoms we call a cold. A stuffy or runny nose, sneezing, headache, cough, fatigue and sore throat are typical house-cleaning symptoms. Remember only sick people get sick. If you are clean and healthy your body would never need a cold to cleanse mucous and other garbage build-up. The doctor within knows when to automatically clean and when he snaps his fingers all 100 trillion cells crack their heels and salute. Your body is a house of order. When told to clean, the cells stop what they are doing and begin cleaning, and as a result you begin draining mucous through the sinuses, lungs etc. Taking cold medicine doesn't fix the problem, it works against what the life-saving doctor within is attempting to do in your behalf.

> **"Disease is nothing else but an attempt on the part of the body to rid itself of morbific matter."**
> Thomas Sydenham - Famous seventeenth century English Physician

A cold develops after we have abused the body with too much junk. Cooked, dead and processed foods acidify the body and lead to constipation, which produces toxicity in the body. When these toxins and mucous accumulate, the body has to punch the red panic button to clean house so the cells are able to function. You know the procedure, you do it in your house. Whenever your house gets dirty and out of order you finally have to stop and say, "I've got to clean up in here so that we can live!" On a simple cellular level that is what your body does when you come down with a cold. The body begins a huge toxin dumping clean up party and during the process you feel stuffy and terrible. Have you ever noticed how good you usually feel after getting over it?

Bacteria, viruses and germs of all types thrive only in a toxic body that attracts them with plenty of garbage for them to feed on along with a mucous-ridden sluggish immune system that can't defend itself any longer in such filth and garbage.

> **"Echinacea and Garlic are the 'one, two punch' for the common cold!"** Dr. Richard Schulze

Attempting to stop a cold with drugs is interfering with the natural cleansing process your intelligence automatically ordered. A cold should be allowed to run its course and you would be wise to support it in its effort to save your life by eliminating congestion. Fruit and vegetable juices, herbal teas, enemas, lymphatic work through massage and bouncing on a rebounder are great tools to assist your body in healing. Proper rest, with lots of good clean water, is a must. Some of the best herbs to take for a cold are; echinacea, garlic, cat's claw and elderberry.

If the bowels are not eliminating properly, then toxins will be reabsorbed into your body and you'll feel terrible as the cold lingers on for days. Allowing a cold to run its course results in you feeling better in the long run. Stopping a cold with drugs results in more health problems and less energy in the future.

Chapter 4
HEALERS OR DRUG DEALERS?

Epilepsy Healed

> **"I am a realist, as long as the profit is in the treatment of symptoms rather than in the search for causes, that's where the medical profession will go for its harvest."** Arthur F. Coca, M.D. - The Pulse Test

The healing power of the human body never ceases to amaze me. To see someone plagued with epileptic seizures, who medical doctors have given up on, come into our clinic and get well is truly awesome. After having been given a drug maintenance plan with no hope for a cure by doctors, they seek a second opinion and come in to Life Essentials Natural Healing Clinic. Some have spent over $300,000 on "the best" medicine in the country, but are still diseased. Like one man said as he brought his son in, "I don't believe in what you do, but I'm here because I have no other options. The best doctors in the state tell me there is no cure for my son. Do you think you could help him?"

After two months of being on a natural detoxifying and cellular nourishment program, the boy's body responded by letting go of toxins. The cells in his body were fed the healing foods they had been crying out for over the last twenty years. The problem was that no doctor had yet to recognize and identify those cries, protests and warning signals given by his out of balance body that ended up manifesting seizures as a symptom. His body was attempting to communicate, but obviously his doctors failed to understand what his body was saying. Like a medical doctor who uses natural remedies once explained, "It's not their fault, they are not taught in medical school to address the cause, they are taught to treat symptoms with drugs." Of course the seizures never got better with drugs, because the seizures were not caused from a deficiency of Depakote, so why prescribe the trash?

> **"Half of what we have taught you is wrong. Unfortunately, we do not know which half."** Dean Burwell, M.D. (Addressing medical students at Harvard University)

Symptoms are your body's way of screaming for help, no different than a child drowning in water. To suppress those symptoms with man-made drugs and never address the cause, is equivalent to plugging your ears so you can't hear a drowning child's screams. It's time to stop ignoring what your body is saying and start understanding that toxins and nutritional deficiencies cause certain symptoms. This insanity in mainstream medicine is killing us. It's time to wake up! Medical doctors who suppress symptoms with drugs without ever finding the cause and correcting it, are setting you up for major health problems in the future. It's no different than you taking the batteries out of your smoke detector in your house so you are no longer annoyed by the high pitch squeal, despite the smoke. Only a fool would do such a thing because he knows that the smoke detector is sounding off for his own safety. It is doing its job, alarming him of danger.

Your body has smoke detectors also, however, we do not refer to the alarms in the body as smoke detectors. When your body's smoke alarms go off, we recognize them as pain, inflammation, headaches, skin rashes, heartburn, fever, low energy, allergies, high blood pressure, high cholesterol, sore throats etc. We have superstitiously been brainwashed to take the batteries out of our alarms and cover up our symptoms with drugs so we are no longer bothered by annoying sirens and symptoms. This insanity practiced by mainstream medicine kills 225,000 Americans each year according to JAMA.

The father who brought his son Mike, in with Epilepsy, narcolepsy, sleep apnea and restless leg syndrome saw a complete reversal in Mike's health. The father became a believer. He witnessed the miracle of healing. Mike was healed from seizures after having had on the average three a week for the last twenty years of his life.

People always ask us, "Can you cure epilepsy, cancer, lupus etc?" The answer is no, we can't cure anything and neither can any other doctor, however, your body can heal itself of any disease once it receives correct nutrition and the toxins are eliminated. When this happens, healing occurs. Through CEDSA we were able to detect which products would detoxify and nourish the body, thus providing a healing environment.

When we matched the herbs, homeopathics and nutritional formulas that resonated well to balance Mike's body then he was able to heal. The results were phenomenal. His symptoms went away and he felt great. The father was left baffled. How in the world could you spend over $300,000 on the "best medicine" in America and have all the tests come back inconclusive and the best they can do is prescribe drugs to maintain dis-ease for the rest of the poor guy's life? And then he brings him in to a natural healing clinic and for approximately $700 worth of products and testing fees, the boy is completely healed of epileptic seizures. The father was angry and was ready to take action against the fraud being perpetrated against Americans who are suffering needlessly. How could insurance cover all the expensive medical testing that failed to help one bit, then refuse to cover a naturopathic approach that allowed his son to be completely healed?

The father wanted to know why insurance does not cover what we do. Most Americans can't fathom why they won't cover something that would eventually reduce medical expenses in the future. When you understand the monopoly that has been formed in this country involving oil, drugs and insurance, then it helps you understand why they do not cover natural medicine, which is competition to their multi-billion dollar empire.

So what were the causes of Mike's seizures? A CEDSA exam identified energetic disturbances in his nervous system, pituitary gland and circulatory system. Mercury poisoning resonated in his body as a major culprit interfering with cellular function, especially with his nervous system, pituitary, thyroid and adrenal glands. Uncovering his symptoms layer by layer like an onion, we also found parasites. As we scanned through our list of parasites we identified nematodes (roundworms) interfering with his health. Toxocara Cati roundworms were the parasites disrupting health. The syphilinum miasm also showed up as a culprit effecting his nervous system. To get right to the point, those were the toxins causing him to manifest epileptic seizure symptoms. Until we detoxified the toxins that were identified through a CEDSA exam he probably would have never healed. Drugs have no power to detoxify cells, but herbs and homeopathic remedies do the job effectively.

Most medical doctors do not test for those causes of dis-ease. As a result healing does not take place, only disease maintenance with drug use. That is the way our current medical system operates here in America. We do things differently here at the clinic. We focus on health, not disease. We balance the body with nutritional and detoxification programs so that healing occurs. So next time you go to another doctor's visit remember, he will only find what he is looking for, not what's causing disease.

When we scanned Mike to check his nutritional levels which includes; all sixty minerals, amino acids, vitamins, fatty acids and enzymes we found him to have a raging magnesium/potassium deficiency. Other nutrients that checked low in his body were calcium, zinc, taurine (amino acids), iodine, choline, inositol and pantothenic acid. His serotonin levels were also extremely out of balance, probably from all his medications. We went to work to detoxify him with homeopathic remedies and herbal drainage tinctures as well as nutritional support formulas. As soon as he started the nutritional/detox program, the seizures ceased completely. Within eight weeks he was healthy and seizure free. Does this sound too good to be true? The doctor within has access to the DNA library that contains all the healing wisdom of the ages and can heal any dis-ease when given the correct nutritional and detoxification tools to work with.

The body is an amazing healer when we pull the toxins out and give it the nourishment it needs to be balanced. Remember, drugs do not balance the body. They further deplete it of vital nutrients and add toxins to the cells. Herbs are foods and when we give the body cell food it awakes, revitalizes, cleanses, heals and it lives. This is life and this is how we heal and experience optimum health.

Nutritional Deficiencies Causing Mike's Seizures		
Magnesium	Potassium	Vitamin A
Iodine	B Vitamins	Zinc
Pantothenic Acid	Calcium	Taurine

Why didn't his previous medical doctors detect any of those toxins and nutritional deficiencies? The answer is very simple. It is very sad, but most of our medical doctors don't check anything that can't be maintained with drugs. They do not check for heavy metals, parasites, pantothenic acid deficiencies etc., on a regular basis. Usually they only check major nutrients like sodium, potassium, calcium and iron (anemia). When doctors do check the blood and the testing shows a problem, it is very serious.

Pathological blood work is usually a poor diagnosis because the body will do everything in its power to maintain homeostasis. When the blood begins to change and deficiencies are detected, then we know the organs and glands have been deprived for a dangerously long time. Waiting for deficiencies to manifest themselves in the blood is about as foolish as you waiting until you feel the wind and rain on your face before you evacuate a town that lies in the path of a hurricane, despite the news warning you to leave twenty-four hours ago.

A wise doctor does not wait until the blood shows signs of deficiencies to start you on nutritional support. Do not be fooled. Just because your blood looks good on a lab report does not necessarily mean that you are nutritionally balanced. A CEDSA exam can identify energetic nutritional deficiencies that can help bring your body back into balance before you start experiencing symptoms.

> "Out of four thousand cases recently examined in a New York hospital, only two were not suffering from a lack of calcium."
> Journal of the American Medical Association

Anyone who wants to invest in their health would be wise to have a CEDSA evaluation once a year to check for possible toxins that could be affecting their health. We live in a toxic world bombarded with pollutants and chemicals in our foods. One glass of store-bought milk is said to contain over a hundred different antibiotics. The majority of all cereal in the USA contains BHT (a preservative) which has been banned in England. It causes chemical changes in the brain. And we wonder why there is so much depression, bipolar disorders, ADD, etc. How many of us start our day off with a bowl of BHT-laced cereal in a bowl of milk containing antibiotics and steroids given to the cow?

You Only Find What You are Looking For

> **"Drugs put a tremendous strain on the liver, the organ responsible for providing enzymes to metabolize the drugs and dispose of their toxic waste products."** Candace B. Pert, Ph.D.

We are surrounded by chemicals in our environment. The United States Office of Technology Assessment informs that the EPA lists more than 65,000 chemicals in its inventory of toxic chemicals. What's even more alarming is that every year they receive more than 1500 notices of intent to manufacture new chemicals. These chemicals build up in your body and cause health problems.

According to Stephen B. Edelson, M.D., *"The liver accumulates rather than eliminates toxins...."* He points out that one of the most serious yet overlooked toxins in our society is mercury. Not only is it found in dental fillings but also in seafood, water, pesticides, fertilizers, paints, solvents, bleached flour, processed foods and even fabric softeners.

When is the last time your doctor checked you for the following toxins that are scientifically proven to cause dis-ease? Most likely your doctor has never found any of the following toxins in you. Why? Because he does not look for them. Does it make sense why one out of every three people are being diagnosed with cancer now? These toxins accumulate in our bodies and medical doctors never recommend a liver cleanse. How do we expect to be healthy if we never do anything to cleanse?

> **"I had a dream. I saw my decaying body torn to shreds by ravenous vultures fighting for every scrap. I struggled to awake from this paralyzing nightmare only to find I was waiting in my doctor's office."** EC Wyndhan

Toxins Your Doctor Should Check You For To Prevent Dis-ease

Heavy metals	Pesticides	Parasites
Chemical Poisoning	Food Allergies	Inhalant Allergies
Viruses	Bacteria	Fungus
Candida Yeast	Molds	Vaccination Toxicity
Radiation Poisoning	Miasms	Prescription Drug Toxins
Aspartame Poisoning	Unloved	Electromagnetic Stress
Herpes	Lyme Disease	Guilt
Silicone Poisoning (implants)	Ulcers	Resentment
Epstein-Barr virus	Coxsackie virus	Mucor Racemosus
Aspergillus Niger	Mercury	Lead Poisoning
MSG Poisoning	Arterial plaquing	Acidosis
Calcium plaquing	Suppressed Emotions	Grudge
Fear	Free Radical Damage	Nicotine Poisoning

This is your health and your life. You deserve a CEDSA exam to check and see if any of these toxins are stressing your organs, glands and systems in any way. If they are, wouldn't you like to get them out? Do you think you might feel better and be healthier if you didn't have to deal with all that toxic trash everyday?

> "Progress is impossible without change, and those who cannot change their minds cannot change anything."
>
> George Bernard Shaw

Pulling toxins out of your body is an investment in your health for the rest of your life. Drugs cannot do this. As a matter of fact, drugs add toxins to the body that cannot be broken down. Most of these end up in your liver and are some of our biggest cancer culprits. Depending upon where the toxins settle and in what fashion they manifest themselves determines the disease they diagnose you as having.

The Right Fuel

> "Out of 2.1 million deaths per year in the United States, 1.6 million are related to poor nutrition."
>
> Dr. C. Everett Koop - Former Surgeon General

Your cells know what to do when they are given the right stuff, no different than when a carburetor in a 1967 Dodge Charger receives 93 high-octane fuel or better yet, nitrous down at the drag strip. Slamming the pedal to the metal will result in "smokin' the tires." When that fuel ignites, a tremendous exchange of energy takes place as the pistons in the engine explode the car into motion. Just as high-octane fuel is what has been created to fuel race cars, so have living plants been created to give your cells fuel to heal. Your cells run at peak performance on fruits, vegetables, whole grains, nuts and seeds.

Only an idiot would pour diet coke in his automobile's gas tank and expect it to run, right? Why? Because that engine was not engineered to burn Diet Coke as fuel. It will not ignite and power the car down the road period. Is the fact that we have to discuss such nonsense ridiculous? Of course it is and the purpose for writing such material is to bring Americans back to their common sense, logical thinking minds. We fill our tanks with junk and then wonder why we can't breathe, have headaches, allergies, no energy, depression, and can't lose weight.

> "One-quarter of what you eat keeps you alive. The other three-quarters keeps your doctor alive."
> Hieroglyph found in an ancient Egyptian Tomb

Everything you put in your mouth is either promoting health or causing dis-ease. Next time you get that cheap ice cream that has twenty-five artificial ingredients in it that you can't even pronounce and you eat it because it tastes so good, but are all stuffed up during the night and then wake up with a sore throat the next morning, you may want to take note that it probably was an unwise food to eat. Your tonsils swelled and a dull headache throbbed as your body retaliated to the toxic trash you forced it deal with. This burden put on your digestive system to break these additives and preservatives down demand a price to be paid. The price paid is made manifest in all of your symptoms. After twenty years of filling your tank with junky gas everyday, your engine blows up, no different than your body breaking down with a heart attack, stroke, arthritis, cancer, diabetes etc.

> "Know ye not that ye are the temple of God, and that the Spirit of God dwelleth in you? If any man defile the temple of God, him shall God destroy; for the temple of God is Holy, which temple ye are."
> 1 Corinthians 3:16-17

Defile the temple, the body that God created for you and He warns us that we will be destroyed. Most Americans disregard that little piece of advice because it doesn't fit into their convenient fast food diet, containing hot dogs, French fries and Diet Coke. The Lord never told us how long the process would take to destroy the temple if we defile it. Perhaps chronic degenerate diseases like arthritis are ways He keeps his word to destroy those who have chosen to defile their bodies He has given them?

You Reap What You Sow

We are created in God's image. God has laws. One of those laws is gravity. Jump off a 100-foot cliff and the gravitational pull on your body will cause you to land so hard it will kill. Understand that there is a law irrevocably decreed from on high and when we receive a blessing of good health, it is by obedience to that law upon which all health is predicated.

> **"Life in all its fullness is Mother Nature obeyed."** Dr. Weston Price

Everything you do has a consequence. Fail to pay your power bill and you'll be shivering all winter long when they cut your power off and you are without heat. Consume liberal amounts of junk food and you'll be sick. Your body will break down and you'll be plagued with a list of symptoms longer than my five-year-old's Christmas wish-list for Santa Claus.

Since mainstream medicine has a tendency to ignore diet (just look at the trash they feed patients in hospitals), it's time to pay attention to what goes in our mouths. In naturopathy we take heed to the laws of cause and effect. Everything you eat, drink and think either promotes health or disease. If you plant tomatoes in the garden, you will not harvest carrots. You reap what you sow.

Good health is something you can claim if you invest in it and throw away the credit cards (drugs) that get you into trouble. The feel good now and pay the price tomorrow is killing Americans and very few people ever connect the dots. We fail to make that connection between suppressing symptoms with drugs today and our newly diagnosed diseases of tomorrow.

> **"We live in an overmedicated society. More Americans are hooked on drugs by their physicians than by all the pushers on the street. It is estimated that one billion prescriptions are written in the United States every year. In my judgement, a majority of them are unnecessary and – as the staff in any hospital emergency room can tell you - many of them are dangerous and even deadly."**
>
> Robert Mendelsohn, M.D.

| A + B = C | A + B = Smoke | Fire + Wood = Smoke |

If you build a fire it will produce smoke. Smoke is a by-product of fire burning wood. When you eat meat, uric acid is produced. If you have sore stiff joints, arthritis or gout, you need to stop eating meat.

| A + B = Uric Acid | Cooked Meat + Consumption = Uric Acid |

| Uric Acid = Inflammation   &   Inflammation = Arthritis (Joint Pain) |

> "Ammonia, which is produced in great amounts as a by-product of meat metabolism, is highly carcinogenic and can cause cancer development. A high protein diet also breaks down the pancreas and lowers resistance to cancer as well as contributes to the development of diabetes." Dr. Willard J. Visek - Cornell University

One of the reasons alternative medicine is put down by pro-drug users is because natural healing puts responsibility upon the patient. This book teaches "response-ability," which is your ability to respond to life in a health-promoting way. Most drug users silently worship their doctor and put 100 percent faith in what he says. People put poisonous drugs in their bodies that cause worse symptoms than what they are taking the drug for in the first place, because that's what "my doctor told me to do." They stop thinking and follow blindly. They become poor victims of such and such a disease. How many so-smart doctors gave their patients Vioxx and other health destroying drugs that have harmed and killed good Americans so many times that the FDA finally pulled the killer from the market? You trusted him with Vioxx, what drugs are you trusting him with now that will be recalled next year?

Our current medical system puts doctors in charge of people's health so that the patient can be a poor victim. This way the person can still go out and eat doughnuts, Pop-Tarts, Captain Crunch, coffee, a thirty-two ounce Diet Coke, French fries and all the other typical trash we Americans liberally consume and when we come down with a debilitating disease, we get to be the poor victim. We are never at fault this way.

So why in the world would someone want to go to a naturopathic doctor who may recommend dietary changes, colonics, exercise, fasting, colon and liver cleanses etc. That sounds like work doesn't it? Remember faith without work is dead. Perhaps that is why we Americans are in such poor health. We stand in the welfare line wanting something for free. We sit in the doctor's office waiting for him to "fix us." We max out our credit cards by buying what we want today with no regards as to how we will pay for it tomorrow and can't even pay the interest. After digging ourselves into debt so deep, we end up filing bankruptcy. Then we throw our hands up and plead for a second chance. We want others to be responsible, to take care of us so we can do as little as possible and still feel good. The bottom line is, natural medicine requires effort on our part and then the blessings from on high will be bestowed upon us. As Hanna Kroeger says, "God helps those who help themselves."

> "What things soever ye desire, when ye pray, believe that ye receive them, and ye shall have them." Mark 11:24

Like going through the drive through at McDonalds for lunch, your health is in the express lane with your doctor dishing out the prescriptions as fast as Lanny can wrap Big Macs. To go home and make a soup with chopped vegetables with some fresh garlic, ginger and onions is what would nourish your body but for some, this is too much work.

> "Indeed, most doctors fail to offer hope because they do not have confidence in their own treatments. In that lack of hope lies the seeds of death. Perhaps it is for the patient to be his/her own doctor, and to seek for the cure until it is found. Pythagoras said, 'Physician heal thyself,' and I say, 'Patient heal thyself, through the powers of purity, Love and intuition.'" Richard Anderson, N.D., N.M.D.

Some time ago a friend of the family had a heart attack. He wasn't aware that we teach people how to avoid such disasters so he had never been to see me. He wasn't very healthy and like a typical seventy-five year old American his doctor had him on a long list of drugs, suppressing his symptoms. I went to visit him in the hospital. As I was there visiting, hospital staff brought his lunch in. Here is a man who just had a heart attack and what do you think they were feeding him for lunch? Fried chicken with grease dripping off of it, potatoes and gravy, a slab of red Jell-O and milk to wash it down. For dessert he had a piece of cheesecake topped with whipped cream.

What kind of hospital serves someone who just had a heart attack the same types of junky foods that have created the dis-ease in the first place? It's obvious that they either don't know or don't care about healing foods for sick people. If you want to do another by-pass surgery in a couple of years, you might as well get him back on those types of foods right away that caused him to have the heart attack in the first place. Feed him greasy fried meats, hydrogenated fats and pasteurized homogenized milk and it will just be a matter of time before he is ready for round two. And of course the surgeon will be there ready to do another by-pass so everyone can call him the hero that saved a life, yet he never mentions a thing about preventing the next attack through correct eating habits and nutritional support. There's no money in prevention, it's all in waiting until something breaks down before they begin treatment. If they really cared about this man's health, wouldn't they invest in prevention? Wouldn't they put him on some circulation support, something to deplaque his arteries?

> **"From birth to old age, the average individual never experiences the taste of real natural food. He is poisoning himself day by day with the food he eats. Few people know the right kind of food to place in their bodies to keep them well and strong, or take the trouble to select this food if they do know."** Paul C. Bragg

There is no doubt that we have some of the greatest emergency room doctors in the world who can save lives and put mangled bodies back together, but when it comes to chronic degenerate dis-eased conditions we are losing the war. Some doctors can't understand how people with chronic diseases and cancer who haven't been helped by their drugs can change their diet, start taking some natural remedies and be completely healed. Why is it so hard for them to believe this? Because their medical training has indoctrinated them to believe that only expensive, patented drugs are to be used in treating disease, despite herbs being used effectively for thousands of years worldwide. Most doctors have been browbeaten into believing that herbs are for the poor, uneducated backwoods, less fortunate people. And to scare their patients, they throw in a warning that some of those herbs can harm you; despite their 3500 page PDR listing the possible harmful side affects from the drugs they prescribe. Who should be warning who?

> **"Two things are infinite: the universe and human stupidity and I'm not sure about the universe."** Albert Einstein

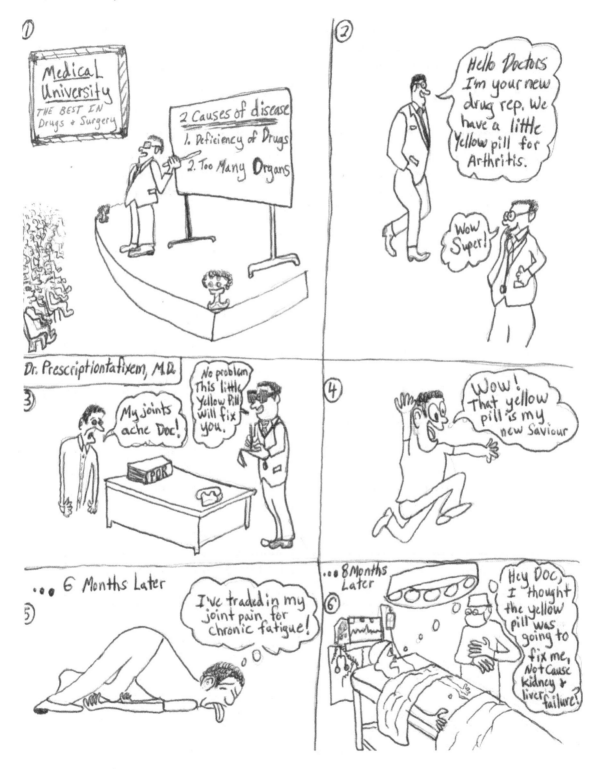

Healing Poisoned Medicine

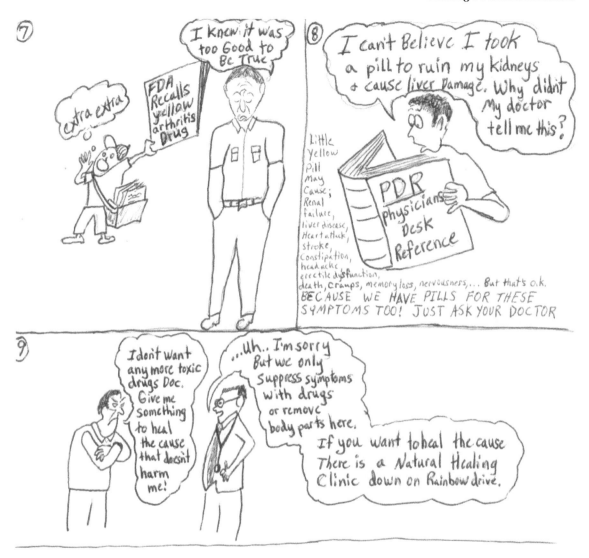

"All great truths begin as blasphemies." George Bernard Shaw

Is Your Car Worth More Than Your Health?

To service a car we change the oil, spark plugs, air filter, and maybe put some fuel injector cleaner in the gas tank. This usually helps a sluggish sputtering car run smoothly again. Like a car that requires a high quality gasoline and oil to run well, so does your body. To service your body use the herbs that God has created and ordained for the service of man. When we put the right stuff in your body, it heals no differently than when you put the right fuel in your car to run smoothly.

Every engine, radio, computer, TV etc., requires the right fuel or power source in order to function. Whether it be gasoline, diesel, two-stroke engine gas/oil mix, 110 electrical outlet or AA batteries there is a specific fuel/power source to make the thing work.

In order for you to empower your body to heal, it requires the correct fuel also. You knew that all along didn't you? Most of us don't want to believe it because we don't want to give up the junk foods that we are addicted to eating.

> "I do not feel obliged to believe that same God who has endowed us with sense, reason, and intellect has intended us to forgo their use."
> Galileo Galilei

If we want to heal, we have to take our heads out of the sand and start looking at what is causing dis-ease, not what little purple pill might make our symptoms disappear for a short while. To say it very simply, drugs are similar to credit cards, what symptoms we suppress today, we will pay for tomorrow. Sometimes it's cancer, other times it's fibromyalgia, but none-the-less, we reap what we sow. Don't kid yourself, the credit card debt must be paid sometime. Your body will let you know without hesitation when that time comes.

Words of Wisdom

> "The Lord God causes the grass to grow for the cattle, and the herb for the service of man." Psalms 104:14

That is a pretty plain and simple statement; God causes herbs to grow for the service of man. The only problem with that statement is there's no dollar attached to it like "high rolling" drugs that reel in over 500 billion dollars a year in sales receipts. It doesn't matter if the plant can cure every disease in the world with just three doses, the masses will not be prescribed something of so little value no matter how effective and safe it proves to be. No patents means no payoffs, and if there are no payoffs then there is no research and no marketing. The pharmaceutical companies do what they do to make money. They maintain disease, they do not heal it. These drug giants don't have time to mess around with a product that doesn't produce revenue like the 2.5 billion dollar seller Vioxx reeled in with its five years of glory thanks to our doctors prescribing it like tickets for the Alabama vs. Auburn "Iron Bowl" football game.

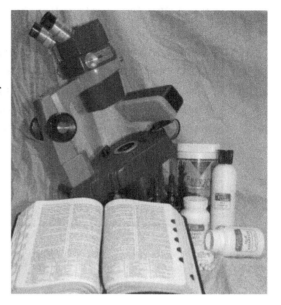

> "The key to health is simple: If we do not eat the kind of food, prepared properly, which will nourish the body constructively, we not only die prematurely, we suffer along the way."
> Norman Walker, D.Sc.

Clever business men who don't have a clue about how the body has been engineered to heal, have educated their pawns in the game to become their sales reps to sell their new expensive, patented, synthetic, adverse-reaction-causing fuel. More money has been spent on advertising drugs than on actual research and the evidence is sick people everywhere continuing to get sicker each year. Cancer and every other disease you can think of is on the rise every single day. Think about it, if drugs really worked, cancer and other diseases would be declining right? Common sense tells us 2 + 2 = 4. Drugs maintaining dis-ease = increased disease.

There is more wisdom and intelligence encoded in the DNA of living plants than in any chemist's concoctions touted as miracle drugs that create a whole new set of yet to be discovered problems at the cellular level.

> "Disease, if you call it something long enough, true or not, the masses will believe it. Just give it enough time." Sagarius

Are you like some people who come in our clinic and after two hours of testing say, "Well, let me ask my medical doctor about these herbs and if he doesn't tell me to use them then I won't. If he doesn't tell me to stop drinking Diet Cokes, eating doughnuts, and French fries then I won't. He tells me one bowel movement a week is perfectly fine. So as long as I take my drugs for high blood pressure, high cholesterol, depression, headaches, birth control, something to help me sleep and one for my low thyroid then I'm perfectly healthy right?"

> "The best of our popular physicians are the ones who do the least harm. But unfortunately some poison their patients with mercury, and others purge or bleed them to death. There are some who have learned so much that their learning has driven out all common sense; and there are others who care a great deal more for their own profit than for the health of their patient—a physician should be the servant of Nature, not his enemy; he should be able to guide and direct her in her struggle for life, and not throw by his unreasonable influences fresh obstacles in the way of recovery."
>
> Paracelsus – Swiss doctor 1493-1541

Ask the Right Person

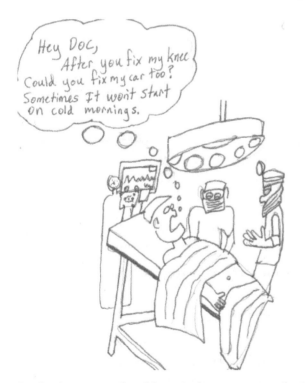

Let's suppose you are in a terrible automobile accident and you need knee surgery to repair your damaged leg, obviously you would consult an orthopedic surgeon, not a naturopath or chiropractor, right? Why? Because that's what the surgeon does everyday for a living. He is an expert in repairing damaged joints. When you are in surgery, you wouldn't raise up on the operating table and say, "Hey doc, while you are fixing things, after you finish my knee could you fix my car too because every time I turn the wheel to the left I hear a terrible knocking sound?" How ridiculous would that be?

As ridiculous as it sounds, we Americans sometimes play the ridiculous consulting game by asking people who know very little about certain modalities. For example, if you are interested in how your body can heal, then you should consult a naturopath. Why? Because that is his field of expertise. He studies how the body heals using, nutrition, whole foods, herbs, homeopathy, massage, colonics, emotional release, etc. Asking a medical doctor who has no training in homeopathy, herbology, nutrition, etc., about natural healing is about as ridiculous as asking a prostitute to come give a talk in church on Sunday morning on morality.

If you want to treat symptoms with drugs and surgically remove body parts then consult a medical doctor. That is what they do, it is their field of expertise.

A friend who has cancer came to consult with me. Her oncologist wants to start radiation and chemotherapy soon. When she went to her appointment she saw the cancer patients in the hospital eating doughnuts for breakfast. What kind of treatment program allows cancer patients to continue to eat garbage foods? Obviously they disregard nutrition when it comes to health.

> **"Most doctors don't know anything about nutrition, because medical schools are so oriented toward intervention that they virtually ignore nutrition as an element in the prevention or cure of disease."** Robert Mendelsohn, M.D.

Case Study – January, 2005

Most of my adult life I have had numerous health problems. About 14 years ago I was stricken with a strange flu-like virus that would not go away. After seeing 2 or 3 medical doctors and 6 months later, I was finally diagnosed with Chronic Epstein-Barr. I was told there was no known treatment. For many years I had experienced chronic fatigue, especially after overexertion or periods of stress.

I was diagnosed with Hypothyroidism in the early 1960's. In this last decade I have been diagnosed with Chronic Fatigue Syndrome, mini-stroke, osteoporosis, food and inhalant allergies, gastrointestinal problems, high triglycerides, anxiety attacks, depression, TMJ, and Fibromyalgia. The fibromyalgia contributed to many of my problems. The debilitating fatigue was probably the hardest to deal with. Household activities were very limited, while church and social events were practically nonexistent.

The medical doctors only knew to keep adding prescription drugs for treatment of all my medical problems. The cost of treatment for my medical problems, along with menopause and hypothyroidism was a $600 - $700 pharmacy bill a month. As I was taking all the medication prescribed by the medical doctors, I realized that the drugs were slowly killing me. I was in constant pain and discomfort, I couldn't sleep and riding in a car was almost unbearable. My digestive system was extremely messed up, and I got very little relief with any medication prescribed for the stomach.

For all my medical problems, I was sent from doctor to doctor and had scans, X-rays, MRIs, Echo-cardiograms, colonoscopies, endoscopies, neurological testing, and blood work of every type. With all the testing, evaluations and medication nothing corrected my problems. I have been under the care of several different chiropractors during the last decade. I am not a "doctor hopper" as it may sound, but several of the doctors who treated me, threw up their hands and gave up on me.

My latest doctor of internal medicine, who I have been seeing for the last 4-5 years, knew **I was developing an interest in alternative medicine since the medical field gave me no hope or lasting help.** In April of 2004, my medical doctor admitted medical science had no cure for me and she suggested I seek other means of help If I chose to do so. She said that if I found a naturopathic doctor whom I felt comfortable with, to go with her blessings. This was a big change of direction for me, because I was indoctrinated to follow only mainstream medical practice.

I checked several places of alternative medicine within driving distances, but was not satisfied that they were right for me. My present chiropractor, Dr. Jon Alan Smith, recommended I see a naturopathic doctor in Gadsden. After talking with Dr. Sainsbury on the phone, I knew that I was being led in the right direction. On June 3, 2004, I had my first visit Dr. Sainsbury. I went with some hesitation, but I knew if I were to have a better life, or life at all, I had to try a different approach. I carried a bag full of medication (9 prescription drugs plus over the counter stuff). Dr. Sainsbury cued in on my multitude of problems and began addressing the most pressing problems by addressing the cause with natural supplements.

Since Dr. Sainsbury has been working with me, replacing drugs with natural supplements I have shown remarkable improvement physically, emotionally and mentally. At the present, I am taking 2-3 very small doses of prescription drugs and before long, I hope to be off all the chemicals. The last two months my pharmacy bill has been $35 instead of $600 - $700. My internist is elated with my state of health. My weight has dropped 20 plus pounds and all my blood work and physical exams are good. Although medical insurance does not cover Dr. Sainsbury's programs, as I told my medical doctor, I would rather be where I am health-wise today, than have the amount of money used for the programs. To quote her, "There is no price you can place on good health."

I am far from where I was health-wise in June 2004 and on January 18, 2005, I am not where I want to be. By God's grace and using Dr. Sainsbury as His instrument, I will be where I want to be health-wise soon.

I now have a "HOPE" for some quality years ahead. Jeremiah 29:11

Thank God for Dr. Reed Sainsbury
B. R., Albertville, Alabama

> "Doctors are men who prescribe medicines of which they know little, to cure diseases of which they know less, in human beings of whom they know nothing." Voltaire

Motivation to Win

My High School football coach had a motivational saying he quoted often when we were battered and fatigued during practice. I have never forgotten it. To this day I still remember being drenched in sweat and beat up from hitting drills, lined up on the goal line with my heart pounding and lungs feeling like they were ready to explode through my chest. Gasping for air and dreading the sound of the whistle to send us racing in another forty yard sprint, I can still hear Coach Hymes demanding us to push ourselves harder, through the fatigue and past the pain barrier by saying, "men, NEVER BE SATISFIED."

The problem with some Americans is that they are satisfied. They rely upon a man-made drug to function and live. They have no drive, ambition or motivation to improve life. They have little self-discipline to stop eating junk food because it tastes so goooood!!! They are slaves to the flesh. They make themselves poor victims of their circumstances and quick to blame others. I can not help those who choose not to help themselves.

If you do not have the will power and drive to make improvements in your life, then this book is not for you. When a football or wrestling coach takes a team of volunteers, players who are all there by choice with a desire to win, then championship status is obtainable. In other words, when people are involved in something because they want to be (it's in their hearts), success will be a lot higher than a group who is there to milk the clock and pick up a paycheck. Those who are involved by choice are committed to sacrifice and hard work everyday to improve themselves in hope of achieving championship status. It would be difficult to coach a team of quitters, people who have no desire to practice to improve their current status. Where there is no sacrifice (guts) there is no glory. You reap what you sow. Are you willing to invest the time and effort into your own health so you can win? Are you willing to do what it takes to be free? Are you motivated and enthusiastic or are you trudging your way through life hoping for the end to arrive because you feel it just isn't worth it?

> "Ability is what you're capable of doing. Motivation determines what you do. Attitude determines how well you do it."
> Lou Holtz - Notre Dame Football Coach

Wrestling is a grueling sport. I have the utmost respect for Olympic gold medalist wrestlers. If you lose, you have no one to blame but yourself. I remember conditioning at the end of practice for thirty minutes solid. My wrestling coach, Ron Seibel would say during those grueling workouts, *"If you quit on me here, you'll quit in life."* No one wanted to be a quitter. No one in life wants to be a quitter. It is our human nature to crave success. We live for admiration and to work hard and achieve a goal is a fulfilling accomplishment. It helps add that spark to life.

If you want to get well, you need a purpose to get out of bed every morning. You need something that moves, inspires and motivates you. Find something you can get excited about, whatever it is, and do it. Go out and make a difference in the world. Be part of the solution, not part of the problem. If you fail to do this, you are selling yourself short.

My father-in-law, Daniel Browning, is a shining example of how enthusiasm promotes good health. He owns and operates Browning Enterprise, a steel fabrication plant in Northeast Alabama. He loves production. He can make almost anything with steel. He is constantly searching for more efficient ways to be productive. He loves what he does and stays busy. His enthusiasm and fulfillment in life is what I believe contributes to his good health. He very rarely ever catches colds.

To achieve optimum health, you need to find your talents and use them. To receive empowerment for health means you are totally free of dis-ease. If you are a slave to man-made chemicals then you are not free. To be healthy means you are balanced; mentally, physically, emotionally and spiritually.

The word doctor means to teach. Many good people are suffering needlessly because of a lack of understanding by the majority of our present health care practitioners in this country. They merely guess as to which prescription drug they'll recommend to hush your bodies cry for help. No doctor has the authority to tell you when you will die or that you'll just have to learn to live with your disease. You can do whatever you believe you can do. Get that in your mind and believe it and feel it with all your heart and you'll conquer any obstacle.

> **"No physician can ever say that any disease is incurable. To say so blasphemes God, blasphemes Nature, and depreciates the great architect of Creation. The disease does not exist, regardless of how terrible it may be, for which God has not provided the corresponding cure."** Paracelsus

In this mortal existence you only have one body, one mind and one life. It is up to you to be in charge of it. No doctor, preacher, family member, boss, enemy or friend has the power to make you do anything. You may allow them to influence you, but the reality is, you are in charge. You steer the ship and take it where you want to go. You are the source. You are power. You are energy. You are alive and that is the miracle that you are. Set yourself free of the shackles that have you bound. Be still and know who you are. Experience life in its fullness, for this is living. To merely wake up every day feeling bad and taking drugs to suppress God-given symptoms is only surviving. Why choose a life like that? Wake up and stop crawling on your belly with the worms and start soaring with the eagles in the blue sky. The power is within you! But you have to want it, see it, feel it and then believe you can achieve it. The physical body always manifests the energetic blueprint laid out in your mind. Our thoughts create the world we live in. If you are sick, it is time to recreate.

> **"And ye shall know the truth, and the truth shall make you free."**
> St. John 8:32

My First Eye Opener to Health

When I was a young teenager, my Dad took my brother and me to meet Scott and Gladys Forsyth in Moses Lake, Washington. They were health enthusiasts who grew wheat grass and juiced it along with other healthy practices, such as composting their own soil for gardening. Many years ago Gladys was diagnosed with cancer and Scott had previously suffered from a heart attack. Like most Americans, they sought the best help available and began chemotherapy treatments for Gladys. Her body did the natural thing; rejected the poison chemotherapy. In an effort to get rid of the toxins, she began vomiting frequently and her hair fell out. Something within her told her that there was a better way.

One night as her dear husband sat by her side, she told him that she couldn't stand feeling sick like this anymore and if this is how her life was going to be, then she would rather go home and die in her own house. She didn't want to suffer in this awful state any longer. She didn't want to take this medicine that was making her so sick and weak.

Being very religious people, they decided to get on their knees and pour out their hearts to God for help. They prayed for deliverance from the hell they were experiencing. "Father, if there be a way to heal this cancer will Thou please show us now," was their desperate plead for help. A short time later they learned from a friend about the Ann Wigmore Living Food Foundation in Boston, Massachusetts. This natural healing center is built upon the principal and belief;

> *"THE NAME OF THE DISEASE IS NOT IMPORTANT. IF YOU PUT NOTHING BUT LIVING FOOD INTO YOUR BODY IT WILL HEAL ITSELF."*

"My doctor became extremely upset and said, 'you'll die' if you don't take this chemotherapy," explained Gladys. Since her doctor admitted to her that he couldn't promise the chemotherapy would work and allow her to live, she chose something different. Going against her doctor's orders, she left with her husband and flew to Boston to The Ann Wigmore Living Food Foundation. They stayed for two weeks and lived this way of life to see if it was effective for healing cancer. They felt strongly that God had heard and answered their prayers. For more information on The Ann Wigmore Foundation that is now operated in San Fidel, New Mexico, go online to www.wigmore.org.

The days went by and Scott and Gladys continued making and drinking "Rejuvelac" (fermented sprouted wheat water). Wheat grass juice and all manner of whole, raw living fruits and vegetables is what they ate. These raw living foods are high in enzymes, chlorophyll and easy to digest. They are cell foods, meaning they feed, nourish and cleanse the cells of the body. This is what your body has been engineered to burn for fuel to receive energy and health despite not being practiced by mainstream medicine due to obvious financial reasons.

The Forsyths began to feel better and their quality of life drastically improved. Three months later, still being on their whole foods diet and drinking freshly squeezed wheat grass juice daily, they went back to their doctor to check the status of the cancer. The doctors ran tests and rechecked their previous reports to see if perhaps they had made a mistake in diagnosing Gladys with uterine cancer. They couldn't believe it, but the cancer was completely gone! Not a single trace of it showed up! It had been healed completely. This healing experience happened twenty one years ago. Gladys is ninety years old now and still in good health, cancer free. She lives at home and continues to teach others how the body heals with the miracles of living foods. And for the medical doctor who told her she would die if she didn't take the chemotherapy, well, he lied. Has your doctor given you a death sentence? Do you believe him or do you want to live like Gladys has shown us?

> "Strive to preserve your health, and in this you will the better succeed in proportion as you keep clear of the physicians."
> Leonardo Da Vinci – 1451

If only other cancer patients knew this simple little health secret, what healing miracles could occur without all the chemotherapy and radiation. Was it a miracle? Absolutely not! That is just how God created your immune system to work when you get sick. Stop poisoning it and start feeding it living foods that cleanse and rebuild and dis-ease cannot exist.

Now, how your body functions and does what it does is a miracle in the sense that science can't even begin to understand the complexity of cells. Just as trees have an intelligence that knows how and when to lose their leaves every fall and lay dormant during the winter and appear to be dead and then magically come back to life again every spring is a miracle. But the fact that your body already knows what to do in every given situation, with every disease, when the right cellular nutrients and detoxifiers are taken in, is definitely a mind-baffling phenomenon.

Life force is intelligence. No man-made substance can even compare to it. When you take the life force in living foods and give them to the life force of the body, healing occurs. Why doesn't every doctor in the country know and practice this? **Because there is no money to be made at healing. Money is made by treating disease and maintaining it, not healing and eradicating it.**

The Forsyth's prayer was answered. Through obedience to the laws of nature they discovered a health secret not taught in our mainstream medical system. You can be assured that the pharmaceutical giants will make double sure that all of their financial grants given to educate the next generation of their legalized drug dealers will exclude all natural healing wisdom. None of this will be taught to our young new doctors, but the introduction of "magical wonder pills" will be taunted as the best medicine for every disease you can shake a stick at.

If every American understood that healing such as Gladys' was possible, then most Americans would "just say no to drugs" and turn to inexpensive natural remedies. Drugs would be reserved mostly for acute emergency situations.

After healing cancer, the Forsyths were eager to share their healing experience with others. They grew wheat grass in their basement, composted their own garden soil and taught health classes. I was a sports-driven teenager the first time I met the Forsyths and I didn't think too much of Scott Forsyth when he challenged me to a contest. He said, "Stand with your arms stretched out to your sides and spin around as fast as you can for thirty seconds." So my brother Scott and I both gave it a try. After a few seconds we were laughing at how stupid we looked and how incredibly dizzy we were. We only lasted about ten seconds before we staggered around like drunks coming out of the Ripple Tavern on a Saturday night.

Then Scott said, "now watch me," as he assumed the helicopter position and began spinning like a drill. He kept going and going and going like the Energizer Bunny without staggering or moving his feet from where he started. It was amazing! My brother and I both laughed and joked at the thought of him blasting off into space at any moment. After thirty seconds of continual spinning, he stopped and walked a perfect sober line without any deviation. He put his finger in my face, and asked, "Now why can I, an old man do that without getting dizzy and you, a young athlete can't?" I was absolutely baffled. I didn't know and I wanted the answer. I hungered for this knowledge and what Scott Forsyth told me, a young punk teenager that day, I never forgot. He said *"Your body is toxic and mine isn't."*

Naturally, I burned with a desire to understand true health and healing, not the phony calorie counting, eat your four basic food groups type that is offered at our universities. Our universities in this country offer degrees in health that fail to teach what the body needs to truly heal, prevent disease and experience optimum health.

My older brother Scott later went on to earn a degree in health and informs me that his degree is a joke when it comes to understanding how the body heals and what to do to achieve optimum health. His education taught him nothing about the foods and plants that cleanse, feed, and strengthen the body's cells so that healing can occur.

> **"The cure of many diseases remains unknown to the physician of Hello (Greece) because they do not study the whole person."**
> — Socrates

Living Foods for Living People

You are a living person. If you want to live and be healthy, you must eat living foods. Only living foods sustain life. Dead foods lead towards death. Are you feeling bad? Has your doctor slapped a dis-ease label on you? How much of your diet comes from a package, box or can? What percentage of your diet comes from Mother Nature?

> **"Let thy food be your medicine and your medicine be your food."**
> — Hippocrates

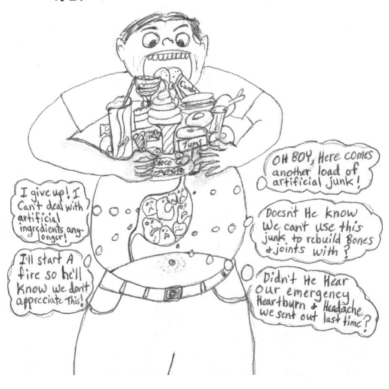

Here are some common cell food healers and effective techniques that can make a difference between life and death used throughout the world:

Healing Foods and Supplements		
Wheat grass	Barley greens	Alfalfa
Blue green algae	Spirulina	Chlorella
Kelp	Bee pollen	Apple cider vinegar
Una de Gato	Evening primrose oil	Garlic
Ginkgo Biloba	Zinc	Vitamin C
Noni juice	Olive leaf extract	MSM
Maitake mushrooms	Colostrum	Flaxseed oil
Graviola	Sprouts	Fruits
Vegetables	Cod liver oil	Oregano oil
Colloidal silver	Protease (enzymes)	Sangre de drago
Essiac tea	Shark cartilage	Laetrile (Amygdalin)
Thymus extract	Melatonin	Reishi mushrooms
Shiitake mushrooms	Aloe Vera	Coenzyme Q10
Coffee enemas	Ortho-phosphoric acid	Bentonite clay
DMSO	Green tea	EDTA
DMSA	Hoxsey formula	Body Balance
Black salve	Haelan	Beta Glucans
Probiotics	Colloidal minerals	Camu Camu
Sea Cucumber	Wild Yam serum	Royal Jelly
Pacific Yew tips	Grapeseed extract	Ginger
Kamut	Goji juice	Aloe Vera
Mangosteen	Red Rooibos tea	Ganoderma

> **"God in his infinite wisdom neglected nothing, and if we would eat our food without trying to improve, change or refine it, thereby destroying its life-giving elements, it would meet all requirements of the body."** Jethro Kloss – Author of Back To Eden

Medical doctors who fail to become educated about the above "natural cures" that have helped millions of people worldwide are doing their patients a great injustice. Some doctors don't want to step on any toes and risk losing their license by doing the "forbidden" and prescribe something other than a toxic drug. It can be hard to take a stand when you know that the consequences may cost you your job.

There have been many natural remedies help millions of people heal in this country but the reality is that their competition, the pharmaceutical companies with their billion dollar advertising investments, pay to squash out any unpatented remedy from being used. Reports are falsified and control groups are cleverly selected to prove the remedy ineffective.

> **"All scientific evidence is bought and paid for by the company that will benefit from a particular finding."** Kevin Trudeau - Author of Natural Cures "They" Don't Want You To Know About

Corrupt statistics and slick attorneys can prove just about anything, especially if large sums of money for their benefit are involved. Most doctors, scientists and especially businessmen have a price. And when the price is right, they sign up on the team that pays the most, no different than NFL football players who sign for twenty-five million dollars to play the next three years with such and such team. It really doesn't matter what you do for a living, the bottom line is most Americans are bought and paid off to do a job. Just ask Jimmy Hoffa or any of the "Good Fellas." By the way, how many jobs have you quit to work somewhere else because the pay is better?

> **"There are three kinds of lies: lies, damned lies and statistics."**
> Benjamin Disraeli

Just this morning on the radio a man was begging for donations to be made for cancer research at a local hospital. Does he have a clue as to how much has been spent on research in the last thirty years since Nixon declared his phony war on cancer? What a joke. Wake up boy, we are losing the war. We are being slaughtered. Every week more and more people are coming down with cancer. The problem intensifies every year because of the false illusion of finding a magic drug cure.

> **"Preventive oncology is an oxymoron. We have so much information on cancer prevention, which we are not using. I wouldn't give a damn if we didn't do any more research for the next fifty years."**
> Samuel Epstein, M.D. - Professor of Environment and Occupational medicine – The School of Public Health, University of Chicago

Cancer researchers are looking for a cure in the wrong place. It would be like scuba divers searching for a sunken ship in the Rocky Mountains. Would someone please be kind enough to explain to such gullible people as they walk down ski slopes with their flippers, snorkels and diving masks, that they will probably not find a sunken ship in Breckenridge or a magic little green, purple, red or blue wonder drug for the cure of cancer or any other disease for that matter.

This money being raised and collected for cancer and other diseases for research is paying for researchers and administrators to receive their large comfortable salaries. Never forget, disease is big business that provides millions of people with comfortable, high paying jobs.

You scratch my back and I'll scratch yours is how our medical system operates. The AMA, FDA, FTC, insurance companies and pharmaceutical kings not only scratch each other's backs, but take turns looking the other way as well. Some people worship money, it is the god they bow down to and will do just about anything to obtain more and more.

Research the money trails in this country so that you understand why our medical system works the way it does.

- How much money is given by drug companies to FDA employees?
- How much money is given to medical schools by drug companies?
- How many FDA and FTC members own stock in drug companies?
- How many members of Congress own stock in drug companies?
- How much money is donated by drug companies for election campaigns?

> "The thing that bugs me is that the people think the FDA is protecting them. It isn't. What the FDA is doing and what the public thinks it's doing are as different as night and day."
> Herbert Ley, M.D. - Former FDA Commissioner

Dr. James Walker in his book, *Holocaust American Style,* blows the whistle on the corruption in America's disease maintenance system. He feels there should be criminal indictment against the medical cartel led by the FDA, FTC and congress whose responsibility is to over see the activities of the FDA and FTC, for allowing over a million people to die each year when it could have been prevented.

> "The worldwide cancer epidemic is primarily the responsibility of the cancer establishment, comprised of the American and Canadian Cancer Societies and the National Institutes of Health of both countries. On their boards sit people who are directly connected to the very industries that are known to produce carcinogens."
> Samuel Epstein, M.D.

Chemotherapy is what medical doctors use to treat cancer in this country, not because it has been proven to heal the best, but because it pays the most. For example non-small cell lung cancer kills more people than any other cancer. Do you know how much is spent on the average cancer treatment a year? It is estimated that approximately $175,000 is spent a year for each cancer patient to be treated with conventional medicine with over half of that payment going directly to the cost of chemotherapy drugs. The big drug manufactures are laughing up a storm to know they have bamboozled the whole nation, doctors and all, into putting this poison in to people's bodies in a sorry attempt to "make them healthy," with their kill, kill, kill drug approach.

In 1985 medical costs for cancer were 71.5 billion dollars, according to the National Center for Health Statistics. By 1990 the total cost of cancer soared to 104 billion, as reported by the National Cancer Institute.

Healing Energy of Plants

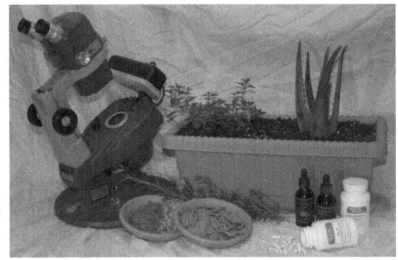

The magnetic polarity of the North and South Pole generates a tremendous amount of energy. Next time you are at the beach notice how powerful the earth's magnetic fields are as they pull the tide in and out, sending huge waves crashing onto the shore. Energy is everywhere in the universe but most of the time you can't see, hear or feel it, unless you are at the ocean.

> **"In every atom, there are worlds within worlds."** Yoga Vasishtha

Another example of subtle energy power is radio and TV. Most of us listen to the radio and watch TV and when we get tired of it we turn it off. But have you ever slowed down enough to think that as you read these words right now those radio waves are everywhere? If you turn on your radio and tune the frequency to the right station, you can pick up whatever is in the air being transmitted from the broadcast studio/radio tower.

The invisible subtle frequencies are everywhere, but you can't hear, see or feel them unless you have a radio or TV tuned in to capture those frequencies. Amazing isn't it? Could you imagine going back in time 500 years and explaining the technological advancement that we humans are going to make to the King of England? Why, they would hang you for such nonsense and witchcraft ideas, or either label you as a raving lunatic and you would be ridiculed by the masses.

> **"First, a new theory is attacked as absurd; then it is admitted to be true, but obvious and insignificant; finally it is seen to be so important that its adversaries claim that they themselves discovered it."**
> William James

Most medical doctors have never studied the healing universe of plants. They are oblivious to the fact that herbs are ingeniously created in a perfect balance far beyond any scientist's comprehension. Despite the fact that most medical doctor are uneducated about herbs does not mean that they are not effective remedies. These healing entities are balanced with minerals, vitamins, amino acids, essential fatty acids and enzymes. The best kept secret and most important ingredient in herbs is the living intelligent life force. This healing vibrational energy is what your cells need to cleanse, nourish and rebuild healthy cells in order to achieve optimum health.

It is important to understand that many drugs originate in some form from herbs. For example, Digitalis, a heart drug, comes from the foxglove herb. Aspirin contains salacin a derivative from willow bark. An ingredient in Taxol which is used for cancer is obtained from the yew tree. An anti-clotting agent called Coumarol is made from sweet clover plants. For thousands of years in India snakeroot herb has been used to help calm people down and the pharmaceutical industry makes a tranquilizer drug from this called Reserpine. Quinine has been used as a fever reducer in cases of malaria and it is extracted from Peruvian bark. Vinblastine used for treating leukemia is derived from periwinkle plants. The list goes on and on.

> **"Keep in mind that twenty-five percent of our conventional prescription drugs are derived directly or indirectly from plants and these twenty five percent of drugs furnish the template for ninety percent of modern synthetic drugs."**
> Varro Tyler, Ph.D. – Professor Emeritus at Purdue University

Scientists rearrange molecular structures of plants and isolate certain ingredients to manufacture drugs. Once they finalize their concoction, they can put a patent on it and sell it for big bucks. If they would leave the ingredients alone, just how Mother Nature created them in the first place, there wouldn't be adverse side effects. But then again, without the opportunity to make billions of dollars, the motivation fizzles out like a bottle of coke with the lid left off over night.

The ingredients in herbs are synergistic, meaning they work well together. Man comes along and messes everything up by tearing the plant apart. God put all those ingredients together in the plant for a reason. It is far healthier to take the plant as a whole, which usually contains vitamins, minerals, amino acids and enzymes. All of these nutrients work together like a well trained team to heal you. Sometimes we do more harm than good by taking isolated vitamins because we read a book by a doctor who recommends large amounts of vitamin E or A.

Why do they tear the plant apart? Because you can't put a patent on echinacea growing wild in the woods. Isolate an ingredient and mix it with some other substances and *voilà* we have a magic drug formula to be sold by a pharmacist for $180 a bottle. It is estimated that less than ten percent of some 300,000 plants have actually been researched. Fifty years from now we will look back on medicine and think of how ignorant and foolish we were for poisoning our bodies with man-made drugs just as we do now about the foolishness of the past practice of bloodletting.

Mother Nature's Intelligence

> **"Man does not weave this web of life. He is merely a strand of it. Whatever he does to the web, he does to himself."** Chief Seattle

In the northwestern tip of Washington State there is one of God's most beautiful creations, The Olympic National Rainforest. Some of the world's largest trees are nestled in sacred groves, which are estimated to be 400 to 700 years old. Among these massive giants are Western Hemlock, Douglas Fir, and Sitka Spruce. Some of the largest trees measure eight feet in diameter and over 200 feet tall. In this paradise is also the world's largest Western Red Cedar, which measures nineteen feet wide and 178 feet tall. It is humbling to stand next to these massive sentinels. An aura of wisdom, peace and serenity resonates in this sacred forest. It is a godly place to visit, that commands respect upon your arrival.

Thick green vegetation blankets the Rainforest as crystal clear waterfalls and streams magically cut through the landscape of ferns and other luscious green shrubs. As you stand in the midst of this living plant kingdom, you can feel the life energy resonating everywhere. It is alive, rejuvenating, powerful and divine. As you stand next to these forest patriarchs

Healing Poisoned Medicine

and look up the trunk of these mighty trees towering up into the blue sky, you develop an appreciation for life.

Plants and herbs are miracles. Push a tiny seed that appears to be lifeless in the dirt and within a short time, it magically springs up a green stem. With the help of a little water and sunshine from on high, little green stems are shooting up everywhere. Within a few weeks a beautiful thriving garden is producing nourishing and delicious vegetables. Soon hundreds of tomatoes, corn, peppers, carrots etc., are ripe enough to eat. That is magic. I say magic because man's mind doesn't fully understand how it all works, nor does he need to in order to enjoy the fruits of Mother Nature's labor.

The miracle of life surrounds us everywhere, yet we are indoctrinated to believe that somehow man's products are better than God's. Take an acorn the size of a thimble and in fifty years it grows into a massive 80-foot tall 4-foot wide oak tree. What is in that little seed that has the potential to evolve into something that massive? Can a scientist duplicate that?

What is contained in that seed is the secret to life. It also contains the secret to healing. It is the secret "unseen" universe that man has only yet to begin to scratch the surface. Science has a long way to go to even begin to get a glimpse into the complexity of life.

Inside every seed is life-force intelligence. It knows what to do when it comes in contact with dirt and water. Intelligence directs it which way to send its roots and which way to push to get sunlight. Plants know how to lay dormant in the long cold winter months and magically come back to life in springtime. How do they do all that? They just know. God created them with intelligence. If the intelligence contained in seeds and plants have enough knowledge to do all this, then does it not make sense that when we eat these living foods and herbs, we are providing our bodies with a tremendous amount of powerful intelligent wisdom? Even more miraculously, these herbs know how to heal when they go into your body. Only a fool would argue against the fact that one little apple seed, if planted in dirt, will grow into a massive tree that will produce possibly thousands of delicious apples every year. The apple tree is intelligent. No programming is necessary, it just produces naturally. That intelligence is what provides your body with the tools necessary to heal imbalances or dis-eases.

The body is far too complex for any doctor or scientist to figure out. They are just now scratching the surface on DNA. For scientists to take their limited knowledge that is constantly being revised (because time proves their conclusions to be false), and put that into man-made synthetic drugs, and then put those drugs into the human body and hope they don't react adversely with the billions of other cellular activities occurring, is about as ridiculous as me banging on my car engine with a sledgehammer hoping to improve my engine's horsepower. Why would you mess around with man's synthetic junk when you could have living intelligence in the form of herbs go into your body and do what they know how to do? The intelligence God programmed in them from the beginning was created for healing purposes. Are we evolving or regressing? Mother Nature's pharmacy is packed with intelligence from on high. Man's chemical drugs have no life force or intelligence, but they sure do have plenty of adverse side effects, enough to kill 225,000 Americans each year.

> **"Perhaps in time the so-called Dark Ages will be thought of as including our own."** George C. Lichtenberg

A computer on my desk has never reproduced another computer. Why? Because it is not living intelligence. It is just an accumulation of man-made plastic with man's knowledge programmed into some software which allows us to do some amazing things but none-the-less it is dead and can do nothing without someone operating it. Intelligence is found in all living things that reproduce in order to continue life. These living entities we call herbs contain intelligent healing elements that know how to feed, cleanse and revive cells. Some herbs like Graviola know how to attack cancer cells while leaving healthy cells alone. Chemotherapy drugs do not know how to do that. Try planting a drug in the ground and we'll see how much intelligent life force it has. Let's see if it has sense enough to come up out of the dirt and live. This whole conversation is ridiculous isn't it? Of course the drug won't grow and neither will optimum health be achieved by ingesting the man-made toxic poison into your body.

> **"And God said, Behold, I have given you every herb bearing seed, which is upon the face of all the earth, and every tree, in the which is the fruit of a tree yielding seed; to you it shall be for meat. ...I have given you every green herb for meat." Genesis 1:29, 30**

Some people, who have the best of intentions, walk around giving Jesus all of the responsibility for their lives. They proclaim, "If it's God's will, then I will die of cancer." Is it God's will that you ate three doughnuts fried in grease for breakfast, two hotdogs made out of left over scraps in a slaughterhouse for lunch and a preservative packed TV dinner radiated in your microwave for supper? Come on people, think! God has given you free agency. You are free to do what you choose. If you drink a bottle of fingernail polish remover and die, I sure hope your family isn't stupid enough to stand around mourning your death in the cemetery saying, "It was God's will that she died." Whatever you eat and drink has consequences. Everything you put in your mouth either promotes health or contributes to disease. Be responsible for what goes in your mouth.

Digestion and the Bowels

> "Every tissue is fed by the blood, which is supplied by the bowel. When the bowel is dirty, the blood is dirty, and so on to the organs and tissues....it is the bowel that invariably has to be cared for first before any effective healing can take place."
>
> Bernard Jensen D.C., N.D., Ph.D.

If you eat three times a day, you should have three bowel movements per day. Let's analyze this for one moment. You eat lunch. You chew your food and mix it with saliva which contains the enzyme ptyalin. This is the first step in digestion. It's important for you to chew your food and completely break it down to a smooth liquid before swallowing. The longer you chew your food, the more digestible it becomes.

After you swallow food, hydrochloric acid (0.8 pH) and pepsinogen enzymes are secreted by parietal cells to mix and break it down in the stomach which usually takes about four hours. The stomach is one area of the body that needs to be acidic (pH of 1.5-2) for proper digestion. These stomach acids are powerful enough to dissolve a thin metal bar. Hydrochloric acid also acts as a natural disinfectant that kills any bacteria that we may eat or drink, so if your digestive system is out of balance or you are taking an acid blocker then you may be at high risk for infection. A mucous lining coating the stomach provides protection from these powerful acids that are necessary to properly break down foods and destroy unwanted bacteria that we may ingest.

If the mucous lining in the stomach isn't able to keep the acid away from the stomach wall, then it can become irritated and ulcers can form. People who are under lots of stress have a tendency to get ulcers because their body uses up its magnesium and potassium reserves to balance out the nervous system. Once depleted, the stomach is unable to manufacture its needed digestive juices, including the mucous, to protect against the strong stomach acids. This leaves us susceptible to ulcerative conditions and infections such as Helicobacter pylori bacteria.

If the stomach isn't acid enough, then it cannot pick up (absorb) calcium and iron. This can cause anemia. Calcium and iron have a positive charge as does the lining of the intestinal tract. Minerals will go right through the intestinal tract without being absorbed because like repels like. However, when the stomach has enough acid, then the minerals pick up an extra positive charge from the acid which allows them to bind with a protein so that they can be properly assimilated.

Once the food in the stomach has been mixed and churned properly with gastric juices and broken down into what is known as chyme, then the pyloric valve opens to release the food into the duodenum, the first part of the small intestine. This acidic liquid activates the pancreas to release enzymes to breakdown proteins (protease), carbohydrates (amylase) and fats (lipase). Alkaline digestive juices (sodium bicarbonate) and enzymes are secreted to further break the food down. Bile is secreted from the gallbladder to help break down fats and lubricate the intestines.

The surface of the small intestine, if stretched out, would cover an area the size of a tennis court. The small intestines are covered with millions of fingerlike villi that constantly sway back and forth sucking up digested food. The villi have lymph vessels that suck up the fat. They also have veins that pick up food and take it to the main transport vessel called the portal vein which carries the food up to the liver for the processing of nutrients.

Waves of muscular contractions in the intestinal tract, also known as peristalsis pushes food through the intestines and eventually into the colon. By the time your food reaches the colon, it is largely made up of unwanted materials and water commonly known as stool. Water is needed to mix with waste to form stool. Without enough water, your bowels do not move. Many constipated people simply need to increase their water consumption in order to hydrate the bowels, so that they can empty.

If an individual is highly stressed or eating a highly acidic diet which is typical of many Americans, then it is common for the magnesium and potassium levels to become depleted as mentioned above. These minerals along with zinc are needed to produce hydrochloric acid to properly breakdown food. As we age, the production of hydrochloric acid is reduced. Indigestion symptoms such as heartburn, gas and bloating can all be caused from this imbalance.

Heartburn is most often caused by the flow of gastric juices up the esophagus. This causes a burning discomfort that is usually made worse by lying down. When someone begins having heartburn or acid reflux, they usually take a chalky antacid like Rolaids or Tums which neutralizes the acids and stops the burning, but creates a major disturbance in the digestive process. The stomach, which needs to be highly acidic, has now just been flooded with a medicine to neutralize the acids. Think about it. The body wants the food in the stomach acidic in order to digest it and we swallow medicine to neutralize it. Why do we work against what the body is doing? This disrupts digestion and consequently, you do not properly break your food down.

Some of the doctor-prescribed acid blockers, like Prilosec or Prevacid, work like a charm at stopping heartburn and the individual sings praises to their doctor for giving them something that relieves their discomfort. However, what the patient isn't taught, is that now we have just shut down the secretion of digestive juices, and foods will not be properly broken down. The body will become malnourished. Bones will become brittle. Organs and glands will be deprived of nutrients. The patient is basically trading in his or her heartburn for arthritis and other diseases if the medication is continued long enough.

The solution for healing heartburn or acid reflux is to get the pH of the body in the 6.8-7.0 range. As mentioned earlier, magnesium, potassium and zinc are crucial for proper digestion.

Taking betaine hydrochloric acid and Pepsogin supplements with meals will ensure that your stomach has what it needs to mix your foods. Once the stomach has your food at the right acidic ratio, then a signal is sent out to close the valves so the stomach can churn your food like a washing machine washing clothes after an adequate amount of soap has been added with the water. When there's a deficiency of hydrochloric acid in your stomach, then the stomach will keep the valves open trying to receive more hydrochloric acid. Burning sensations, acid reflux and heartburn are usually symptoms of your digestive system not having enough hydrochloric acid to mix and break down foods properly. Most Americans have been misled to believe that heartburn is the result of too much acid, when in actuality, it is the result of too little.

Your body takes in nutrients and expels wastes, similar to an automobile. On a car, the engine burns the fuel, uses it to push the pistons, which accelerates the car into motion and then expels the leftovers as exhaust. What happens if you shove a tennis ball in the exhaust pipe of your car? It builds pressure and backfires. Your body is no different. All 100 trillion cells are nourished by what your digestive system is capable of breaking down. So if you are not properly breaking down your foods and eliminating the wastes through bowel movements, where are they going? This fecal waste material accumulates in the intestinal tract and is reabsorbed into the blood through the portal vein. This stresses the body, weakens the immune system, and leaves you highly susceptible to illness. Mucoid plaque, which is another way of saying undigested food, accumulates in your intestinal tract.

Have you ever seen someone who looks perfectly normal except for a bulge right below the navel area? Depending upon the individual, that bulge could be an accumulation of perhaps thirty to even seventy pounds of undigested food. Some obese people have bulges hanging down rubbing on their thighs. This could very well be a ballooned colon carrying a tremendous amount of backed up fecal matter.

Many Americans who appear healthy and not overweight can still be carrying many pounds of mucoid plaque in their colons and could benefit from a colon cleanse. Fasting, and taking psyllium husk, bentonite clay and other herbs are highly effective for cleansing the intestinal area.

> "There is no natural death. All deaths that come from so-called natural causes are merely the end point of progressive acid saturation. Many people go so far as to consider that sickness and disease are just a 'cross' or an element which God gave them to bear here on this earth. However, if they would take care of their body and cleanse their colon and intestines, their problems would be pretty much eliminated and they could eliminate their 'cross' by proper diet, proper exercise, and in general, proper living."
> George C. Crile, M.D. - Head of the Crile Clinic in Cleveland
> (One of the world's greatest surgeons)

The bowels need to move two or three times every day. If a person has eaten three meals a day for seven days, equaling twenty-one meals without a bowel movement, where do you suppose all of that material is accumulating? If each meal weighs a pound, that is twenty-one pounds of food going in with nothing coming out. All the trash backed up in the intestinal tract is causing toxicity throughout the whole body, producing symptoms like fatigue, headaches and skin rashes. Sure, you can treat the symptoms with painkillers, caffeine and cortisone cream but does that make any sense? Why not just clean house and get rid of some crap, literally? Expelling old fecal matter from the body gives your cells room to work, takes pressure off capillaries and organs which reduces inflammation and many symptoms go away.

The colon is like a balloon. When it gets full it keeps expanding and stretching. Any toxic substance left in the colon has the capability of being put right back into your blood stream through the portal vein. A clean colon, liver, kidneys and spleen results in clean blood. Clean blood equals a healthy immune system. A healthy immune system allows you to be around sick people and remain healthy. This is an extremely important key to health. Keep the colon clean and you'll eliminate ninety percent of your health problems.

Toxins in the bowel = toxins in the blood = toxins in organs & glands = toxins in the cells = DIS-EASE.
Where the toxins settle, and the form in which they come out is the disease you are diagnosed as having.

> "Of the 22,000 operations that I have personally performed, I have never found a single normal colon, and of the 100,000 that were performed under my jurisdiction, not over 6% were normal."
> Harvey Kellogg, M.D.

According to many health experts, like Dr. Bernard Jenson, digestion is the great secret of life. Many people we see that have arthritis are suffering due to poor digestion. They aren't absorbing the nutrients they need to build strong bones, tendons and ligaments. Their discs deteriorate because they are literally starving for nutrition. Meat takes 32-72 hours to move through your colon. Have you ever noticed how tired and sluggish you feel after stuffing yourself at Thanksgiving dinner with meat and all the goodies? That's because you have just overloaded your system with way too much protein. All your energy is needed to break down the meal you've just consumed, leaving you exhausted.

A good example is the engine in your car. Everyone knows that the carburetor needs the perfect gas/air mixture in order to run smoothly in stop-and-go traffic. Not enough gas and your car dies. Too much gas and you flood it. It won't run at all. Your body is much more complex than a carburetor, but basically its function is to produce energy to live life. Do you want a fine tuned Mercedes or a backfiring, sluggish, sputtering Dodge Dart? Pay attention to the gas (food) that you put in your tank (mouth).

> **"Life expectancy would grow by leaps and bounds if green vegetables smelled as good as bacon."** Doug Larson

Diarrhea is often constipation in disguise. When the bowels are so toxic that they can't function in a normal fashion then the cells call a special type of cleansing party. Your body, governed by divine intelligence, cleans house in order to save your life and the results are diarrhea, which is a natural way the body eliminates toxins. It's no different than when you eat out and get food poisoning. What does the body do? In all of its wisdom, it causes your stomach to become nauseated and then you vomit. You will usually feel much better after the poisons are out. When it comes out both ends at the same time, that's when you know you have a serious house cleaning party going on.

A Headache Healed

Case Study – October 30, 2007

Since the time I was about 13, I have been plagued with migraines. As I got older, not only did the migraines worsen in severity but also frequency. I would sometimes get them 3-6 times a month and they would last anywhere from 1 day to 4 days, not including the 24 hour recovery time needed to get all the drugs out of my system.

I tried every migraine drug I could get my hands on and when all else failed I was prescribed strong pain killers. About 3 times a year I was taken to the ER or my doctor's office for a shot because nothing would take the pain away. I was terrified of becoming addicted to pain killers, but even more terrified of the horrendous pain of the migraines that disabled me. I remember so many times that the pain was so excruciating that I would crawl to the bathroom, lay my head on the toilet to throw up and just lay on the floor with my hands clutching my head sobbing in pain.

I felt as though every time I got a migraine I lost a part of my life that I could not get back. It seemed as though I revolved around my pain, most days I woke up in pain from a "normal" headache, afraid that this would turn into a migraine. After a change in my typical pattern of migraines I was sent once again for a MRI/MRA. This time an abnormality showed up which sent me once again to a neurologist. The abnormality turned out to be scarring in the brain matter, similar to people who have MS or who have had a stroke. I was put on several different types of medicine, the last being a nerve medicine used to treat shingles.

I finally had enough of all the doctor's appointments, the therapy, and especially all the medicine. At this point I was on 9 various types of medications and began to wonder if I had a serious medical problem. All the treatments had failed.

In July 2007, I got serious and started flying from Michigan to Alabama to see Dr. Sainsbury every 8-10 weeks. He did a CEDSA exam and found many imbalances in my body causing the migraines. He found allergies and I was given remedies to desensitize them. Chemical poisoning showed up causing an imbalance in my liver. My pituitary gland was way out of balance as well. He put me on nutritional support and detoxification formulas and I began to improve.

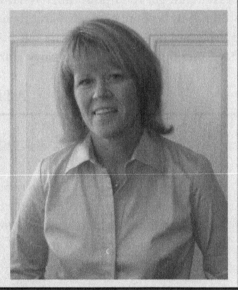

I have now been 3 months without a headache or migraine. I am invigorated when I wake up every morning, without even a trace of pain. I am now down to only 2 prescriptions on a regular basis instead of 9. It is wonderful that I no longer need pain killers, migraine medicine or anti-depressants. This experience has been a life altering event for me!

Annette Morgan
Clinton Township, Michigan

> **"There is no such thing as an incurable disease, only incurable people."** Dr. John R. Christopher

One of the first things we do when someone comes in to our clinic, especially with headaches, is to simply ask how many bowel movements they are having on the average. Then we check the colon, ileo-cecal valve and small intestines with a CEDSA exam. When someone says they only go once a week, then we have a good clue as to what ninety-five percent of their problem is right off the bat. It is appalling that most medical doctors don't even acknowledge a person's bowel habits. We get a large number of people come in to our clinic with headaches after their medical doctor's drugs fail to solve the problem. When asked what their medical doctor said about the fact that they only eliminate through the bowels once a week the response has always been, "My doctor never asked how many times I go." What kind of doctors fail to check common sense stuff? It shows that most doctors are not looking for the cause, just a simple quick fix with a symptom suppressing drug.

> **"When doctors learn to do more educating, they will be able to do less medicating."** Bernard Jensen D.C., Ph.D., N.D.

A throbbing, nonstop headache has suddenly come upon twenty-two year old Lauren. She is a first year teacher straight out of college and up until now she has had nearly perfect health her whole life. But for six days now she has been bogged down by a nagging, relentless headache. The pain in her head is unbearable and she can't stand it anymore. She goes in to see her medical doctor. She explains the very uncomfortable pain that she is having. In less then two minutes he sends her out the door with three prescriptions, two painkillers and one for sinus congestion, despite her not having any congestion at all. When she questions him about it, he says it is just in case there is some congestion triggering the headache. No testing of any kind is performed to determine the cause of the headache. And once again he does not ask about her bowel movements. He merely guesses as to which magic drug to give her. Folks, this is not health care. It is drug dealing to mask symptoms. On the streets he is called a pimp. In an office, he is called a doctor.

Skeptical about taking these three drugs, she calls our clinic and makes an appointment to get a second opinion. In naturopathy we use vitamins, minerals, amino acids, enzymes, homeopathy and herbs to bring the body back into balance, which alleviates illness by correcting the cause. We perform a CEDSA test that is noninvasive and painless. Within fifteen minutes of testing the root cause of the headache is found.

When Lauren is tested, a simple nutritional deficiency is found. No, it's not a deficiency of Tylenol, antibiotic or any other man-made substance. Her gallbladder, uterus and adenoids do not need to be taken out and thrown in the trash or some other radical surgical procedure as if to say, "Sorry God but the human body really doesn't need all those things you put in there so I'm going to fix what you didn't get right." The culprit for Lauren's headache is a simple magnesium deficiency along with some low amino acid levels. For a thirteen dollar bottle of Magnesium and potassium, the nagging headache is completely gone by the next morning and has not been back. The prescriptions were never taken and Lauren is back to feeling good again. Problem solved through simple and cost effective, natural medicine. No drugs or painkillers were ever needed and no adverse side effects were experienced. And best of all, no vicious cycle of drugs was ever started to leach vital nutrients out of her already deficient body.

Lauren is a typical American who demands a little more than a two-minute prescription drug recommendation. Common sense told her that the headaches were probably not caused from a deficiency of drugs so why should she take them? Common sense caused her to ask the question, "Wouldn't it be wiser, healthier to find someone who could find the cause of the headache and correct it with something that won't harm my cells and skip the drug plug for every illness game?

Lauren and thousands of others have been helped by taking safe, effective natural medicine that nourishes and detoxifies at the cellular level without negative side affects. By addressing the cause of disease we give the body what it needs to heal. This is called health. Unfortunately, this is not taught in our universities to our medical doctors.

> **"There is a true glory, the glory of duty done."** General Robert E. Lee

If Americans started demanding that their doctors look for the cause of the cancer or any other disease and stop administering poisonous drugs that kill, then we might start making some progress with cancer and other supposedly incurable diseases. How are you going to cure a disease if you don't find the cause? It's time for change. It's time to start finding the cause of dis-ease and then fix the problem.

> **"Remember, it is pure food, simply and appetizingly prepared, and not drugs that bring back the glow of health to the cheek, and maintain maximum health in those who are well."**
> Hans Anderson – Author of The New Food Therapy

Remodeling Your House

There are no short cuts to health; there are no magic wonder pills to cure you. Your lifestyle is directly related to your health. What tools you provide your body with determines whether or not you get well.

Take for example a hundred-year-old home. Let's suppose this house is in terrible shape, but it has a lot of sentimental value, so you decide to hire a carpenter to remodel it. What is the

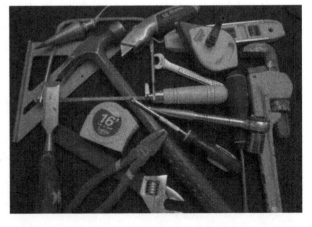

first thing he does? He draws up blueprints, an over-all plan on how you want the finished product to look and function.

The next step in remodeling is the carpenter needs the correct tools. Without them, he can't do much. Your body needs effective elimination routes and lymphatic drainage. It needs correct plant derived nutrition at the cellular level. Just as a carpenter needs a good hammer, saw, level etc., to build or remodel a house, so do the cells of your body. What are the tools your cells need? Good wholesome nutrition. Raw living foods that contain all sixty plant derived minerals, sixteen vitamins, twelve essential amino acids and three essential fatty acids. Of course our foods today don't always contain these nutrients, because the soils are depleted of minerals. Supplementation with a good plant derived mineral/vitamin formula ensures that we obtain these elements. Once we supply the body with these tools, the God-programmed intelligence that runs your body can go to work and heal. The great thing about your immune system and healing capacity is the autopilot feature. It knows what to do. Given time with correct nutrition, proper elimination and detoxification routes, the body is self-healing.

> **"Intelligence makes the difference between a house designed by an architect and a pile of bricks."** Deepak Chropra, M.D.

Your self-healing carpenter is the innate intelligence encoded in every cell of your DNA. It is the blueprint that tells you to have red or brown hair. It instructed your body to form two eyes instead of one. It created you with ten fingers and ten toes. Is it making sense? This intelligence knew how to create you in your mother's womb and it certainly knows how to heal you now. It reproduces new red blood cells without you consciously thinking anything. It knows. It's the intelligence that runs your body. It is part of the intelligence that runs the universe and allows the sun to rise every morning. Yes, it is awesome. It is divine. It is a manifestation of the infinite glory of God and **YOU** are a part of it.

Naturally, we need good positive thought patterns as well as emotional balance. It is vital that you feel spiritually connected and feel worthy of life, good health and God's love and blessings. This is the basic concrete foundation needed to support your structure, or physical body. You need to feel grounded and understand that you are part of the universe and without you, the universe wouldn't be complete. But with you, the universe is complete and God's creation is perfect and complete. You matter. You play an important role in this universe. God created you. How could you not be important and essential? Is the Grand Canyon important? How about Niagara Falls or The Rocky Mountains? Yes they are important but God has given you dominion over them. That means something special, never forget it.

> **"I have said, Ye are gods; and all of you are children of the most High."** Psalms 82:6

Just as the carpenter presents you with a beautiful remodeled home with everything in good working order, so can your body repair and rebuild. Give it the right tools and it performs miracles. You can hire five postal-workers to come and remodel your house and supply them with blueprints, lumber, sheetrock, paint, hammers, nails, saws, drills etc., and all the tools necessary to remodel. Most likely they will not be able to do the job you want done, because they don't know how, despite having all the tools and raw materials available.

Postal workers have been trained to sort mail, and get letters and packages from one place to another. They are experts in delivering the mail, not remodeling a house. If you haven't been trained in how to build a house, you will probably not be very successful in your remodeling efforts.

Chapter 5
YOUR AMAZING BODY

Dr. Paul Brand (surgeon 1914-2003) and Philip Yancey (best-selling writer) have done an outstanding job in helping us to understand the miracle of the human body. It truly is The Temple of God. The next few pages will enlighten, educate and humble you about the gift you have been given, your body. After reading about the complexity of your body's organs, glands and systems, you'll develop a sense of reverence and respect for the greatest creation in the universe-you. You are intelligent, organized matter manifesting the glory of God.

Excerpts from a two volume study by Dr. Paul Brand and Philip Yancey, "Fearfully & Wonderfully Made" and "In His Image"

The Incredible Miracle Of Birth

This amazing human body grows from the fertilization of a single egg. People make a fuss about test-tube babies, but the true miracle is the common union of a sperm and egg in a process that ultimately produces a human being. Lewis Thomas writes, *"The mere existence of that cell should be one of the greatest astonishments of the earth. People ought to be walking around all day, all through their waking hours, calling to each other in endless wonderment, talking of nothing except that cell. If anyone does succeed in explaining it, within my lifetime, I will charter a skywriting airplane, maybe a whole fleet of them, and send them aloft to write one great exclamation point after another, around the whole sky, until all my money runs out."*

Over nine months our cells divide up functions in exquisite ways. Billions of blood cells appear millions of rods and cones—in all, up to one hundred million, million (trillion) cells form a single fertilized ovum. And finally we were born, glistening with liquid. Already our cells are cooperating. Our muscles limber up in jerky, awkward movements; our face recoils from the harsh lights and dry air of the new environment; our lungs and vocal chords join a first air-gulp to yell.

Our life will include the joy of seeing our mother's approval at his first clumsy words, the discovery of our own unique talents and gifts; the fulfillment of sharing with other humans. We are many cells, but we are one organism. All of our hundred trillion cells know this.

What is a Trillion?

We speak of millions, billions and trillions so casually, yet these numbers are so huge that we cannot start to comprehend them. So let us take an example. If you had two million dollars, you would be a multimillionaire. One of the things you could do with half of your money would be to give it to your spouse. So let's imagine that you told your spouse to go out and have a good time and spend a thousand dollars every day and not come back until all those million dollars were used up. Your spouse wouldn't be back for three years. That would be quite a trip. Now, let's try it with one trillion dollars, at a thousand a day. In this case, your spouse would not return for two million years.

So when we are told that our body contains a hundred trillion cells, and that each cell is supplied and nourished directly by our blood, we can get a little glimpse of the magnitude of what it takes to provide the life we can take so easily for granted.

The Ecstasy of Community

Each of our individual cells shares in what we can call the ecstasy of community. No scientist can even measure how a sense of security or peace is communicated to the cells of the body, but individual cells certainly participate in our emotional reactions. Hormones and enzymes bathe them, bringing on a quickening breath, a trembling of muscles, a flapping in the stomach. But if you look for a pleasure nerve in the human body, you will come away disappointed. There is none. There are nerves for pain and cold and heat and touch, but no nerve gives a sensation of pleasure. Pleasure appears as a by-product of cooperation by many cells.

Inside our stomach, spleen, Liver, pancreas and kidneys, each packed with millions of loyal cells, are working so efficiently we have no way of perceiving their presence. Fine hairs in our inner ears are monitoring a swishing fluid, ready to alert us if we were suddenly to tilt off balance.

When our cells work, we are hardly conscious of their individual presence. What we feel is the composite of their activity known as the self that each of us is. Our body, composed of many parts, is one.

Wherever we look, it seems community is the order of the day. Our earth is not the center of the universe, but rather a speck of dust in a boundless community of planets, stars, and galaxies, all of which interact with and affect each other. The tiny atom, once thought indivisible, now appears as a universe of its own, with whirling electrons and mesons and quarks and glimmers of reality that last a scant nanosecond.

Living matter ushers in new levels of unpredictability. The smallest living unit, the cell, comprises a nucleus jammed with chromosomes as well as an Irish stew of various organelles, mitochondria, sacs, tubes, cilia, all squirming around in near-chaotic freedom. This book concerns a community of such cells, one hundred trillion in all, which must cooperate together to produce a functioning human body.

Diversity of Cells

Our body employs a bewildering array of cells, none of which individually resembles the body that others see as "you." We are first struck by the incredible diversity of our cells. Chemically our great variety of cells are almost all alike, but visually and functionally they are as different as the animals in the zoo. There are over a thousand uniquely structured, different types of cells, each numbering in the millions, many in the billions, making up the body. This great diversity of cells combines to make up the many massive collections of cells, organs, like the eye, brain, ear, liver, pancreas, spleen, and on and on.

Individually they seem puny and oddly designed, but we know these invisible parts cooperate to lavish us with the phenomenon of life. Every second our smooth muscle cells modulate the width of our blood vessels, gently push matter through our intestines, open and close the pumping in our kidneys. When things are going well—our heart contracting rhythmically, our brain humming with knowledge, our lymph nurturing tired cells—we never have to give these cells a passing thought. So in the sections to follow, we will want to take one group at a time and reverently acknowledge their miraculous contribution to our life.

Cells Making Up The Reproductive Organs

The aristocrats of our cellular world are the sex cells. A woman's contribution, the egg, is one of the largest cells in the human body, its oval-shape just visible to the unaided eye. It is fitting that all the other cells in the body should derive from this elegant and primordial structure. In great contrast to the egg's quiet repose, the male's tiny sperm cells are furiously flagellating tadpoles with distended heads and skinny tails. They scramble for position, as if competitively aware that only one of billions will gain the honor of fertilization.

The Eyes

To make up just the retina of each eye, it takes 127,000,000 cells. Seven million are cones, each loaded to fire off a message to the brain when a few photons of light cross them. The cones give us the full band of color awareness, and because of them, we can easily distinguish a thousand shades of color. The graceful tentacles that reach out toward light. They are the backup cells for use in low light. These rods are so sensitive that the smallest measurable unit of light, one photon, can excite them. Under optimum conditions, the eye can detect a candle at a distance of fifteen miles. Yet when only rods are operating, we do not see color (as on a moonlit night when everything looms in shades of gray), but we can distinguish a spectrum of light so broad that the brightest light we perceive is a billion times brighter than the dimmest.

Each of these rods and cones are responsive to only a single wavelength of light, and when triggered, sends an electrical response through the optical nerve back to the brain. The optical nerve is a coaxial cable containing over a million fibers. The brain does not receive photographic images of anything. Instead, it must absorb a composite set of yes or no messages from the 127 million rods and cones. Impulses from the retina race along the fibers of the optic nerve, fan out in the brain and finally slam into the visual cortex, stimulating the miracle of sight. It sorts and organizes them all and gives us an image of the world outside the eyes. The cortex of the brain has no easy task, since one billion messages a second stream in from each retina. Out of this combination, it can detect in three dimensions, in full color, in a marvelous, seamless picture of the outside world.

The rest of the eye is no less marvelous. The lens that perfectly focuses the light, regardless of the distance. The iris which controls the amount of light reaching the retina. Then there is the cornea, the collection of cells covering the eye. These billions of cells made themselves absolutely transparent, like glass, through which we "look."

The Ears

Compared to some animal protuberances, our ears seem small and underdeveloped. They capture a smaller share of the auditory range than a dog's or horse's ear, and offer no competition to those animals' talents for ear expressiveness as we can with our lips.

Even so, the human faculty of hearing is impressive. Ordinary conversation causes air molecules to vibrate and move the eardrum mere twenty-five-thousandths of an inch, but with enough precision for us to differentiate all the sounds of human speech. The eardrum membrane has the flexibility to register the drop of a straight pin as well as the noise of a jet aircraft taking off, which is one hundred trillion times louder.

Three Bones In The Ear That Never Grow

After the eardrum vibrates, three tiny bones, known as the hammer, anvil and stirrup, transfer that vibration into the middle ear. Of all the bones in the body none are more remarkable than these three, which are the very smallest. Unlike all the other bones, these do not grow with age—as a one-day-old infant, these bones were already fully developed to the size they are right now. Since every sound that reaches us causes these bones to swing into action, they are in constant, unrelieved motion. Working together, they magnify the force that vibrated the eardrum until it is twenty times greater in the inner ear than when it entered the outer ear.

The Liquid Inner Ear

The inner ear is an inch-long, sealed chamber filled with viscous liquid. The vibration that began with molecules of air and was converted to a mechanical pounding finally ends up as a turbulent fluid force. The action of the three bones sets up pulsating waves. Everything we know as sound depends on this seismic chamber of the inner ear.

How do we distinguish two different sounds, such as the buzz of a fly droning about in the room and the rumble of the lawnmower a block away? Every distinct sound has a "signature" of vibrations per second. A tuning fork shows the process clearly. When struck, its tines visibly move back and forth. If we hear a wave of molecules oscillating 256 times per second, for example, we are hearing the musical "middle C." As an average person, we can detect vibrations of 20 to 20,000 cycles per second.

Inside the inner ear, 25,000 unique and specially tuned receptor cells are lined up to receive these vibrations, like strings of a huge piano waiting to be struck. This mass of cells in each ear is similar to the rods and cones in the retina of the eyes, but in the ear they transmit specific messages of sound to the brain. Seen through a scanning electron microscope, the cells resemble rows of baseball bats standing upright together. Each cell is designed and specifically tuned to respond to a certain pattern of sound. A few of these cells will fire off signals to the brain when a 256-cycle vibration reaches them, and we "hear" a middle C. The others will await their own programmed frequency. We can only imagine the massive chaos of cell activity when we sit in front of a full orchestra and hear twelve different notes at once, as well as the variety of musical "textures" from the different instruments. In all, the ear distinguishes some 300,000 tones. In addition to listening, the brain combines these messages with other factors—how well we like classical music, how familiar we are with it—and offers the combination of impulses in a form we perceive as pleasure.

Only The Brain Can Hear

Again, just as the eyes do not "see" but, rather, just transmit information, neither do the ears "hear." The brain does the seeing and the brain does the hearing. The most important fact about hearing is that the vibration itself never reaches the brain. The process resembles a cassette tape which absorbs sound not as mechanical vibration but as a series of electrical and magnetic codes. Once the vibration excites its appropriate sound receptor cell, the force inside our head changes from mechanical to electrical. Thousands of wires, or neurons, lead from the patch of 25,000 sound-sensitive cells into the auditory part of the brain. There the frequencies are received in a sequence of on-or-off blips. The experience of sound depends on which of these cells transmits its signal, how often, and in cooperation with what other cells. The brain pieces together these messages and we "hear." After receiving the electrical code from the sound receptors, the brain makes its own contributions of meaning and emotion.

We find in even greater amazement on a further phenomenon of the brain. If we let our mind contemplate, we can "hear" in our mind the four crashing chords of Beethoven's Fifth Symphony, the melodious voice of someone singing Silent Night, the piercing tones of a London air raid siren complete with its unbidden sense of anxiety. There is no force, no vibration of molecule, no firing of sounds out of what exists only in the complex nerve cells jammed into every cubic inch of white matter.

Smell

I write of hearing with a sense of wonder but I write about the gift of smell with near incredulity. Smell leaves the world of quantifiable physics and approaches mystery.

The amount of substance needed to trigger smell defies belief. No Du-Pont laboratory can perform an analysis with one-hundredth the speed and accuracy of a bloodhound's nose. A detective holds a sock before the baleful dog. He sniff's deeply a few times, sorting out stale cigarette smoke, the artificial odor of Dr. Scholl's footpads, the complex history of a piece of leather, traces of bacterial action and, somewhere, pieces of the man himself, the criminal. He finds a trail through the woods and shuffles along, snorting and evaluating. Suddenly a yelp. He has sniffed in another piece. The pine needles, the dust, the men around him, the thousand smells of the forest floor—none of these interfere with his singular determination to follow the one molecular structure imprinted on his brain. He will follow that spoor through creeks and swamps, across logs, down city sidewalks, up apartment stairs—wherever it leads—one day, two days, even a week after the criminal has left the telltale bits.

The human nose is not so gifted, yet is still miraculous in its own way. We humans possess baffling powers capable of discriminating some 10,000 different odors. Because of this, the nose is also an organ of nostalgia. The smell of frying bacon, wood burning, a whiff of briny seashore, the faintest lingering trace of a certain perfume, or the esthetic order of a hospital corridor can stop us like a bullet. We can relive that former moment in a flash, jerked backward in time by the memory of that fragrance locked away in the brain.

The brain faithfully squelches odors after an initial heightened period. Smell is primarily a sentinel warning, and once warned, the brain, refuses to be troubled with redundancy. Fish merchants, tanners, garbage collectors and paper mill employees gratefully accept this mercy of habituation. "You get used to it," they say with total accuracy.

Taste

Taste deserves mention, of course, as one of the five great senses. But taste suffers in comparison to smell and, in fact, relies mostly on smell, as any of us with a stopped-up nose can confirm.

An electron microscope scan of the tongue's dense mat of taste buds reveals splendid structures: dramatic cliffs and caverns, cactus flowers, clusters of tall, waving stalks, exotic leaves. They work well enough to afflict most of us with lavish appetites and insatiable cravings. But it takes twenty-five thousand times as much of a substance to register on a stubby taste bud as it does to register on a smell receptor. And for some mysterious reason, taste buds live a mere three to five days, then die off, so the only "experienced" taste exist in the fortress of the brain.

What we taste and smell is much more than conscious recognition. Through the brain, tastes affect many body functions as they stimulate a programmed response, such as the ringing of the bell with Pavlov's dogs. For example, when a patient is receiving food directly into the stomach or intravenously, the body will absorb more nourishment if the patient "primes" it by tasting food first. The experience of taste stimulates the gastric juices in the same way the smell of sizzling steak or frying bacon can awaken in us a sudden, unexpected hunger.

Blood

Like most of us, the organ of blood, if we can think of this fluid mass as an organ, comes to consciousness mainly when we begin to lose it. We miss the dramatic sense of blood's power that is the true miracle of life that flows through our veins and arteries.

What does our blood do all day? Perhaps a technological metaphor would serve to give us a clue. Imagine an enormous tube that weaves in and out of every city, town and home throughout the world. Throughout the Southern Hemisphere of Australia, South America and Africa, throughout the Northern Hemisphere of India, Russia, Europe, North America, China and all the islands of the sea. This pipe, millions of miles long, would link every person worldwide. Inside this tube would be an endless supply of treasures which float along on rafts—mangoes, coconuts, asparagus, produce, and products from every continent; including watches, computers, automobiles, furniture, all styles and sizes of clothes, the contents of thousands of shopping center, supply stations and everything else one could think of. Six billion people would have direct access, at a moment of need or want. All they simply do is reach into the tube and seize whatever products suit them. In return, they load onto the rafts all of their trash waste and refuge. Then, somewhere far down the pipeline the refuge is taken off, the rafts scrubbed and cleaned, and replacements are supplied so that nothing is lacking.

Our Internal Pipeline

Such a pipeline exists inside of the body, servicing not six billion but one hundred trillion cells in the body, each cell being as complex as a modern city of 100,000 people. An endless supply of oxygen, amino acids, nitrogen, sodium, potassium, calcium, magnesium, sugar, lipids, cholesterol and magical hormones surge past each of the cells, carried on blood cell rafts or suspended in the fluid. Each cell has a special withdrawal privileges to gather the resources needed to fuel its complex engine for all of its chemical functions.

In addition, that same pipeline ferries away refuse, exhaust gases and worn-out chemicals. In the interest of economical transport, the body dissolves its vital substances into a liquid just like coal is shipped more efficiently through a slurry pipeline than by truck or train. Five or six quarts of the all-purpose fluid suffice for the body's hundred trillion cells.

The Make-Up of Blood

A view through a microscope clarifies the various components of blood but gives no picture of the daily frenzy encountered by each cell in the blood. What the telescope does to nearby galaxies, the microscope does to a drop of blood to unveil the staggering reality. A speck of blood the size of this letter "o" contains 5,000,000 red cells, 300,000 platelets and 7,000 white cells. The fluid is actually an ocean stocked with living matter. Red cells alone, if removed from the body and laid side by side, would carpet an area of 3,500 square yards, which is the size of a football field.

Red Blood Cells

Red blood cells are by far the most numerous—smooth, shiny discs with centers indented like jelly doughnuts. Uniform size and shape make them seem machine stamped and impersonal. But they work hard and never sit motionless. From their first entrance into the bloodstream from the bone marrow, they are pushed and shoved through rush hour traffic. Beginning the cycle at the heart, they take a short jaunt to the lungs to pick up a heavy load of oxygen.

The blood contains an amazing and complex molecule called hemoglobin which permits twenty times as much oxygen to be ferried around in our blood and gives blood its characteristic red color. In all, 9,508 atoms (3,032 carbon atoms, 4,812 hydrogen atoms, 780 nitrogen atoms, 872 oxygen atoms and 12 sulfur atoms) hook up in an intricate formation around a mere four crucial atoms of iron. This tiny amount of iron in the hemoglobin grabs huge quantities of passing oxygen atoms like a magnet, and the red cells biconcave shape assures the maximum exposure to oxygen in the lungs. Each red cell carries 280 million hemoglobin molecules.

Blood Vessels

The blood, loaded with oxygen, immediately is returned to the heart, which propels it violently over the Niagara Falls of the aortic arch. From there, highways crowded with billions of red cells branch out to the brain, the limbs and vital internal organs. There are, in just one person's body, sixty thousand miles of blood vessels which link every one of the living cells; even the blood vessels themselves are fed by blood vessels. Highways narrow down to one-lane roads, then bike paths, then footpaths, until finally, the red cell must lean sideways and edge through a capillary one-tenth the diameter of a human hair. In such narrow confines the cells are stripped of food and oxygen and loaded down with carbon dioxide and urea. If we were reduced in size to being no bigger than a red cell, we would see them as bloated bags of jelly and iron drifting along in a river until they reach the smallest capillary, where gases fizz and wheeze in and out of surface membranes. From there red cells rush to the kidneys for a thorough scrubbing, then back to the lungs for a refill. Then the journey begins all over again.

Recycling

This pell-mell journey, even to the extremity of the big toe, lasts a mere twenty seconds. An average red cell endures the cycle of loading, unloading and jostling through the body for a half million round trips over four months. In one final journey to the spleen, the battered cell is stripped bare by scavenger cells and recycled into new cells. Three hundred billion such red cells die and are replaced every day, leaving behind various parts to reincarnate in a hair follicle or a taste bud.

The body performs it's janitorial duties with impressive speed and efficiency. No cell lies more than a hair's breadth from a blood capillary, lest poisonous by-products pile up. Through a basic chemical process of gas diffusion and transfer, individual red blood cells drifting along inside narrow capillaries simultaneously release their cargoes of fresh oxygen and absorb waste products of carbon dioxide, urea, uric acid, etc. The red cells then deliver the hazardous waste chemicals to organs that can dump them outside the body.

Blood Platelets

To recall, in a tiny drop of blood the size of this letter "0," there would be 5,000,000 red cells and 7,000 white cells, but there would be 300,000 platelets. Our very survival depends upon these delicate flower-shaped cells. Their function remained hidden until recently. Now scientists recognize that platelets, which survive only six to twelve days in the blood, play a crucial role in the life-saving process of clotting, serving as mobile first-aid boxes detecting leaks, plugging them up and tidying up the debris.

When a blood vessel is cut, the fluid that sustains life begins to leak away. In response, tiny platelets melt, like snowflakes, and spin out a gossamer web of fibers. Red Blood cells collect in this web, like cars and trucks crashing into each other when the road is blocked. Soon the tenuous wall of red cells thickens enough to staunch the flow of blood.

Platelets have a very small margin of error. Any clot that extends beyond the vessel wall and threatens to obstruct the vessel itself will stop the flow of blood through the vessel and perhaps lead to a stroke or coronary thrombosis and possibly death. On the other hand, people whose blood has no ability to clot live short lives, for even a tooth extraction may prove fatal. The body cannily gauges when a clot is large enough to stop the loss of blood but not so large as to impede the flow within the vessel itself.

The White Blood Cells

Even more interesting than the red blood cells are the white blood cells, the armed forces of the body which guard against invaders. They look like blobs of turgid liquid with darkened nuclei. Flattened on a microscope slide, white cells resemble fried eggs sprinkled with pepper, each dot making a deadly chemical weapon. As the white cells circulate in the body they assume roughly spherical shapes and resemble pale glass eyes aimlessly adrift in the blood vessels. When an invasion hits, they abruptly come alive.

Watching the white cells, we can't help thinking of them as sluggish and ineffective at patrolling territory, much less repelling an attack. Until the attack occurs, that is. If a wound appears, an alarm sounds. Muscle cells contract around the damaged capillary walls, damming up the loss of precious blood. Clotting agents halt the flow at the skin's surface. Before long, scavenger cells appear to clean up debris and fibroblasts, the body's reweaving cells, gather around the injury site. But the most dramatic change involves the listless white cells. As if they have a sense of smell, nearby white cells abruptly halt their aimless wandering. Like beagles on the scent of a rabbit, they hone in from all directions to the point of attack. Using their unique shape-changing qualities, they ooze between overlapping cells of capillary walls and hurry through tissue via the most direct route. When they arrive, the battle begins.

How Our Warriors In Our Blood Fight

White blood cells roam through the body by extending a finger-like projection and humping along to follow it. Sometimes they creep along the walls of the veins; sometimes they let go and free-float in the bloodstream. To navigate the smaller capillaries, bulky white cells must elongate their shapes, while impatient red blood cells jostle in line behind them.

As shapeless white cells, resembling science fiction's creature "The Blob," they lumber toward a cluster of luminous green bacterial spheres. Like a blanket pulled over a corpse, the invading cells still glow eerily inside the white cell. But the white cell contains granules that detonate, destroying the invaders. In 30-60 seconds, only the bloated white cell remains. Often its task is a kamikaze one, resulting in the white cell's own death. If an infection is getting out of hand, the dead white corpuses are in such quantity that they must be drained away. We call this massive collection "pus."

During healthy periods, twenty-five billion white cells circulate freely throughout the blood and twenty-five billion more loiter on blood vessel walls. When an infection occurs, billions of reserves leap from the marshes of bone marrow, some in immature form like beardless young recruits pressed into service. In the body's economy, the death of a single white cell is of little consequence. Most only live several days or several weeks, and besides the fifty billion active ones prowling the body, a backup force one hundred times as large lies in reserve in the marrow of the bones. At the cellular level, massive warfare is a daily fact of life. Fifty thousand invaders may lurk on the rim of a drinking glass, and a billion can be found in a half-teaspoon of saliva. Bacteria enshroud the body. Every time we wash our hands, we wash five million of them from the folds of our skin.

Oxygen

We can live a day or two without water and several weeks without food, but only a few minutes without oxygen, the main fuel for the hundred trillion cells. Heavy exercise may increase the demand for oxygen from the normal four gallons up to seventy-five gallons an hour, prompting the heart to double or even triple its rate to speed red cells to the heaving lungs. If the lungs alone cannot overcome the oxygen shortage, the red cells call up reinforcements. Instead of five million red cells in a speck of blood, seven or eight million will gradually appear. After a few months into the rarefied atmosphere of Colorado's mountains, for example, up to ten million red cells fill each drop of blood, compensating for the thinner air.

In the lungs, carbon dioxide collects in small pockets to be exhaled with every breath. The body monitors the expiration cycle and makes instantaneous adjustments. If too much carbon dioxide accumulates, as when we burn more energy by climbing a flight of stairs, and involuntary switch increases the breathing to speed up the process. This is the reason no one can commit suicide by not breathing—the involuntary trigger "forces" one to breathe.

The Blood Purifiers—The Kidneys

Complex chemical wastes are left to a more discriminating organ, the kidney. Some observers judge them second in complexity only to the brain. The body obviously values them greatly, for one-fourth of the blood from each heartbeat courses down the renal artery to the twin kidneys. The artery divides and subdivides into a tracery of tubules so intricate as to bedazzle that finest Venetian glass blower.

Filtering is what the kidney is all about, but in very little space and time. The kidney manages speed by coiling the tubules into a million crystal loops, where chemicals can be picked over one by one. Since red cells are too bulky for those tiny passageways, the kidney extracts the sugars, salts and water from the blood and deals with them separately. The segregation process roughly compares to a master mechanic who has a garage too small to fit a whole car inside. To repair a car engine, he hoists it out of the car, carries it to the garage, disassembles and scours each individual valve, piston and ring, then reassembles the hundreds of parts minus the grime and corrosion.

After the kidney has removed the red cells' entire payload to extract some thirty chemicals, its enzymes promptly reinsert 99% of the volume into the bloodstream. The 1% remaining, mostly urea, is hustled away to the bladder to await expulsion, along with whatever excess water the kidney deems expendable. One second later, the thunder of the heart resounds throughout the body and fresh blood surges in to fill the tubules.

Reed T. Sainsbury

Immune System of Our Blood

Each day we live at the mercy of organisms one-trillionth our size. No matter how we see ourselves, despite all our fantasies of grandeur and dominion, all our fragile human successes, the real struggle has always been against bacteria and viruses, against adversaries never more than seven microns wide.

Battle imagery is particularly appropriate to describe what happens inside our bodies, for with an array of menacing weapons and defenders, our bodies, quite simply, declare war on invaders. At the first sign of invasion, a chemical Paul Revere alarm sounds, and numerous body systems hasten into action. Capillaries dilate, like inflatable tunnels, to allow a swarm of armed defenders into the combat zone. White blood cells of five distinct types form the initial assault zone. Transparent brisling with weapons and possessing a Houdini-like ability to slip between other cells, the white cells are the body's chief fighters.

Some white cells, armed with crude chemicals, serve as shock troops and attempt to overwhelm the invaders through sheer numbers. Others with massively shielded cell walls roll in with heavier ammunition like battle tanks. Attack strategy differs also. Some white cells free-float in the bloodstream, sniping at strays. Some stalk the vital organs, alert for any invader that may slip through initial defenses. Others try to corral invaders into a fortress-like lymph gland for execution. And still other, the sanitary corps, linger until the battlefield is strewn with bits of cells and leaking protoplasm, then move in to clean up after the melee.

Specialized White Cells

The body can quickly mobilize ten times the normal number of white cells. In fact, doctors use a census of them as a diagnostic blood test to judge the severity of infection. We need fast numbers of white cells for one reason, some of them are "specific" defenders, programmed against only one type of disease. In truth the battle within resembles not so much a one-on-one infantry assault as a furious mating dance in which white cells crowd against the bacteria or viruses seeking the right "fit" before calling up reserves. The average white cell lives merely ten hours. But a select few live for sixty or seventy years and preserve the chemical memory of dangerous invader, all the while checking in at their assigned lymph gland every few minutes. These master cells safeguard the chemical secrets that remind the body how to respond to any invader previously encountered.

A white cell must somehow hone-in on the actual invaders who are camouflaged by the chemical smoke-screen of battle and the rubble of bleeding cells, clotting agents, and broken membranes.

Anti-invaders (Anti-Bodies)

Also a part of our blood are tiny anti-invader "molecules" (called inappropriately antibodies) which are only 1/1000 the size of bacteria. These molecules cling to the enemy like a moss to a tree. Softening them up for the approaching white cells and neutralizing their destructive spike shapes. A single type of anti-invader midget protects against only one disease; for example, the measles antibody has no effect against infantile paralysis.

Because of the staggering range of invaders confronting a person in a lifetime, the body must stockpile an enormous arsenal of weapons. This ability of the body to generate so many different types of anti-invader midgets is a process of mystery and chemistry, a combination of physics and grace down at the molecular level.

If we cut our hand, roaming anti-invader molecules tag the known invaders almost immediately. In the event of a new one spotted, a circulating white cell touches it, memorizes its shape, and rushes to the nearest lymph node. There, that white cell transforms itself into a veritable chemical factory and conveys the newly acquired information to thousands of other white cells that in turn produce billions of anti-invader molecules. Once this has been done, the formula is stored so that a subsequent invasion will incite a fast motion repeat of the process.

The Lungs

The animal kingdom lives in utter dependence on this one element, oxygen. Some lower animals' devices for gathering oxygen are inexpressibly beautiful—the jewel-like fonts of marine worms, the fluted gills of tropical fish, the brilliant orange skirt of a flame scallop. Our own lungs come down on the side of function, not form, but they work well enough to make an engineer drool. The lungs crowd all the rest of the organs in our upper torso, spilling into every crevice and cranny. When air is pumped in to stimulate breathing, they seem to want to burst out of the chest cavity.

Bronchial tubes from the throat bisect, narrow down, divide again, and fan into a tree of tubes that culminate in three hundred million sacs. The sacs, only one cell thick, are caught like dewdrops in a spider web of blood vessels that channel blood around the sacs for the all-important oxygen transfer. The folds and convolutions of the lungs result in a surface area forty times larger than the skin's, and area large enough to carpet a small apartment.

The Bones

Bone cells live in rigid structures that exude strength. Cut in cross section, bones resemble tree rings, overlapping strength with strength, offering impalpability and sturdiness.

No Exxon researcher has yet discovered a material as well suited for the body's needs as bone, which comprises only one-fifth of our body weight. Engineers have demonstrated that the arrangement of bone cells forms the lightest structure and made of least material to support the body's weight. As the only hard material in the body besides teeth, bone possesses incredible strength, enough to protect and support every other cell. Sometimes we press our bones together like a steel spring, as when a pole-vaulter lands. Other times we nearly pull a bone apart, as when our arm lifts a heavy suitcase.

In comparisons, wood can withstand even less pulling tension, and could not possibly bear the compression forces that bone can. A wooden pole for the vaulter would quickly snap. Steel, which can absorb forces well, is three times the weight of bone and would burden us down.

Our Stuffed, Hollow Bones

The economical body takes this stress-bearing bone and hollows it out, using a weight-saving architectural principle it took people millennia to discover. It then fills the vacant space in the center with an efficient red blood cell factory that turns out a trillion new cells per day. Bone sheathes life.

We find bone's design most impressive in the tiny, jewel like chips of ivory in the foot. Twenty-six, specifically designed bones line up in each foot, about the same number as in each hand. Even when a soccer player subjects these small bones to a cumulative force of over one thousand tons per foot over the course of a match, his living bones endure the violent stress, maintaining their elasticity. Not all of us leap and kick, but we do walk some sixty-five thousand miles, or more than two and one half times around the world, in a lifetime. Our body weight is evenly spread out through architecturally perfect arches, which serve as springs, and the bending of knees and ankles absorbs stress.

The Muscles

Six hundred different muscles, which comprise fourty percent of our weight (twice as much as bones), burn up much of the energy we ingest as food in order to produce all our movements. Muscle cells, which absorb so much of that nourishment, are sleek and supple, full of coiled energy. Their shinny black nuclei look like bunches of black-eyed peas glued tightly together for strength.

Tiny muscles govern the light permitted into the eye. Muscles barely an inch long allow for a spectrum of subtle expression in the face. Another, much larger muscle, the diaphragm, controls coughing, breathing, sneezing, laughing and sighing. Massive muscles in the buttocks equips the body for a lifetime of walking. Without muscles, bones would collapse in a heap, joints would slip apart and movement would cease.

Muscle cells perform just one action, they contract. They can only pull, not push, as two protein molecules interact and the molecules slide together like teeth of two facing combs. Cells unite in strands called fibers, resembling coils of rope, and fibers report to a further hierarchy called a motor unit group. Muscles rely on an advanced hierarchy to organize the individual cells.

One motor nerve controls a motor unit group, wrapping its end plates around the muscle group as an octopus would encircle a pole. When that nerve gives a signal, all of its muscle fibers immediately become shorter and fatter. Some fibers are "fast-twitch" for short bursts of energy while others, "slow-twitch," are less quickly fatigued. Muscle fibers adhere to what is called the "all or none" principle. They do not have a variable throttle of energy, but a simple on-off switch. Variations of strength, as when a piano player lightly taps a key or pounds it mightily, occur because of the quantity of motor units firing off at any moment.

As the meter records the stream of static flowing from just one muscle area the size of a needle point, hundreds of other muscles go wholly undetected. A large and crucial group of them fire off whether or not we think about them. For example, the automatic muscles controlling our eyelids, breathing, heartbeat and digestion. It is as if the wisdom of the body does not trust the forgetful, erratic free will to handle these life-or-death functions. So protected are they that we cannot voluntarily stop our heartbeat or breathing.

Consider the electrical network linking every home and building in metropolitan New York City. At any given second lights are turned on and off, toasters pop up, microwave ovens begin their digital countdown, water pumps lunge into motion. Yet that enormous interlinking of decisions and activities is marked by randomness. A far more complex switching system is currently operating in your body at this second as you read this book, and it is perfectly controlled and orderly. When you reach the end of this page, you will turn it with your fingers, still only vaguely aware of the complex system that allows such an act.

A harmony of inhibitions synchronizes the whole body, coordinating heartbeats with breathing, and breathing with swallowing, setting muscle tone and adjusting to all changes in movement. In short, inhibition keeps one part of the machine out of the way of the other.

The Skin

There is no organ like the skin, averaging a total of a mere nine pounds. Skin cells form undulating patterns of softness and texture that rise and dip, giving shape and beauty to our bodies. They curve and jut at unpredictable angles so that every person's fingerprint—not to mention his or her face—is unique. It flexes and folds and crinkles around joints, facial crags, gnarled toes and fleshy buttocks. It is smooth as a baby's stomach here, rough like a crocodile there. A bricklayer's hands may be taut, rough and layered with sandpaper, but placid, pliable material may cover his abdomen. Intricate spot-welds fasten a leg's wrap, holding it tautly to the muscle layer, while the elbows droop loosely, like the skin of a cat that can be tossed by the scruff of its neck.

Choose sections of the scalp, the lip, the nipple, the heel, the abdomen and the fingertip to view through a laboratory microscope. They are as different as the skins of a host of species—a patchwork somehow growing in a continuous sheet over the body. On the fingertip, tiny ridges crisscross the skin's surface to provide traction, such as snow tires do. Amazingly, for no apparent reason, each of us is given a different pattern for the ridges, a flourish which the FBI capitalizes on in its fingerprint files. The ridges themselves give texture and power to grasp a slippery object.

The skin does not exist merely to give the body an appearance. It is also a vital, humming source of ceaseless information about our environment. Most of our sense organs—the ears, the eyes, the nose—are confined to one spot. The skin is rolled thin like pie dough and studded with half a million tiny transmitters, like telephones jammed together waiting to inform the brain of important news.

The skin contains molecules of melanin which interact with sunlight to make a tan. The dark skin of blacks is the result of a mere one-thirtieth of an ounce of melanin spread out all over the body. The skin is continually sloughing off, starting as moist, gelatinous cells which gradually march to the surface to flatten out and dry into keratin, a protective, flaky coating, before being shed. It is keratin which produces rigid fingernails.

Sweat

Humans have an efficient cooling system which uses sweat to cool our bodies to a constant internal temperature so that sensitive organs can maintain proper balance. Were it not so, we could hardly function in a climate where temperature exceeds 80 degrees. To heat the body, muscle contractions or shivering produces heat.

Although sweat glands vary by individuals, there are over two million on the average person. A marathon runner may shed three to five quarts of fluid in a three-hour race, but inside his temperature will hardly waver.

The Digestive System

What happens to food after it is eaten? The human body uses various kinds of food for energy and growth. To be used, however, food must be changed into a form that can be carried through the bloodstream. This amazing process, going on day after day, is a marvelous study in itself. Just for example, coiled up in the abdomen are 22 to 25 feet of incredibly marvelous small intestines. The lining of the small intestine contains many folds. These folds increase the surface area that can be in contact with the food product, which is also greatly enlarged by microscopic finger-like projections called villi. The digested food is passed through the cell membranes of the villi into the blood and lymph, which carry it to the cells for both energy and growth.

The Nerves

The king of cells is the nerve cell. It has an aura of wisdom and complexity about it. Spider-like, it branches out and unites the body with a computer network of dazzling sophistication. Individual axons, "wires," carrying distant messages to and from the brain, can reach a yard in length.

A healthy body is a beautiful, singing harmony between the central nervous system and the tissues it controls. Yet in all this harmony, every neuron must determine its own action based on the many impulses that come in. The microscopic computer in each nerve cell gauges our intentions, consults other muscles, analyzes hormones, energy availability and the inhibition of fatigue or pain, and fires a yes or no order to its muscle group.

The body communicates by electricity passing through the nerves. This fact mystified researchers for a long time because nerves are so delicate that a hair-width bundle of them contains 100,000 separate "wires." So instead of the electrical current working like it does in our homes with 110 volts inside each socket, the electrical current inside us passes through the interactions of sodium and potassium ions. That is why our sodium/potassium chemical balance is so important. The ions inside the cells carry the various messages like runners passing a torch in a relay race.

The Brain

The brain, floating in its ivory box in a pool of cerebrospinal fluid, contains the person we are. Every other cell in the body ages and is replaced at least every seven years. The skin, eyes, heart, even bones are entirely different today from those we carried around just one decade ago. In all respects but one, we are now a different person—but for one exception. The exception being the neurons or nerve cells which make up the brain and fan out throughout the entire body. Never replaced, these maintain the continuity of selfhood that keeps alive the physical entity we call ourselves.

For two-way communication outside the brain, there are two groups, "the way in" cells which carry impulses from the organs of the body to the brain, and "the way out," cells which carry instructions from the brain out to the extremities. From the darkness and loneliness of that box, we reach outside the brain with millions of living wires. They extend from the brain like tendrils of a plant, stretching desperately toward impulses of smell, sight, sound and touch into the world of light and matter.

Ninety-nine Percent of The Brain Is For Internal Processing

But almost all of the activity in the brain is for internal processing. In the entire brain, only one in one thousand cells reports in from the extremities to receive visual images, sounds, touch, pain sensations, smells, the monitoring of blood pressure and chemical changes, the sensations of hunger, thirst, and sex drives, muscular tension—all the "noise" from the entire body—occupy one tenth of one percent of the brain's cells. Yet each second those fibers bombard the brain with a hundred million messages. Of those, a few hundred at most are admitted to the small, center brain, called the brain stem.

Another two-tenths of one percent of cells controls all motor activities, the motions involved in playing a piano concert, speaking a language, dancing a ballet, typing a letter or operating a video game. In between these two groups of cells, the way out, lie all the other—enormous numbers of cells cooperating in a vast network of intercommunication to allow the process we know as thought, feeling and free will. We can think of them as a network of ten billion bureaucrats constantly phoning each other about plans and instructions for keeping a country running. Unlike a telephone switchboard that connects single subscribers indirectly through a central switching station, each nerve cell in the brain has up to ten thousand of its own private lines. All along its length dendrites reach out and form connections with other neurons, in effect linking each cell with wires from an entire city. It "listens" for the patterns of impulses at their average rate of arrival and decides whether to continue the message by firing off chemicals along its thousands of other connections.

The Brain's Highly Selective Communication

We want to move our hand. Is the stimulus from the brain strong enough to contract the muscle? How many muscle fibers are necessary for the appropriate strength? Are opposing muscles properly inhibited? The single nerve carries all these electrical messages, up to one thousand separate impulses a second, with an appropriate pause between each. Every impulse is monitored and affected by all the ten thousand synaptic connections along the path. Actually a stupendous crackling wildness surges in all of us at every moment.

Some functions, though, do not fit the rigid, robot-like response of reflex. In the brain stem lies another level of guidance, the subconscious regulators of breathing, digestion, and heart action. These need more attention than reflexes: And the body's requirements change quickly. For example, heartbeat and breathing surge wildly when we race up a stairs.

Where The Brain Does It's Thinking

Highest of all in the hierarchy of the nervous system is the cerebral hemisphere of the brain, the holy of holies of the body—most protected by bone, most vulnerable to injury if the protection is ever breached. They're ten billion nerve cells and one hundred billion glia cells, which provide the biological batteries for brain memories, creating consciousness. In the brain lies our inclination to evil and rage as well as our impetus toward purity and love.

Profound Inter-Communications

Physically speaking, the whole mental process comes down to these two billion cells spitting irritating chemicals at each other across the synapses or gaps. The web of nerve cells defies description or depiction. One tiny section the size of a pinpoint, not a pinhead, contains one billion connections among these cells. A mere gram of brain tissue, the size of a very tiny pill, may contain as many as four hundred billion synaptic junctions. As a result, each cell can communicate with every other cell at lightning speed—as if a population far larger than earth's were linked together so that all inhabitants could talk at once. The brain's total number of connections rivals the stars and galaxies of the universe.

The entire body's primary function is to support the brain, keeping it nourished and protected. The brain uses up one-fourth of all the oxygen we breathe in. A lack of oxygen for five minutes will usually cause death. The brain contains imagination, morality, sensuality, mathematics, memory, humor, judgement, religion, as well as an incredible catalog of facts and theories and the common sense to assign them all priority and significance. In the head, there are forces within forces, as in no other cubic half-foot of the universe that we know. There is nothing on the earth so wonderful. Yet nothing on earth is so fragile.

DNA

The most revolutionary discovery about the body during the later half of this century is DNA. Every 100 trillion cells in your body contains the DNA (blueprint) to make a brand new you. Half of the DNA comes from the sperm of the father and half from the egg of the mother. Once the egg and sperm share their inheritance, the DNA chemical ladder splits down the center of every gene such as the teeth of a zipper pulled apart. DNA re-forms itself each time the cell divides: 2, 4, 8, 16, 32 cells, each with the identical DNA. Along the way cells specialize, but each carries the entire instruction book of one hundred thousand genes. A nerve cell may operate according to instructions from volume four and a kidney cell from volume 372, but both carry the whole compendium. It provides each cell's sealed credential of membership in the body. Every cell possesses a genetic code so complete that the entire body could be reassembled from information in any one of the one hundred trillion cells of the body.

No group of doctors can reproduce a whole new human from one cell but the intelligence in your cells called DNA can do it all day long. Scientists have identified at least six billion steps of DNA in a single cell. The DNA is so narrow and compacted that all the genes in an entire body's cells would fit into an ice cube, yet if the DNA were unwound and joined together end to end, the strand would stretch from the earth to the sun and back more than four hundred times. That is 74 billion, 320 million miles! Trying to understand the complexity and intricate precision of a single cell is humbling to the intellect, to say the least.

According to Dr. Carl Sagan, if all the information contained in the DNA of one cell could be written down in book form, it would take a huge library to hold the complete set. There would be approximately 4,000 books the size of the Bible to hold this information. The DNA in each cell is so complex and precise that it can be compared to the whole entire universe.

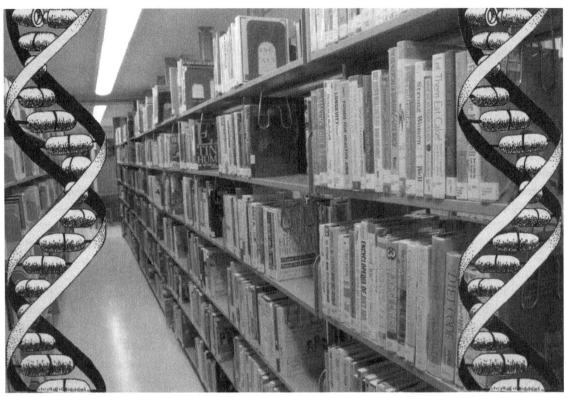

Every cell in the body contains a library of information known as DNA. There is enough DNA in each cell to produce a whole new you.

After learning more about how amazing the human body is one can't help but taking a moment to marvel at the miracle that we are.

> "Each patient carries his own doctor inside him. We are at our best when we give the doctor who resides within a chance to go to work." Albert Schweitzer, M.D. - Nobel Laureate 1940

Chapter 6
MEDICAL MYTHS EXPOSED

Gallbladder – A Necessary Organ or Bio-trash?

Gallbladder surgery is another example of how our medical system maintains disease and fails to prevent illness from getting out of hand. Most Americans go to their medical doctor for routine checkups. Doctors check their blood pressure, cholesterol, blood sugar etc., and they send them home with a prescription if any of those numbers don't fit into their "normal" box. Then one day you have some indigestion, nausea and pain. It gets worse so you go to your doctor. They begin running tests and sure enough, it is the gallbladder. They find it infected, filled with stones and nonfunctioning. "We need to do surgery and remove it as soon as possible," the doctor informs. Why didn't the doctor check the gallbladder last time you were in for your checkup? The answer is obvious. Doctors don't check the gallbladder, liver, appendix, etc., when you are feeling well. They wait until something breaks or malfunctions to start looking at the problem. The only thing left for them to do now is decide which kind of surgery to do or what drug to dope you up with for the rest of your life. Very seldom is there ever any preventative action taken. Does this system make any sense?

When a person comes into our clinic with a headache, chronic fatigue, overweight or arthritis… it doesn't matter what symptoms they have, we are going to check the gallbladder and every other organ, gland and system to see which is functioning properly and which needs support. By correcting imbalances in the body before they turn into full-blown problems that require surgery, we can eliminate problems BEFORE they happen.

Case Study – Oct, 2006

For many years I have had problems with heartburn and indigestion. I had to take antacids after every meal or I would be completely miserable. I thought this was just the way it was for some people.

One day at work I really started having problems with heartburn. It got so bad that I couldn't stand up straight for an extended period of time. I had sharp pains between my shoulder blades and in my chest. I went into the medical clinic at work and they thought that I was having a heart attack. The doctor wanted me to go to the emergency room immediately. I didn't feel like that was what I needed to do. Instead, I called and made an appointment with Dr. Sainsbury.

Dr. Sainsbury did a CEDSA (Computerized Electrodermal Stress Analysis) on me to determine the cause of my symptoms. No energetic disturbances were detected with my heart and circulation. But when he checked my gallbladder it was very high and my stomach and small intestine points checked very sluggish on the computer. Dr. Sainsbury found the supplements that checked the best to flush my liver and gallbladder out. He also recommended digestive enzymes and hydrochloric acid to support my digestive system.

I started taking the products and by the next day I was feeling much better. As the days went by I kept improving. It wasn't long before my heartburn and indigestion stopped altogether. I am now healthy and no longer experience heartburn and indigestion. The products gave my body the tools it needed to heal. Now I don't even have to take antacids after meals and I feel great. I know that if I would have gone to the hospital they would have removed my gallbladder and that would have lead to future health problems.

I have total confidence in Dr. Sainsbury and the way that he addresses the cause of symptoms by giving the body what it needs to heal. I take my wife and children to him whenever any of them have problems. I highly recommend Dr. Sainsbury and his natural healing programs for anyone who has health problems. I am the type of person who has to see or experience something in order to believe it. He made a believer out of me. I am convinced that natural healing works!

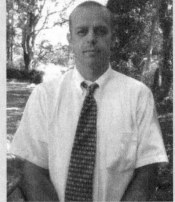

Joey Nelson
Rainbow City, Alabama

> "The most serious potential danger associated with experimental orthodox medicine is that a patient may avoid or delay receipt of safe, natural healing care in a timely fashion leading to irreversible damage caused by toxic drugs, mutilating surgeries and medieval carcinogenic radiation." James Chappell, D.C., N.D., Ph.D.

Gallstones are usually caused by a deficiency of organic sodium in the body. Our high protein, processed food diets cause us to be acidic. When the body is acidic minerals like sodium and calcium are used to buffer the acids thus leaving us depleted of these minerals. The key to preventing gallstones is to eat more alkaline foods such as fruits and vegetables that contain organic sodium. Inorganic sodium (table salt) comes from rock and is not utilized by the body. However, organic sodium found in celery is what your cells need for health.

Gallstones can come in all shapes and sizes. They can be green, white, black, red or tan colored depending upon your body chemistry. As more and more form and accumulate in the bile ducts they put backpressure on the liver which causes it to make less bile.

Gallbladders are like any other appliance; if you don't clean and service them periodically they begin running sluggishly until they no longer work. Being overwhelmed with toxic garbage, they invite infections, parasites, allergies, and all kinds of digestive disturbances. Many times a simple gallbladder cleanse can clear up annoying symptoms such as fatigue, hives, shoulder, upper arm, back and joint pain. Preventative measures need to be employed to maintain health and prevent gallbladder surgery.

What good is a gallbladder anyway? The fact that God put it in the body to begin with tells us a lot. Everyday your liver manufactures 1 to 1 1/2 quarts of bile and then stores it in the gallbladder. When we eat, the gallbladder squeezes itself empty to help us breakdown our foods, especially fats. Dairy products, red meat, mayonnaise, French fries etc., are high in fats. With a clean, healthy liver and gallbladder the body will control the blood fat levels fine. If your cholesterol level is high it is because there is an imbalance in your body. The body manufactures cholesterol for a reason. A sluggish thyroid or toxins in the liver and gallbladder are most likely the culprits. Once again, we don't want to fight what your body is doing, instead we want to understand why it is doing what it is doing and work with it by correcting the cause.

Many heart attacks are caused by liver and gallbladder dysfunction, especially when the gallbladder is removed. Improper digestion allows fat to buildup in the arteries putting more stress on the heart to beat harder to push the blood through the crud. When that pressure is more than what the heart and blood vessels can handle then they have a heart attack.

If you cook hamburgers tonight for dinner and you let the pan sit on the stove and cool off what does it look like? A thick, white layer of grease coats your pan. What do you put in the water to wash that greasy pan with? Dish detergent is what you put in to cut the grease, right? We were camping once and forgot to bring soap. We tried for twenty minutes to scrub the grease off the pan in the river and it just wouldn't come off. Your gallbladder is the dish detergent bottle in your body. Whenever you eat anything fatty, bile (soap) is secreted from the gallbladder to break it down and keep it from building up in your arteries and coating your cells. By taking the gallbladder out, we throw away our bottle of dish 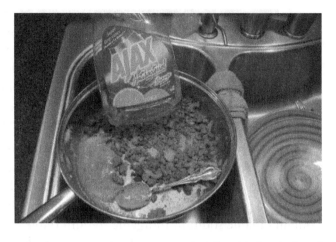 detergent. Now when we eat fats, the liver, which in most Americans is already overloaded and swamped with toxins, has to attempt to deal with this added stress. In most cases, it fails to cope and the results down the road are heart attacks and blood sugar imbalances also known as diabetes.

Most Americans simply do not break down and metabolize their foods correctly. Gallstones form and interfere with the secretion of bile. When the body fails to secrete enough bile (soap) to clean grease off of cells so insulin can secrete through, then blood sugar issues will likely occur. We are seeing an overwhelming amount of people having their gallbladders removed, then being diagnosed with diabetes.

Having no gallbladder is like trying to wash greasy dishes without soap. If your gallbladder has been removed, then we highly recommend supporting your liver to breakdown fats with our Beta Plus formula. Essential fatty acids like flaxseed and evening primrose oil are important for fat metabolism and removing plaque from the arterial walls.

Ignorant people and arrogant doctors like to warn others that natural healing is not scientific and so "you need to watch out and beware." It's quite ironic that there is all kinds of scientific research being done around the world, but their findings are somehow just shoved in the corner and ignored by mainstream doctors. If the research doesn't promote drug sales or expensive surgery, then it seems to have no merit in our capitalistic medical community. The following is an example of this.

> "The yellow pigment in bile that causes the characteristic yellowing of jaundice sufferers may not be simply a body waste after all, scientists say. Bilirubin, long thought to have no value, may be beneficial in thwarting cancer, aging, inflammation and other health problems, researchers from the Berkeley and San Francisco campuses of the University of California have found. The researchers say bilirubin appears to be a powerful antagonist of oxygen compounds that play a role in numerous diseases and conditions. Roland Stocker, the lead investigator in the study, said the results indicate scientists should examine other wastes

from chemical processes in the body to see if they also have other functions. Reporting in the most recent issue of Science, Stocker and his associates said in test-tube studies, bilirubin acted much like anti-oxidants vitamin C and E, neutralizing so-called oxygen radical compounds that destroy beneficial vitamin A and linoleic acid, a common fatty acid that is a major component of cell membranes. 'Instead of spending 95% of our time developing means to get rid of bilirubin, we should spend time on possible beneficial roles of bilirubin,' Stocker said." (Vancouver Sun, March 7, 1987)

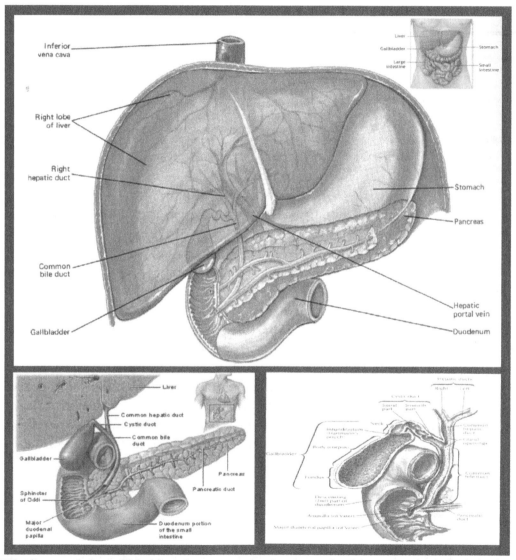

*The liver and the gallbladder play a crucial role in your health. Notice how the bile duct from the gallbladder goes directly to the small intestine. Bile is stored in the gallbladder and then secreted to break down fats. How many hamburgers and French fries do you eat?

> "In my years of medical practice I've seen a lot of surgery performed because surgeons believe that God blundered mightily when He created the human physique. You're supposed to regard it as providential that they're around to repair God's mistakes."
> — Robert Mendelsohn, M.D.

Liver/Gallbladder Flush For Stones
From Hulda Clark, Ph.D., N.D. "The Cure For All Diseases"

Ingredients:
4 tablespoons **Epsom salts**
Half cup **Olive oil** (light olive oil is easier to get down)
1/2 cup fresh (you squeeze yourself) pink **grapefruit juice**
4 – 8 **Ornithine capsules** (amino acids) for sleep. (Don't skip this or you may have the worst night of your life!)
Pint jar with lid
Black Walnut Hull tincture, any strength. (10 to 20 drops, to kill parasites coming from the liver.)

Choose a day like Saturday for the cleanse, since you will be able to rest the next day. Take no medicines, vitamins or pills that you can do without. They could prevent success. Eat a no-fat breakfast and lunch such as cooked cereal, fruit, fruit juice, bread and preserves or honey (no butter or milk), baked potato or other vegetables with salt only. This allows the bile to build up and develop pressure in the liver. Higher pressure pushes out more stones. Limit the amount you eat to the minimum you can get by on. You will get more stones. The earlier you stop eating the better your results will be, too. In fact, stopping fat and protein the night before gets even better results. Finish eating by 12 noon with only sips later.

2:00 p.m. Do not eat or drink after 2 o'clock. If you break this rule you could feel quite ill later.

Get your Epsom salts ready. Mix 4 Tbsp. in three cups water and pour this into a safe jar. This makes four servings, ¾ cup each. Set the jar in the refrigerator to get ice cold (this is for convenience and taste only).

6:00 p.m. Drink one serving (3/4 cup) of ice-cold Epsom salts. If you did not prepare this ahead of time, mix 1 Tbsp. in ¾ cup water now. You may add 1/8 tsp. You may rinse your mouth, but spit out the water.

Get the olive oil and grapefruit out to warm up.

8:00 p.m. Repeat by drinking another ¾ cup of Epsom salts. You haven't eaten since two o'clock, but you won't feel hungry. Get your bedtime chores done. The timing is critical for success.

9:45 p.m. Pour ½ cup (measured) olive oil into the pint jar. Squeeze the grapefruit by hand into the measuring cup. Remove pulp with fork. You should have at least ½ cup, more (up to ¾ cup) is best. You may top it off with lemonade. Add this to the olive oil. Also, add Black Walnut Hull tincture. If you haven't gotten stones out in the last few cleanses, add citric acid to bring success. Also, using 2/3 cup water for Epsom salts instead of ¾ can bring success. Close the jar tightly with the lid and shake hard until watery. (only fresh citrus juice does this).

Now visit the bathroom one or more times, even if it makes you late for your ten o'clock drink. Don't be more than 15 minutes late. You will get fewer stones.

10:00 p.m. Drink the potion you have mixed. Take 4 Ornithine capsules with the first sips to make sure you will sleep through the night. Take eight if you already suffer from insomnia. Drinking through a large plastic straw helps it go down easier. You may use salad dressing, syrup, or straight sweetener to chase it down between sips. Take it to your beside if you wish. Get it down within 5 minutes (15 minutes for very elderly or weak persons). If you had difficulty getting stones out in the past add ½ tsp. citric acid to the potion. You may put it in capsules.

Lie down immediately. You might fail to get stones out if you don't. The sooner you lie down the more stones you will get out. Be ready for bed ahead of time. Don't clean up the kitchen. As soon as the drink is down, walk to your bed and lie down flat on your back with your head up high on the pillow. Try to think about what is happening in the liver. Try to keep perfectly still for at least 20 minutes. You may feel a train of stones traveling along the bile ducts like marbles. There is no pain because the bile duct valves are open. (thank you Epsom salts!) **Go to sleep**, you may fail to get stones out if you don't.

Next Morning. Upon awakening take your third dose of Epsom salts. If you have indigestion or nausea wait until it is gone before drinking the Epsom salts. You may go back to bed. Don't take this potion before 6:00 am.

2 hours later. Take your fourth (the last) dose of Epsom salts. You may go back to bed again.

After 2 more hours you may eat. Start with fruit juice. You may add another ½ tsp. citric acid to it (or capsules) and get even more stones. Half an hour later eat fruit. One hour later you may eat regular food but keep it light. During the day take the parasite-killing herbs. By supper you should feel recovered.

Alternative Schedule 1: Omit the first Epsom salts dose at 6 p.m. Take only one dose, waiting till 8 p.m. Change nothing else. Many people still get stones with one less dose. If you do not, do the full course next time.

Alternative Schedule 2: Add ½ tsp. citric acid to the oil-grapefruit mixture. Stir till dissolved. Next morning, add ½ tsp. citric acid again to the first fruit juice you drink when done with Epsom salts.

Alternative Schedule 3: For brain and spinal cord cancers, caffeic acid is the antigen to be avoided. This includes grapefruit. Blend whole apples instead, Red or Golden Delicious. Strain to get ½ cup juice. Add ½ tsp. citric acid to oil-juice mixture.

If you don't get stones…

* Use slightly less than ¾ cup water for each Epsom salts dose, such as 5/8 or 2/3 cup.

CONGRATULATIONS! You have taken out your gallstones without surgery!

How well did you do? Expect diarrhea in the morning. This is desirable. Use a flashlight to look for the gallstones in the toilet with the bowel movement. Look for the green kind since this is proof that they are genuine gallstones, not food residue. Only bile from the liver is pea green. The bowl movement sinks but gallstones float because of the cholesterol inside. Count them all roughly, whether tan or green. You will need to total 2,000 stones before the liver is clean enough to rid you of allergies or bursitis or upper back pains permanently. The first cleanse may rid you of them for a few days, but as stones from the rear travel forward, they give you the same symptoms again. You may repeat cleanses at two-week intervals. Never cleanse when you are ill.

Sometimes the bile ducts are full of cholesterol crystals that did not form into round stones. They appear as "chaff" floating on top of the toilet bowl water. It may be tan colored, harboring millions of tiny white crystals. Cleansing this chaff is just as important as purging stones.

With gallstones, much less cholesterol leaves the body, and cholesterol levels may rise. Gallstones being porous can pick up all the bacteria, cysts, viruses and parasites that are passing through the liver. In this way "nests" of infection are formed, forever supplying the body with fresh bacteria. No stomach infection such as ulcers or intestinal bloating can be cured permanently without removing these gallstones from the liver.

Epsom salt is not the healthiest thing to put in the body but it sure does help in cleansing gallstones. For those who do not want to use the Epsom salts, there is another cleanse that takes a little longer, but is still effective.

> "The laws of God and Nature are immutable: They can not long be broken without retribution. Life in its fullness is Mother Nature obeyed." Weston Price, D.D.S.

#2 Liver Flush Without Epsom Salts for Gallstones

For this flush, you will need 144 ounces of organic apple juice and 1 bottle of Alpha-Ortho-Phos. This flush is done during 2 days of fasting, so be prepared not to eat (this is best done over a weekend). For the first 2 days, drink 6 12- ounce glasses of the apple juice each containing 50 drops of the Alpha-Ortho-Phos (this is to soften the stones). Make sure to spread the apple juice throughout the day so as to lessen the hunger and blood sugar drop.

On the third day upon arising, take 8 ounces of Extra Virgin olive oil and the juice of one lemon and mix together well. Drink the mixture and go back to bed, lying on the right side with the right knee pulled up to the chest. The olive oil forces the gallbladder to push the stones out. In 2 or 3 hours, you should pass the stones in a bowel movement. They will be greenish-blue in color. There could be very many pieces or one greenish-blue bowel movement. Once the movement has passed, you may resume your normal pattern of eating.

For more information on gallbladder cleansing and to see actual pictures of gallstones go online to curezone.com/gallstones.

The Cholesterol Myth

How would you feel to know that you could make $94,000 a day for the rest of your life? Would you tell your boss, "Take this job and shove it" and go on vacation? Well, the CEO of Pfizer, the manufacturer of Lipitor, cashed in 33.9 million smackers last year. That's 2.8 million a month, which equals $94,000 a day. Not too shabby for a day at the office, while your drug-dealing doctors pedal your dope for you.

> "Why was $150 million spent on cholesterol research involving a drug whose negative effects outweigh the positive? And how did medical science ever get side-tracked with recommending avoidance of dietary cholesterol and saturated fat, a practice which fails to address the basic problem?"
> Stephen E. Langer, M.D. Author of Solved The Riddle of Illness

The moneymaking myth that high cholesterol is a major cause of heart disease and stroke has been strategically orchestrated by the pharmaceutical industry to sell their cholesterol lowering drugs.

Cholesterol is a waxy fat that is attached to a protein for transport in the blood. Most cholesterol in your body is manufactured in the liver and does not come from your diet. Researchers have shown that eighty percent of all cholesterol in the blood serum is produced by the body from foods that do not contain cholesterol. The difference between what is considered "good" cholesterol and "bad" cholesterol is the protein to which the cholesterol is attached.

Low Density Lipoproteins (LDL) is considered "bad cholesterol" (a term invented by the pharmaceutical companies to sell their products) because it is found as plaque in the arteries. If what we are told about high cholesterol causing heart attacks is true, then when people die from heart attacks we would see elevated blood cholesterol levels right? What story do autopsies tell? When autopsies are done, half of all heart attacks and strokes occur in people without elevated cholesterol levels. (Ridker PM. Clinical Cardiology. 2003 April; 26(4 Suppl 3): III39-44)

Cholesterol is not the cause of heart disease and strokes. We have seen people with cholesterol counts over 600 that have no arteriosclerosis, no blockages, no high blood pressure and no heart disease. Turning the other direction, we see people with very low cholesterol counts of 100 who have had heart attacks and required triple bypass surgery.

Dr. Edward Athrens of Rockefeller University has conducted cholesterol research for over forty years. He does not believe that lowering cholesterol levels reduces heart disease and thinks that the lowering cholesterol craze is unscientific and wishful thinking.

Our bodies need cholesterol for health. Cholesterol is not the bad guy everyone makes him out to be. Cholesterol is used in our bodies to make hormones such as blood sugar-regulating hormones, stress hormones and sex hormones. Do you know people who get on cholesterol medication and lose their sex drive, gain weight, become depressed and have no energy? Hmm, maybe the drugs we take to lower cholesterol throw other activities in the body out of balance and cause more health problems? Without enough cholesterol our testosterone, estrogen, and cortisone levels are thrown out of balance. A study published in the Journal of Clinical Pharmacology and Therapeutics (21:89-94, 1996) reported that men taking statin drugs increased the frequency of sexual dysfunction by fifty percent. Don't worry, that same drug company will turn around and be glad to sell you a bottle of Viagra to perk things up. They have you covered.

Cholesterol is necessary for sperm to join with an egg and to create a new life. When this intelligent life process occurs, they bring along their own supply of cholesterol. When a woman becomes pregnant, her blood serum level of cholesterol rises by about fifty percent in order to nourish the fetus's trillions of new developing cells. Dr. Barnes points out how ridiculous the high cholesterol myth is.

> **"If cholesterol were harmful to arteries, as so many have stated, the fetus would have a heart attack before the baby saw the light of day."**
> Broda Barnes, M.D.

Cell membranes, myelin sheath and the brain all need cholesterol in order to be healthy. Without cholesterol your nerve cells cannot transmit signals. Do you know how many people we see in our clinic taking cholesterol-lowering drugs who complain about failing memory? Their doctor never mentioned the fact that cholesterol is the most organic molecule in the brain and makes up seventy-five percent of your brain's weight. NASA astronaut and flight surgeon Dr. Duane Graveline, reports that he lost his memory after six weeks of being on Lipitor. He is the author of *Lipitor – Thief of Memory* and explains how after taking Lipitor he could not recognize his wife and house for six hours at a time.

Dr. Beatrice Golomb, from University of California reiterates how notorious the statin drugs are for causing memory loss. She reports, *"We have people who have lost thinking ability so rapidly, that within the course of a couple of months, they went from being head of major divisions of companies to not being able to balance a checkbook and being fired from their company."* Now isn't that just cute? Get your cholesterol where your doctor wants it and lose your job in the process, because your brain can't function because your medicine is causing more harm than good. Wake up Americans, your doctor's drugs are backfiring on you!

> "Cholesterol is the basic building block to manufacture sex hormones – estrogen and testosterone. Lacking optimal intake of cholesterol, ladies will have hot flashes so bad they can melt steel and guys won't know whether to lead or follow on the dance floor."
> Joel Wallach, D.V.M., N.D.

The fact that many who take cholesterol lowering medications experience adverse side effects should be aware of how dangerous statin drugs are. Inflammation of the liver and the breakdown of muscle tissue are common reactions with these drugs. Do you know why? Because they are poisonous! Why else would your liver swell and muscles deteriorate?

Our immune systems need cholesterol in order to have healthy lymphocytes and T-cells to fight infection. Cholesterol also helps the liver produce bile acids, which help break down fats so that toxins can be eliminated. Most likely, your doctor never mentioned any of this to you, did he? Of course not, because Pfizer has promised him a candy bar if he's real good boy. Doctors are wined and dined and treated like royalty by pharmaceutical reps to prescribe their dope.

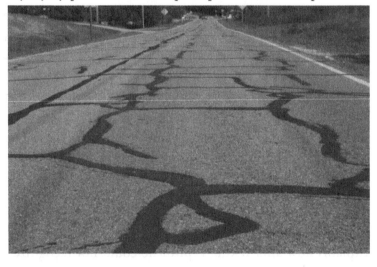

Just as the highway crews go out with hot tar to seal and repair cracks in the roads to prevent them from crumbling to pieces, so does your body manufacture cholesterol to repair cracks in your 70,000 miles of arteries.

Let's suppose scientists studied damaged roads and found that decaying roads contained more tar than healthy roads. Because of this they conclude that tar causes road damage. Would this be completely ridiculous and absurd? A similar ridiculous occurrence is taking place to push Americans to lower their cholesterol with drugs.

Researchers Walsh and Grady from the University of California proclaim that there is NO EVIDENCE from primary prevention trials to prove that lowering cholesterol levels with the use of statin drugs decreases mortality rates from heart disease. (JAMA 1995 Oct 274:1152-1158)

If nothing is done to support the arteries, then plaque/cholesterol can accumulate and attach itself to the artery and restrict blood flow, thus causing a heart attack. When this happens in the brain we call it a stroke.

The key to understanding the cholesterol puzzle is that cholesterol will only attach itself to the artery when the artery is damaged, just like putting a patch on a hole in a tire. It's your body's innate way of healing without you ever, being aware. If your arteries are healthy, then cholesterol goes right through you without any problems.

> "The American public can no longer blindly trust that its vaunted medical journals and world-class medical experts put the interests of patients first." John Abramson, M.D.

Another myth-shattering study was published in JAMA in 1987 entitled, "Cholesterol and Mortality: 30 Years of Follow-up from the Framingham Study." This study is not well liked by the drug companies, because it shows that after the age of 50 there is no increased death rate with elevated cholesterol levels. Even more shocking is the fact that when cholesterol levels did begin dropping lower, then the death rates increased by fourteen percent for every 1 mg/dL drop in total cholesterol every year! Basically, what this study reveals is the fact that when we start messing things up with drugs we die sooner. (JAMA 1987 Apr 24; 257(16):2176-80)

The European Heart Journal reports a study done with 11,500 patients. Behar and associates discovered that people with cholesterol lower than 160 mg/dL increased their risk of death by 2.27 times higher than those with higher cholesterol. The risk of heart attack was the same in both groups. The report also revealed that people with lower cholesterol increased their risk of cancer.

Would anyone in his or her right mind trade high cholesterol that isn't even proven to decrease heart disease for cancer? JAMA published a shocking report by Thomas B. Newman, M.D, MPH that reveals how two-faced drugs are. Cholesterol lowering drugs (fibrates and statins) cause cancer in rodents. ("Carcinogenicity of Lipid-Lowering Drugs." JAMA Jan 3, 1996-Vol 275, No. 1.) You know what? We have enough problems with cancer, without taking a medicine that causes cells to act like rebellious teenagers. It's about time to stop this medical insanity. It's time to just say no to drugs.

The Journal of Cardiac Failure published a study for those who have had heart failure. The conclusion after analyzing 1,134 patients is, "Low serum total cholesterol is associated with marked increase in mortality in advanced heart failure." In other words, by lowering your cholesterol, you are at higher risks for more complications and a lower survival rate. Are they murdering our people with cholesterol-lowering prescriptions?

> "Conventional medicine is limited to treating the symptoms of secondary risk factors. Drugs blocking the synthesis of cholesterol and other lipid-lowering agents are now being prescribed to millions of people. These drugs are known to cause cancer and have other severe side effects. You should avoid them whenever you can."
> Matthias Rath, M.D. – Author of Why Animals Don't Get Heart Attacks …But People Do

What happens when a medical doctor begins researching "the research?" He begins to untangle a web of lies that have been deliberately told in order for the pharmaceutical industry to sell more drugs. John Abramson, M.D., instructor at Harvard Medical School exposes enough corruption in what is called "medical science" to make you think twice before you pop your next pill. The financial links between FDA officials and drug companies explains how and why dangerous killer drugs are prescribed in the USA when they haven't been proven safe or more effective than placebos. For those who are not afraid to stare corruption in the face read his book, *Overdosed America The Broken Promise Of American Medicine – HOW THE PHARMACUETICAL COMPANIES ARE CORRUPTING SCIENCE, MISLEADING DOCTORS, AND THREATENING YOUR HEALTH.*

After seeing how corrupt pharmaceutical companies are with their outright lies in order to sell more drugs, Roni Rabin from Newsday.com retaliates by saying, "We've been bamboozled about cholesterol risks." How many drugs have you taken or are taking right now, that have been lied about?

> "There are multiple layers of people engaged in a conspiracy of not telling the truth."
> Dr. Mary G. Enig - Biochemist, University of Maryland

One major cause of high cholesterol can be a low functioning thyroid gland (hypothyroidism). When the body thermostat is set lower than 97.8-98.2 degrees, then the body has a tough time regulating cholesterol levels. The solution is to support the thyroid nutritionally. Kelp, which is high in iodine, amino acids and raw desiccated thyroid extract help balance the thyroid. When the thyroid is functioning at a healthy level, then cholesterol levels will often times balance out.

Deadly Hydrogenated Oils

So what are the culprits that cause arteriosclerosis? Hydrogenated oils are our worst enemies. Most of our processed foods contain this man-made, indigestible, artery-damaging trash. Start reading labels and you'll find crackers, chips, cookies and almost anything you buy in a package or box contain these trans fats. Any food you have that lists hydrogenated oil, partially hydrogenated oil or the butter substitute margarine should be shunned like the plague. Most Americans like the way trans fats taste, but are we willingly committing suicide by eating this health destroying junk? If we want to be healthy, we have to start paying attention to what we put in our mouths. We reap what we sow. Go online to www.bantransfats.com for more information.

Another big artery damaging terrorist we willingly invite into our bodies is homogenized and pasteurized dairy products. When dairy products are homogenized, they are sent through cylinders that beat the molecules up so badly that the cream will no longer float to the top of the milk. It's very convenient for people who don't want to mess around with cream, but now your body has to attempt to break down another made man product that has been taken from nature and altered.

Pasteurization is the process of boiling milk and dairy products to kill bacteria. Put a few drops of formaldehyde in it and the grocery store can keep it on the shelf longer before it spoils. By pasteurizing milk we destroy all the enzymes and most of the vitamins, amino acids and calcium bioavailability. After man destroys what nature creates, we then force our bodies to deal with the nutrient-depleted trash. What's the result? Kidney stones, bone spurs, congestion, ear infections, mucous, colds and arthritis are common symptoms with those who are large dairy consumers.

It is interesting to note that osteoporosis is most common in the United States, England, Israel, Sweden, and Finland where large quantities of dairy products and calcium supplements are consumed. On the other hand, osteoporosis is rare in Africa and Asia where milk consumption is very low.

Humans are the only animals on the planet that continues drinking milk past childhood. All other animals are weaned off of mother's milk shortly after birth and they do not drink milk from other animals, but we humans do.

Store-bought milk does not do a body good. It causes a lot of illness. If you feel you must drink milk then try to get milk straight from the farmer in its whole, raw form with everything Mother Nature put in there, you'll be far better off. Goat's milk is superior to cow's milk. It's easier for humans to digest.

The Appendix

The appendix, according to Dr. Mendelsohn, is regarded by most surgeons as another one of God's mistakes. He explains, "I can't tell you the number of times I have heard a surgeon tell a woman that the appendix is "a useless, vestigial organ – some of God's leftover physiological junk."

It is worth noting that in 1975, 784,000 appendectomies were performed in the USA and approximately 3,000 of those patients died. These surgeries were considered emergency situations, but when the appendixes reached the pathology lab, one out of four were found to be perfectly healthy. Oops! Oh well, a man's got to do something for a living, right?

Every organ and gland has a function in your body. Just because medical science doesn't understand this does not mean we should allow organs to be cut out and thrown away. The appendix is part of your immune system. It helps fight infection. Studies have proven that people who have had their appendixes removed were twice as likely to develop cancer of the bowel. Furthermore, you are left at high risk for other infections as well. The appendix acts as an overflow valve to keep impacted fecal matter from pushing back into the small intestines and being reabsorbed into the blood.

> "Surgeons are trained to do surgery, not avoid it."
> Robert Mendelsohn, M.D.

Don't be mistaken, in some instances, when people have neglected their health and they are in the emergency room because the appendix is on the verge of bursting, then of course surgery is required. The point is, let's avoid that by keeping your digestive system balanced and your bowels moving. A CEDSA exam once a year will indicate what areas of your body need cleansing and toning. A parasite detox may be needed. The appendix and gallbladder are favorite hiding places for parasites. A wise person does not wait until he or she has symptoms to take their health serious.

No Incurable Diseases

> "We are the physical manifestation of the essence of our collective consciousness. We are the I AM. To see us is to see that which sent us."
> James Chappell D.C., N.D., Ph.D.

Understand that you have the power to depart this world when you are ready and when you choose. The Taramahara Indians in Mexico die peacefully when they are ready. When they feel they have accomplished what they came to do on earth, they say goodbye to everyone and walk out in the woods. Do you know what they do to die? Nothing. They simply sit down and stop moving and mentally let go and give up. Once the mind gives the body permission to go there is no struggle. The lymphatic system shuts down and within twenty-four hours they are dead.

Some Americans do nothing all day long. They sit in front of the TV all day, lifeless. They have no reason to get out of bed in the mornings and the Prozac they are on has them in a foggy haze. They have given up on health and trudge out the rest of their life subconsciously just waiting to die. What a waste. On top of all that, they get very little exercise and the arthritis gets worse and worse. Like a chain on a bicycle that is never used that becomes so rusty and stiff that it freezes up, so are some of our joints because we stop moving them.

Circulation is a key to life. Get up and move! Swing your arms around. Squat up and down and exercise all the muscles in the body daily. Move your body in all the directions it was meant to be moved in order to stay limber. If Americans would do ten minutes of simple exercising everyday, then most could avoid wheelchairs and walkers. How many Americans can't do a full squat with just their body weight? If we were to train our youth to do twenty-five full squats everyday, then by the time they were seventy-five they would still be able to do them perfectly and pain free. When we stop moving, joints become calcified, like rust on a bicycle chain. Dis-ease sets in and then we die.

> "Most of the things worth doing in the world had been declared impossible before they were done."
> Louis D. Brandeis - American Judge 1856-1941

Case Study – May, 2006

Dear Dr. Sainsbury,

First I want to thank you for all that you have done for me. You have helped me to help myself both physically and emotionally.

Initially, when I contacted you I was unable to get through the day without constant tears, unbelievable fatigue, and severe anxiety. I had been diagnosed with lupus, osteoarthritis, disc bulges, had injections of epidurals (to no avail) and was considered a candidate for back surgery as well as severe bone loss. My fatigue was such that I could not get through the day without at least two naps. Almost immediately after seeing you, the tears stopped, my anxiety decreased, to almost non-existence and my energy has returned to a point such as I experienced many years ago. More importantly, through your affirmation CD, I have discovered my much needed spiritual rebirth. I am now healthy, energized, happy, joyful, and certainly in harmony with the flow of life.

Again, I want to thank you for helping me return to a joyful, balanced, harmonized and healthy life style. In my opinion, your efforts have contributed more to my health than any other professional that I have contacted.

Please keep up the good work, I pray this will help enlighten anyone who may have any doubts as to the benefits that can be obtained through your natural remedies and counseling.

Sincerely,

Doris O'Neil
Collinsville, Alabama

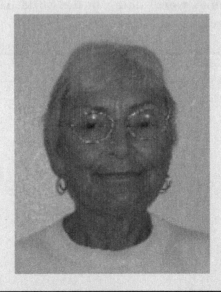

Crohn's Disease Healed

Mainstream medicine claims Crohn's disease is incurable. They are absolutely right, if all you have to work with is their drugs and antibiotics, while never addressing the cause or the terrain of the body. Jordan Rubin, N.D. healed himself of Crohn's and Colitis, but he didn't do it using a medical doctor's drugs. He looked like a concentration camp inmate after spending months in hospitals and being treated with drugs. He almost died, but finally found what his body needed to change the terrain that was favoring his dis-ease.

By eating live, fermented, probiotic rich foods and soil-based organisms his body began to heal. He conquered Crohn's disease naturally. His books are sold in Wal-Mart and he has a thriving business called "Garden Of Life." He has some great products to replace good bacteria in the gut that help change the terrain so that the body can heal.

Dis-ease: Your Body's Way of Filing Bankruptcy

Age is an excuse many use to be a poor victim. They hobble around sore, stiff and arthritic. Some have the ignorant belief that arthritis is just part of getting old. In the book *Chemistry of Man* by Dr. Bernard Jensen, he relates the following story, *"There is a myth going around that arthritis is a disease of old age. An elderly lady, so the story goes, went to see her doctor about arthritis pains in her left knee. "How old are you?" the doctor asked. "I'm 65," she said. "I'm 65 and I have arthritis, too," the doctor told her. "There's no cure for it. Just go home and chalk it up to old age." And this little old lady looked at the doctor and said, "I want to tell you something. My right knee is the same age as my left knee, and it doesn't have arthritis!"* Body chemistry is what determines the health of your joints, not your age.

Remember what was said earlier about Dr. Alexis Carrel keeping the chicken heart alive for twenty-nine years? He concluded that the cell is immortal. It is the fluid that surrounds the cell that creates dis-ease and death. In other words, our lymphatic system and an alkaline pH are key in keeping us healthy and alive.

Anyway you slice it, your health has a price and every disease is earned. You can pay now or pay later. It's not much different than a credit card. Buy anything you want now and worry about paying for it later. This type of carefree over spending usually digs a pit so deep that many Americans end up filing bankruptcy. Cancer is your body's way of filing bankruptcy. All the reserves have been spent and there is nothing left over to sustain life. Cells begin to mutate. Death is going back to the dust from whence you came and letting the bank take over.

Earning Your Cancer Trophy

Many of us play the credit card spending game with our health. We take, take, take and never put back and then wonder why our bank account is overdrawn and our health has fallen apart. We take Advil for headaches, Claritin for allergies, Cortisone shots for back pain, Tums for indigestion, Prozac for depression, Synthroid for thyroid and Lipitor for high cholesterol and then wonder why we are the poor victims of cancer twenty years later. The sad reality is, congratulations, you just earned your cancer trophy. It's yours. This is your award for doing all that you have to create the environment for cancer to exist. Cancer is your new trophy for consistently swallowing your lymphatic blocking, liver clogging, acidifying, toxic drugs religiously for the last fifteen years. As soon as you felt that first twinge of discomfort, the second that you had one single symptom, you ran to the kitchen cabinet to grab your magic pill to make you all better. And magic it has been for all these years, however, now the piper must be paid. How much do you have in your account? Do you have enough left to pay the debt or is it going to put you six feet under?

> "Be not deceived; God is not mocked: for whatsoever a man soweth that shall he also reap." Galatians 6:7

It's time to call it how it is and stop making excuses. We get what we earn. The good news about our newly earned cancer trophy is, if we created it, then we have the power to uncreate it. God gave us that healing ability within. We are free to choose to suffer or heal, die or live.

> "Disease is never acquired. It is always earned. Disease is a natural result obtained from an unnatural lifestyle. ... Disease occurs only when one's internal environment is favorable for disease growth. We create our internal environments. ... As you never see flies in a clean garbage can, you also never see disease in a completely pure being."
> Richard Anderson, N.M.D.

The Antibiotic Paradox

Antibiotics are being prescribed faster than flies can buzz around watermelon rinds and corncobs at a picnic. Pediatricians and family physicians prescribe over $500 million worth of antibiotics each year to treat ear infections in children. That's only half of the story. Another $500 million smackers is dished out on antibiotics to treat other pediatric problems. Over the last fifteen years, antibiotic prescriptions for our children have soared to over a whopping fifty-one percent!

> "No antibiotic can be said to have proven successful in truly eradicating any infectious disease in modern times."
> Marc Lappe, Ph.D. - Professor at University of Illinois

Children are not the only victims of antibiotic overdose. Obstetricians and gynecologists write 2,645,000 antibiotic prescriptions every week. Women get on these intestinal flora destroyers and then are plagued with vaginal yeast infections caused from the antibiotics! Like children playing tag out on recess, we trade one illness for another. After candida yeast gets in the blood stream from taking antibiotics that kill off the good bacteria, then the joints begin to ache, we have rashes, headaches and no energy. Does this sound like you? Have you been diagnosed with fibromyalgia or lupus? Have you taken antibiotics in the past? Now the puzzle pieces start to line up and we can see why you have these symptoms.

Solving Your Dis-ease Puzzle

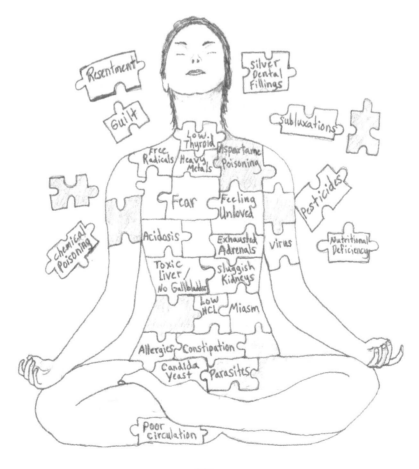

> "Candidiasis is basically a twentieth-century disease, a disease resulting from medical developments like antibiotics, birth control pills and estrogen replacement therapy." Leyardia Black, M.D.

Most medical experts and even the AMA admit that antibiotics are absolutely worthless for colds, influenza and upper respiratory tract infections. It's a fact that antibiotics are useless against viruses. It's important to understand that antibiotics don't cure disease, they cause it. In some instances, antibiotics can save a life and help us get over an infection, if it is caused by bacteria, but most of the time our immune system becomes stronger by letting nature run her course.

> "Not only are antibiotics powerless against the viruses that cause colds and flu, but misuse of antibiotics can actually do more harm than good." Fred Rubin, M.D. - Associate Clinical Professor of Medicine at the University of Pittsburgh and contributor to the Merck Manual

Our immune systems are like children. If every time our child fell or bumped his arm, and we grabbed him and said, from now on I'll carry you so you won't ever get hurt again, how would he ever grow up? He learns and grows by falling. He learns balance and he learns what to avoid. Of course we don't want him to do anything out of reason, but the bottom line is, through adversity he grows up. Similar to a child maturing, so are our immune systems growing and being strengthened as they are challenged.

Another analogy can be made by comparing our immune systems to muscles. Our immune systems become stronger from workouts like muscles do when we lift weights and exercise. The muscle adapts to its environment by becoming bigger and stronger to meet the demands placed upon it. Put your leg in a cast and don't walk or move it for two years and see what happens. The muscles begin to atrophy. What we don't use, we lose. Our immune system could be compared to a giant muscle. Any time we ingest antibiotics, we are allowing it to skip a workout that will cost us in the championship match when we need the strength and stamina to win. How many people do you know who lost their championship fight to cancer or some other disease because their immune system was weak from skipping workouts?

> "There may be a time down the road when 80% to 90% of infections will be resistant to all known antibiotics."
> Alexander Fleming - Discoverer of Penicillin

Fleming warned us that what appears to be great may also prove our fate. Experts are concerned about our future because of the massive amounts of antibiotics we have taken are beginning to backfire. In other words, the microbes are beginning to become stronger and resistant to our current antibiotics. Darwin's theory "survival of the fittest" is proving true in the microscopic world of bacteria.

If you do choose to take an antibiotic as a last resort or in an emergency, make sure and take some acidophilus to replace the good bacteria that the antibiotic will kill off. This will prevent candida yeast from getting in the blood and becoming systemic.

> "Antibiotics are indiscriminate killers; they kill bacteria that are required for our survival as efficiently as they kill harmful bacteria."
> — Bruce Lipton, Ph.D.

Acidosis – The Terrain That Favors Dis-ease

When it comes to health, we must look at the pH (potential of Hydrogen) of the body. A pH scale runs from 0 to 14. On the low end of the scale, 0 means complete acidity. On the high end, 14 indicates complete alkalinity. Obviously a 7 on the scale is right in the middle, neutral. Healthy individuals have a pH (saliva) that hovers in the 6.8-7.0 range. Healthy urine pH runs somewhere between 5.5-5.8. Foods eaten in the same day of testing your pH will greatly influence the results, which could be misleading.

pH Scale

Acidity		
	0	battery acid
	1	hydrochloric acid secreted by stomach
	2	lemon juice, vinegar
	3	orange juice, grapefruit, soft drinks, wine
	4	beer, acid rain
	5	black coffee, soft drinking water
	6	urine, saliva, egg yolks, cow's milk
Neutral	7	pure water
	8	sea water
	9	baking soda
	10	Great Salt Lake, detergent, milk of magnesia
	11	ammonia, household cleaners
	12	soapy water, baking soda
	13	household lye, oven cleaners, bleaches
	14	liquid drain cleaner
Alkalinity		

Do you want to simplify the mystery of health? Most health problems are maintained by the body's pH being too acidic. Yeast (Candida), viruses, bacteria, arthritis, cancer, fibromyalgia, diabetes etc., love an acidic atmosphere. If you have a dis-ease, analyze what you ate yesterday, last week, and have been eating for the last year and that will give you a good clue as to what caused it. If we want to heal, we must change the terrain of the body by eating alkaline forming foods.

It's important to understand that some foods like lemons and grapefruits are acidic in nature but once consumed and metabolized in your body they leave an alkaline ash. That is why we call most fruits and vegetables alkaline forming foods, while high protein foods such as meats, poultry, fish, and grains are acid ash producing foods.

> "Germs, bacteria, viruses and alike, are scavengers and can live only on wasting-away cells, mucous and toxic conditions. They can never exist in a healthy and clean cell structure or body."
> John Christopher, N.D.

The theory that germs cause disease is a myth. Louis Pasteur was famous for discovering that bacteria can cause illness. He subsequently developed the pasteurization process for milk, in which milk is heated up and boiled. Hence, according to his theory all the bacteria would be destroyed thus preventing disease. Pasteur spent his life studying how germs cause illness but on his deathbed he confessed the following.

> "I have been wrong. The germ is nothing. The 'terrain' is everything."
> Louis Pasteur

Consider this simple illustration. If you have a tree in your back yard with moss growing all over it and you want to get rid of the moss, because let's suppose it is cancer, then what must you do? Oh sure, you can have a doctor pull out a scalpel and perform surgery and cut it off. You could also have him burn it off with poisonous chemicals. He could freeze it off with dry ice. Or he could burn it off with a laser. All of these are possibilities to treating moss (cancer) on the tree, however, what's going to happen in eight months or so? Of course the moss will grow right back, because we have failed to remove the cause. We have done nothing to change the terrain that favored the moss (cancer) to grow in the first place.

> "The idea of a microbe as a primary cause of disease is the greatest scientific silliness of the age."
> Pierre Antoine Bechamp - France 1816-1908

> **There are two primary causes for moss growing on trees.**
>
> 1. Moisture &
> 2. Shade

Without moisture and shade, moss can not and will not grow. This is the terrain or environment required for moss to live. That is why it usually grows on the north side of trees, houses etc. If we were to take a moss-laden tree and transplant it in the Arizona Desert what would happen? The hot, dry, sunny climate would kill the moss. Are you starting to get the point? Do you see why killing things in the body with antibiotics and chemotherapy is a foolish attempt to achieve optimum health? If we don't want yeast infections, fibromyalgia, arthritis, cancer etc., then we have to change the terrain or environment that has allowed it to grow in the first place. That is addressing the cause of dis-ease so the body can heal and be made whole. It is called health.

> "If I could live my life over again I would devote it to proving that germs seek their natural habitat-diseased tissue-rather than being the cause of diseased tissue...."
> Rudolph Virchow - The Father of Cellular Pathology

Mainstream medicine treats dis-ease. In Naturopathy we correct the cause of disease. We are not interested in a quick fix procedure to get rid of the cancer or moss, because we know it's just a matter of time before it grows right back. If we want to heal dis-ease, then we have to remove the cause that allowed it to grow in the first place. Think about it, something fed the tumor and caused it to grow.

> "If the germ theory were founded on facts, there would be no living being to read what's written." Dr. George White

Chemotherapy and radiation do nothing to change the terrain that has favored cancer to exist in the first place. Sure, this poison and radiation can very well get rid of cancer, but it also poisons the rest of our cells. Without changing our diet, thoughts, emotions and lifestyle, it is just a matter of time before the cancer comes right back to the environment that nourished it to grow in the first place. The only difference is that when it comes back, it returns with a vengeance to a body whose immune system is even weaker than before, after undergoing the cell damaging procedures of radiation and chemotherapy.

> "Our way of life is related to our way of death."
> The Framingham Study, Harvard University

> **So what is the terrain that causes cancer to exist?**
> 1. Acidosis
> 2. Malnutrition
> 3. Toxins
> 4. Poor Circulation
> 5. Miasms
> 6. Emotional Issues

In order to change the terrain of the body, we need to pay attention to the acidic and alkaline foods and drinks that we consume. Yellow vegetables have a natural calming, laxative effect. Green vegetables help build the blood and are excellent for anemia, which causes a sluggish, tired feeling. The green chlorophyll in vegetables is also anti-inflammatory and helps the body heal faster. The red fruits and vegetables stimulate the body and are good for circulation.

Nearly all fruits and vegetables are alkaline. Most proteins and starches are acidic. Intuition will tell you what foods your body needs. Eat the fruits and vegetables that sound good to you on that particular day. Most people do very well to consume 75 percent of their diet from the alkaline food list while limiting their consumption of acidic foods to only 25 percent.

Alkaline Forming Foods – (Healthy Foods)

Alfalfa Sprouts	Apple Cider Vinegar	Limes	Prunes
Almonds	Collard Greens	Love	Quinoa
Apples	Corn, Fresh	Mangoes	Radishes
Apricots	Cucumbers	Maple Syrup	Raisins
Bananas	Dates, Dried	Melons, All	Raspberries
Barley Juice	Dulse	Milk, Goat (Raw)	Rhubarb
Beans, Dried	Figs, Dried	Millet	Rutabagas
Bee Pollen	Garlic	Molasses	Sauerkraut
Beet Greens	Ginger	Mushrooms	Soybeans, Green
Beets	Goat Whey	Mustard Greens	Spirulina
Berries (most)	Grapefruit	Okra	Spinach, Raw
Blackberries	Grapes	Onions	Sprouts
Broccoli	Green Beans	Oranges	Squash
Brussels Sprouts	Green Peas	Parsley	Strawberries
Cabbage	Herbs (All)	Parsnips	Stevia
Cantaloupe	Kale	Peaches	Tangerines
Carrots	Kelp	Pears	Tomatoes
Cauliflower	Leech Nuts	Peppers	Turnip Greens
Celery	Lemons	Pineapple	Watercress
Chard Leaves	Lettuce	Plums	Watermelon
Cherries, Sour	Lima Beans, Dried	Potatoes, Sweet	Wheat Grass Juice
Cinnamon	Lima Beans, Green	Potatoes, White	Yams

Acid Forming Foods – (Avoid or Eat Sparingly)			
Alcohol	Cornstarch	Lentils, dried*	Sardines
Anger	Corn Syrup	Lobster	Sausage
Aspirin	Corn Oil	Macaroni	Scallops
Aspartame	Corned Beef	Mayonnaise	Seeds*
Bacon	Crackers	Milk (cow)	Soft Drinks
Beer	Currants	Niacin	Soybeans
Blueberries*	Dairy Products	Nuts*	Soymilk
Bran, Wheat	Drugs (Medicinal)	Oatmeal*	Spaghetti
Bran, Oat	Eggs*	Olives*	Squash*
Bread, Wheat	Flour, Whole Wheat	Pasta	Sugar -
Butter	Fish (All)*	Peanuts	(Refined)
Cake	French Fries	Peanut Butter	Tea, Black
Carob	Fruits, Canned	Pepper, Black	Turkey*
Cereals (All)	Fruits, Glazed	Peas, Dried*	Vinegar -
Cheese	Fruits, Sulfured	Popcorn	(Distilled)
Chicken*	Hamburgers	Pork	Walnuts*
Chickpeas*	Honey*	Rice, Brown*	Wheat
Chips	Hotdogs	Rice, White	Wheat Germ
Chocolate	Ketchup	Rice Milk	Wine
Coffee	Legumes*	Salmon*	Yogurt
Corn, Canned	Unforgiveness	Worry	Vitamin C

*Healthy Foods But Acidic

****

Remember, moderation is the key to balancing the body. Eating meat sparingly is all right for some, others do very well to avoid it completely. All of us are different and some of us do better on certain diets. Remember, this is a very general list to help the majority of Americans heal. There are exceptions to the rule. If you listen closely, your body will let you know what works best for you by how you feel when you feed it certain things. Experiment and find out what works best for you.

Some people do well to follow the *Eat Right For Your Type* or *Blood Type Diet* by Peter D'Adamo, N.D. He claims that people are healthier when tailoring their diets according to their specific blood types. For example,

Blood type A should basically stick to fruits and vegetables. He advises them to stay away from dairy products, animal fats and meats. These people have sensitive immune systems and are at high risk for cardiovascular disease, diabetes and cancer.

Blood type B should consume a balanced diet of fruits, vegetables, grains, fish, dairy, meat but avoid chicken. These people have the best chance of avoiding or overcoming disease.

Blood type AB does best consuming mostly a vegetarian diet. Only on rare occasions should they eat fish, meat or dairy, but no chicken.

Blood type O should eat a high protein diet including red meat and restrict their carbohydrate intake. Fruits and vegetables should be a part of their regular diet, but they should limit their intake of whole wheat products, corn, and avoid dairy products and most nuts. These people are at higher risk for hypothyroidism, ulcers and blood clotting issues.

> "Acid wastes buildup in the body in the form of cholesterol, gallstones, kidney stones, arterial plaque, urates, phosphates, and sulfates. These acidic waste products are the direct cause of premature aging and the onset of chronic disease."
>
> Dr. Stefan Kuprowsky

It is extremely important for us to understand that the way foods are prepared before we put them in our mouth makes a world of difference. For example, raw milk, straight from the cow or goat is alkaline forming, however once it has been pasteurized (boiled), it becomes acid forming. The same goes for cheese, butter, yogurt etc.

What the dairy industry fails to mention is the fact that once milk has been pasteurized (cooked to kill bacteria), then it takes more calcium to digest it than it gives back to your bones. It leaves your body acidic and in order to buffer the acids the body will use up its mineral reserves. Sodium, calcium, magnesium, potassium and iron will be depleted from you body as your innate intelligence strives to keep the pH of the fluids inside and outside your cells at 7.0.

Almonds are alkaline from Mother Nature, but when they have been roasted they become acidic and very hard on the digestive system. Most grains are acidic until they are sprouted. When the enzymes in them spring to life, they become alkaline and full of living nutrition.

After analyzing all the acidic foods you have been feeding your body for most of your life, doesn't it make sense as to why you have symptoms and maybe don't feel 100 percent? Most Americans eat 80 percent acidic foods and 20 percent alkaline. If we want to heal, then we need to reverse that. A healing environment is provided when 80 percent of our diet comes from the alkaline group and 20 percent from the acidic side.

If you are very sick, then perhaps we need an even stricter diet, however that is a two-edged sword. Sick people sometimes complain about how they don't like fruits and vegetables. No wonder they are sick. Fruits and vegetables are cell foods. They cleanse, feed and nourish cells. They should be the staple of our diets, if we want to be healthy.

If these types of people, who aren't accustomed to eating living foods, drastically change their diets too fast, the body starts dumping toxins. They can become very sick and feel even worse. This is called a healing crisis, however, the patient doesn't have a clue what their body is doing. All they see is that they attempted to follow the natural way by eating God's food and taking His herbs, and all of a sudden they feel worse. So they quit and mistakenly conclude that natural healing doesn't work. They become anti-anything-natural because they didn't understand what the body was attempting to do. The point is, if a 400 pound person who has been eating junk food his whole life, suddenly stops poisoning his body and starts eating whole foods his cells will automatically go into a cleanse mode. Each person needs to go at their own pace. Be smart and remember, moderation in all things.

The key is to slowly detoxify so you feel good as you cleanse. Use caution as you go through this life changing process. Find a naturopathic doctor or some other holistic practitioner to consult. Most of us do a lousy job at treating ourselves. We need a coach to help us, just as an athlete needs a coach to help him overcome obstacles and improve his performance to be his best.

A major problem with modern medicine is that we split everything up and go to specialists. The body works as a whole, and if we want to heal we must support the whole body. As mentioned earlier, the thyroid needs iodine to function properly. When the thyroid is deficient in iodine, then most likely the calcium levels will be out of solution because iodine controls calcium in the body. This leads to arthritis. Cataracts in the eyes are another symptom produced when calcium is out of balance.

Neutralizing Acids in the Body

> **"The countless names of illnesses do not really matter. What does matter is that they all come from the same root cause... to much acid in the body!"** Theodore A. Baroody, D.C., N.D., Ph.D.

When we eat cooked, dead, processed, junk foods the body becomes very acidic. Acids build up in the body and must be buffered or neutralized before being eliminated through the kidneys. In order to function, the body begins to neutralize the acids with our mineral reserves which include; **sodium, calcium, potassium, magnesium** and **iron**. Through this buffering system, vital minerals are lost through the kidneys and bowels. When these minerals are not replaced, then our body begins leaching minerals, especially calcium from our own bones to buffer the acids. The bones are our biggest calcium supply. The hips are our largest bone structure and a rich calcium source. This is where the body usually robs calcium from first to buffer the acids. In the meantime, we are being diagnosed with osteoporosis and brittle bones break from the slightest trauma. The solution to reversing arthritis is to eat more fruits and vegetables and get the body more alkaline. Supplementing the diet with minerals can be very helpful..

Many sick people are so acidic that their alkaline reserves have been completely depleted. When there's no money in the bank, you can't make a withdrawal. In simple terms, when there's no alkaline mineral reserves left in the body, then the body becomes saturated with acid-wastes. The kidneys then produce ammonia (9.25 pH) to buffer the acids, after the alkaline reserves have been exhausted. This is the body's way of dealing with our poor eating habits in an effort to keep us alive. When someone complains of burning sensations when they urinate, then you know they are eliminating a tremendous amount of acids. This is the body's innate fire-alarm warning us to put the fire out with alkaline foods and minerals before we burn up inside from acids.

> **"Nobody you know is 100% acidic. Nobody alive, that is! The fact is, 100% acidity is the very definition of death and decay!"**
> Michael Culter, M.D.

When our saliva pH hovers in the 6.8-7.0 area, then our body can build back our mineral reserves and reverse dis-ease. The so-called "incurable diseases" like arthritis and fibromyalgia all of a sudden become reversible, because we have changed the environment that caused those dis-eases in the first place. Of course, if the foods we are eating are lacking in minerals, then we'll still have deficiencies. That is why most of us need to supplement our diets with a good mineral supplement.

> **"You can trace every sickness... and every ailment to a mineral deficiency."** Dr. Linus Pauling, Nobel Prize-Winning Scientist

When we are acidic and calcium is robbed from the bones to neutralize acids, then the stage for dis-ease is set. The calcium leached from the bones to buffer acids is many times deposited at the joints and can cause arthritic knots, bone spurs and kidney stones.

Organic plant-derived sodium is what keeps the joints healthy, limber and moveable. It also helps regulate fluid levels throughout the body. Spirulina is an excellent source of sodium to take in tablet form. Powdered whey, okra, celery, spinach, figs, raw goat's milk, chicken and turkey gizzards are all high in sodium.

The body was designed and usually does best to use minerals that have passed through the plant kingdom. Sodium chloride (table salt), is not utilized by the body because the sodium and chloride are held together by ionic bonds. This form of salt is toxic and cannot be used to buffer acids.

Mother Nature's Foods – Healing Light Energy

> "Man, the alchemizer, transfers color and vibration from his food to himself—and that is his aliveness, his vitality. A corpse has all the chemical elements, but you can't bring him back to life. The essential life of man is in the vibration that is man, and this life force is carried with the mineral elements in their response to the light of the sun." Bernard Jensen, D.C., Ph.D., N.D.

Dr. Oz's Green Drink (As seen on Oprah)

2 cups spinach
2 cups cucumber
1 head of celery
½ inch or 1 teaspoon fresh ginger root
1 bunch parsley
2 apples
Juice of 1 lime
Juice of ½ lemon

Combine all ingredients in a juicer. This recipe makes 28 to 30 ounces or 3 to 4 servings.

When light from the sun is refracted through a prism, it splits up into seven clear colors. Foods are nothing more than color materialized by the plant. Plants take sun light, which is color, and through photosynthesis make food. Fruits, vegetables, nuts, seeds, grains and flowers are manifestations of light energy transformed into physical edible matter. When we eat food and digest it, we break down the physical solid food material and change it back into light and color, which is energy to feed the body.

A great way to alkalize your body and provide it with a tremendous amount of nutrition is juicing. Fresh carrot, celery and one apple juiced is a healthy way to start your day. Another great juice recipe is Dr. Mehmet Oz's green drink as seen on Oprah Winfrey.

Color therapy is powerful. Restaurant owners understand this. Have you ever gone out to eat in a dark restaurant, except for the glow of red lights in the lamps on tables? Red stimulates you to eat. How many times do we associate colors with how we feel? The following are some examples of common statements involving color to express how they feel. Were you feeling blue last year when your mother died? It made him so mad when he found out about the dishonesty at the office that he saw red. Listen to some mellow yellow music to calm you down. That movie was about black magic. We use colors to express feelings and moods, but rarely see actual colors.

Color is energy. The frequencies contained in colors make up life. Red, orange, yellow, green, blue, indigo and violet are the seven colors of life. It is interesting to note that we also have seven energy centers in the body called the endocrine system. Ayruvedic medicine that originated in India over 2500 years ago, refers to these energy centers as chakras.

> "The power of meditation can be ten times greater under violet light falling through the stained glass window of a quiet church."
> — Leonardo da Vinci

Chakra	Endocrine Gland	Color
7 Crown	Pineal	Violet
6 Brow	Pituitary	Indigo
5 Throat	Thyroid	Blue
4 Heart	Thymus	Green
3 Solar Plexus	Pancreas	Yellow
2 Sacral	Gonads	Orange
1 Base	Adrenals	Red

> "The spirit down here in man and the spirit up there in the sun, in reality are only one spirit, and there is no other one."
> — The Upanishads

Let's Be Practical

Hundreds of books have been written by very wise doctors who have had great success in helping people heal. The problem with most of these books is that they are not practical for most Americans. We live in a toxic world. That doesn't mean we have to live life in a plastic bubble and not breathe the toxic air or touch any man-made chemical; that is ridiculous.

Remember, balance is the key to health and it is also the key to life. You don't have to become a fanatic. It's good to use common sense and avoid obvious pitfalls.

Most of us don't want our life to be consumed with thinking about health. We all want to be able to go about our lives and enjoy our families, hobbies, jobs, etc. We don't want to have to think about every morsel of food we put into our mouths. Moderation in all things is important to remember. Let's keep it as simple as possible, so that we feel good and are able to live life to the fullest.

An occasional treat of some sweets and processed foods is probably not going to kill us. As long as we don't consume junk food every day, then we can occasionally splurge and still be all right. However, most Americans splurge everyday with every meal. We are way out of balance. As a result, we are using prescription drugs to cover up every warning symptom our body has to get our attention. When they wear off, we reach for more and more until we need a higher dosage, and then eventually a new more powerful drug to stimulate the body to do things against its will. The price will be paid sooner or later, don't kid yourself.

Most Americans will see improvements in their health if they eliminate coffee, white sugar, white flour, soft drinks and artificial sweeteners. Start drinking water instead of cokes and snack on fresh fruits and vegetables instead of candy bars, chips, crackers etc. This alone can turn many health problems around.

Here are the basic guidelines for being healthy. Keep in mind that if you are terminally ill with cancer or some other disease, then it is time to become a fanatic for a while so your body has the best chance to heal. On the other hand, for someone who is fairly healthy, with perhaps a few minor symptoms or maybe you just want to prevent disease, then these are basic healthy recommendations.

Dr. Sainsbury's Health Plan

1. **Eat Mother Nature's food**
   Whole grains
   * Ezekiel bread (from sprouted grains) and yeast-free sourdough bread are good choices.
   * Raw, unsalted nuts and seeds. Almonds are best. Soak a few almonds in water overnight and eat them for breakfast. This activates enzymes and is very healthy.
   * Dairy products are mucous forming. Try eliminating all dairy for a week and see if your health improves. Goat's milk is better than cow's milk. If you can't get dairy products from a farmer in its natural raw state, you may want to

leave them off the grocery list. Homogenized and pasteurized dairy products are big culprits for respiratory illnesses and allergies, especially for children.
* Substitute your table salt with sea salt.
* Eat meat in moderation-not everyday. Fish (that have scales and fins), chicken, turkey, lean steak from organic sources are best.
* Organic eggs are good.
* Beans, lentils and peas are healthy.
* Raw honey, molasses and stevia are good sweeteners. Use stevia if you have blood sugar issues.

> "...White sugar, white bread, pasta, and pastry that Americans eat have given them more chronic diseases than any other nation in the world. The reason they don't spoil is that they are so doped up with potentially hazardous artificial chemicals that they are virtually embalmed. One of the characteristics of wholesome food is that if it gets old it spoils so you won't hurt yourself by eating it."
>
> Dr. David Reuben

2. **75% of your diet should consist of nature's food**
Fruits and vegetables (organic if possible), should be the staple of your diet. Eat foods made by nature, not man. If it won't spoil, nature didn't make it. Living foods contain enzymes. Cooking over 118 degrees destroys nutritional value and enzymes needed for digestion. If you keep two meals and your snacks in the "Nature's Food" category, then you can afford to splurge on one meal.

3. **Keep your pH (Saliva) balanced**
Your body functions best when the pH of the saliva is 6.8-7.0. Eating raw fruits and vegetables will help you achieve this. All herbs are alkaline forming foods. Fresh squeezed lemon in your water is alkalizing. Use our pH Enhancer formula in your drinking water to ensure you are drinking alkalized healthy water. It contains modified sodium silicate and just a few drops really helps get the pH up. Everybody knows that their body needs lots of water, but we want healthy alkalized water. Most bottled water is acidic.

4. **Proper elimination**
The body will be dis-eased if it doesn't eliminate the wastes efficiently and regularly. For optimum health, you should have 2-3 bowel movements every day. No energy and headaches are common when the bowels are sluggish. Raisins and prunes are

natural laxatives. All fresh fruit helps the bowels move, especially when consumed in the morning for breakfast. Many people do well to eat fresh fruit until 12 noon. This keeps the bowels healthy. Eating heavy cooked foods like biscuits, muffins, pancakes, French toast, milk with cereal, causes the bowels to become sluggish. Your body goes through an elimination cycle every morning and fresh fruits assist in cleansing. Cooked foods clog up the bowels. Chronic diarrhea is often times constipation in disguise. Aloe vera juice, cascara sagrada, senna and psyllium husk powder are good natural laxatives.

5. **No soft or diet drinks or artificial sweeteners**
Use raw honey or molasses for sweeteners. If you have diabetes or blood sugar issues, you need to use stevia for a sweetener. Stevia is an herb from South America that is 200 times sweeter than sugar with 0 calories. It actually helps regulate the blood sugar. Artificial sweeteners cause cancer by interfering with cellular activity. They also cause blood sugar disturbances. Carbonated drinks block calcium absorption in the body and are very acidic (pH 2). If you have arthritis, get off carbonated beverages.

6. **No microwaves**
Radiation causes cancer. That is why there are warning signs in X-ray rooms and radiation clinics for cancer. Microwaves are radiation ovens that destroy nutritional value of food. Eating microwaved food has been shown to alter your blood chemistry, favoring cancer. Unnatural radiolytic compounds are formed from using microwaves. Dr. Hans Hertzel has proven microwaving food to be dangerous and a risk for cancer. For more information look up http://www.mercola.com/article/mircowave/hazards2.htm.

Do not radiate your food and then ask God to bless it to nourish and strengthen your body. You might as well set a gallon of gasoline on the table and ask him to turn it into grape juice as long as you have that kind of faith! Think before you swallow. We can't make stupid decisions like jumping off the roof of a building and then pray to God to save us. We live in a world of cause and effect. The way your food is prepared affects your health. Be responsible.

7. **Drink clean, purified water**
Don't drink tap water containing chlorine and fluoride. Natural spring water is best. Reverse osmosis is a better solution than tap water. Distilled water is good when doing a cleanse.

8. **Limit your consumption of sugar & processed food**
Read labels and stay away from ingredients you can't pronounce. (Breyers Ice cream–vanilla for example has five ingredients whereas some of the cheaper stuff lists twenty-five artificial ingredients. These chemicals were never meant to be put in the body. After years of consumption, they accumulate in the body and interfere with cellular activity. If you choose to eat some sweets and processed foods occasionally, then eat the ones that have ingredients in them that you know are foods and can pronounce, like Breyers. Balance is the key to health and if you eat lots of fresh fruits and vegetables, then you can probably tolerate some processed foods occasionally and do fine. Remember, respect the temple God has given you. It is sacred and you only have one. There are no trade–ins, like we are privileged of doing with automobiles, when they no longer meet our expectations. Be wise, live long and prosper!

9. **Cook with garlic, ginger, turmeric & onions often**
These foods are powerful immune system chargers and help maintain health and prevent imbalances that result in illness. They are food medicines that keep you strong, healthy and balanced. They are Mother Nature's antibiotics without the adverse side effects. They are antiviral, antibacterial and antifungal. In parts of Russia where people can't afford medicine, garlic is referred to as "Penicillin." Eating a couple of cloves a day keeps the doctor away and maybe your friends too. Ha! Eat it liberally when cold and flu season hits. A vegetable stew with lots of garlic keeps the immune system healthy and balanced, ready to fight any trouble maker that comes to your neighborhood.

10. **Eat meat sparingly**
Meat takes a lot of energy to break down and it produces uric acid. If you have arthritis or gout, stay away from meat. Eat lots of vegetables and fruits, especially fresh cherries. Uric acid can accumulate in the joints and cause inflammation and pain. Many Americans get up in the morning and have a sausage biscuit for breakfast, a hamburger for lunch, and spaghetti and meatballs for dinner. They eat meat three times a day. This is way too much. Eating meat two or three times a week is a healthier choice. Some diabetics, who can't tolerate fruit because of the sugars, do well by eating fish or other lean meats and vegetables daily. Some people do very well leaving meat out completely. Other people tend to do better with some meat in moderation. There are exceptions to every rule. We focus on finding what works best for you as an individual. The "Eat Right 4 Your Type - Blood Type Diet" can be very valuable wisdom for some.

11. **Breathe deeply**

    Oxygenate those 100 trillion cells in your body. Breathe in through your nose as deep as you can fifty times a day. Dr. Otto Warburg won the Nobel Prize for discovering that cancer cells can't survive where there is oxygen.

    > "All chronic pain, suffering and diseases are caused from a lack of oxygen at the cell level." Arthur C. Guyton, M.D.

12. **Avoid drinking with meals**

    Drinking water, juice etc., with meals dilutes digestive juices. Wait thirty minutes before or after a meal to drink liquids. Chew each bite of food at least thirty times before swallowing. Chewing your food and mixing it with enzymes in your saliva is the first step in digestion.

13. **Get enough sleep**

    Most people need eight hours every night. Give your body what it needs. Remember sleep is healing. Get up when you are rested and go to bed when you are tired. Exercise and hard labor makes you sleep well at night. Some Americans don't sleep well because they don't do anything all day long. Sorry, but watching TV is in the same category of not doing anything. Usually, the earlier you go to bed the better. The body rests best before midnight. Sleep studies indicate that for every hour you sleep before midnight, it is equivalent to two hours of sleep after midnight. Remember, early to bed and early to rise, makes one wise.

14. **Avoid aluminum cookware**

    Aluminum is linked to Alzheimer's and nervous system disorders. Most restaurants cook with aluminum pots and pans.

15. **Do a liver, kidney, gallbladder & spleen cleanse once a year**

    You take your car in and change the oil every 3,000 miles and tune it up right? How about giving your body a tune-up? Dandelion, nettles, goldenrod, milk thistle, artichoke leaf, boldo, uva ursi, juniper, corn silk, burdock and parsley are good for these organs. A thirty day cleanse, with fifty drops three times a day with our KLS-Plus formula, tunes things up. This is preventative medicine.

16. **Fast once a month (no food for 24 hours, water only)**

    After God created the earth in six days, He then rested of His labors. Sunday is a good day to let your digestive system rest of their labor by fasting for twenty-four hours. Control the desires of the flesh by giving up food for a day and be spiritually enlightened. This keeps your priorities in check and realigns what goals you have. Give your digestive system and body a break from working so hard all the time. If your cells could talk, they would tell us that they are over-worked and underpaid. They need a break occasionally, just like you do. Fasting gives them a rest. Be glad you don't have to fast fourty days like Christ did.

17. **Fast and do a colon cleanse every year**
It is believed that all disease starts in the colon. Eat only fresh fruits and vegetables. Juicing is very healthy. Dr. Richard Anderson's Arise & Shine Cleansing program is very effective. Take psyllium husk and bentonite clay shakes several times a day along with Chomper and Herbal Nutrition herbal formulas. Most of us do well to cleanse for twenty-one days, with the last three days having water only, no food. This takes self-discipline, but you reap what you sow. This is a good insurance policy for the body. It's a great way to lose a few extra pounds put on over the holidays and boost up your immune system, so you don't catch the next onslaught of cold viruses that come your way.

When I did my first cleanse, I had eight large bowel movements every day. The old fecal matter (mucoid plaque) that came out looked like black strips of tire from off of the highway. I thought I was healthy and in good shape. Little did I know my intestinal tract was way overdue for a cleanse. See ariseandshine.com for more information

18. **Do a parasite cleanse every year**
Microscopic parasites are everywhere. These little guys set up shop in your body and steal your nutrition. They can interfere with the functions of organs and glands, especially the liver, gallbladder, ileo-cecal valve, intestinal tract and appendix. We de-worm our pets and animals, but somehow think we humans are immune. If you had a microscope everywhere you went to see the "unseen" universe of microbes everywhere, it would shock you. No one is 100 percent immune to parasites. If you have pets, you are at high risk. Pets lick their hind ends and some eat fecal matter. Then, you come home from work and kiss and love on them, because the two of you have missed each other so much. Animals clean themselves with their tongues, they are not civilized. The bottom line is animals and humans get parasites. Do a parasite cleanse once a year.

19. **Get chiropractic adjustments regularly**
Adjustments keep your spine aligned. Life is traumatic and a good adjustment keeps pressure off nerves that correspond to every organ and gland in the body. Headaches can be triggered by pinched nerves as well as every other symptom you

20. **Get a massage periodically**
Massage is a great stress releaser. Most of us need stress release and a massage can help you relax. It is very effective for helping the lymphatic system drain toxins as well. Some headaches and joint pain are caused by tight muscles. Relaxing those muscles with massage can sometimes be the magic touch that heals. The laying on of hands is healing. A good massage and chiropractic adjustment can make you feel like a new person. Pain disappears when vertebrae line up and tight muscles are relaxed.

21. **Use real butter, not margarine**
Once again, stay away from artificial junk that the body can't metabolize. These artificial ingredients were never meant to be put in the body. Margarine is one molecule away from plastic and probably just as toxic. Read the ingredients on what you buy. If it says hydrogenated oil or partially hydrogenated oil, avoid it. If it is solid at room temperature, then it stays solid in the body. Artificial fats and oils are what block arteries and cause heart disease. They cause an immune response that in turn leads to arteriosclerosis, plaque build-up, etc. Use real butter, organic of course, is better. Coconut oil is an excellent oil in which to cook your food. Olive and Canola oil are next best.

22. **Drink 16 ounces of water upon arising every morning**
Hydrate your 100 trillion cells after sleeping all night. They need water to function and clean up. Try washing your car or the dishes without water. Water is a cleanser and most Americans are severely dehydrated. If you wait until you are thirsty to drink water, you are way too late. The bowels have a tough time moving when they are dried up. Give your body water so it can function and clean with. Imagine living in a house with no running water. Your toilets and sinks need water to clean and so do all 100 trillion cells in your body.

23. **Do not use nonstick cookware**
These chemicals absorb into your food from the pan and cause health problems. Use stainless steal or earthen cookware. Use coconut oil, real butter, olive or canola oil.

24. **Stay away from "fat free" products**
Fat-free and sugar-free means they have created a chemical to taste like what you want it to, but it's actually just a combination of chemicals that cause stress and interfere with cellular function. There's a price to be paid for everything you choose to put in your mouth. What you don't know may kill you if you keep doing it ignorantly.

25. **Forgive those who have trespassed you**
By holding on to anger, resentment, bitterness, hurt or a grudge of any sort you are not hurting the other person, you are only hurting yourself. We are commanded to forgive so we can set ourselves free. It is good to forgive others and be nice and kind for their benefit, however, it is more important to forgive so that we liberate ourselves from negative emotions. By holding on to negativity, we usually hurt ourselves the most. Quit worrying about what others say and do and release your own trash. Or better said, take the beam out of your own eye first and stop making others wrong.

The Awakening

There is a movement taking place in this country. Go into any bookstore and see how many books are in the alternative medicine section. Medical doctors who are tired of not seeing results wake up from their dream-drug-fairly-tale. They don't sleep well at nights because the nightmare has them all riled up. What nightmare? No, not the one on Elm Street with long-fingered Freddie Krueger tormenting innocent teenagers slumbering the night away, but, the real one that kills good people everyday (225,000 a year). The one that has him riddled with guilt because deep down inside, underneath all the years of medical indoctrination, he knows that cells can't heal with drugs. Years of prescribing countless numbers of the man-made chemicals makes him want to hide his face back under the covers and pretend it never happened. The whole medical system built upon this fraudulent illusion of man made chemicals healing cells is preposterous and ignorantly ridiculous. Any true doctor understands and knows that cells need nourishment in the blood through circulation and cleansing through the lymphatic system.

> **"Follow principle and the knot unties itself."** Thomas Jefferson

The honest doctor gets disgusted seeing his patients do great one month and then crash the next, yo-yoing from the adverse side effects of prescription drugs. He is sickened by the prescribing of more and more drugs to combat adverse side effects and observing kidney and liver damage from the drugs. He comes to the frightening realization that what he is doing is not healthcare, but disease maintenance. It bothers him to the point that he can't stand it any longer, so his integrity compels him to do something about it. This awakening to the horrid thought that maybe there is a better way to alleviate symptoms than poisonous prescription drugs compels him to begin a crusade of investigating natural healing modalities. What he discovers is what he has known all along, but was not taught in medical school. The discovery made is this: herbs cleanse, feed and nourish cells. Drugs do not cleanse, feed or nourish cells.

The choice is simple. Do doctors want to be drug dealers or give the body what it needs to heal?

Smart doctors realize that they have been used like a pawn in a chess game set up by the multi-billion dollar pharmaceutical industry to con medical doctors into being their legalized drug dealers. Doctors with integrity, guts and common sense, who are not already bought off, lose their desire to mask symptoms with drugs. They shift their interest in identifying and correcting the cause with natural remedies that do not harm cells in the process. They begin working with each patient's own natural healing abilities by recommending homeopathic detoxifiers, herbal blends, vitamins, minerals and enzymes. These doctors may even do chelation therapy, hydrogen peroxide, mineral IVs etc.

> "The necessity of teaching mankind not to take drugs and medicines, is a duty incumbent upon all who know their uncertainty and injurious effects; and the time is not far distant when the drug system will be abandoned." Charles Armbruster, M.D.

If natural healing didn't work, then patients wouldn't come back for natural treatments, especially when their insurance won't cover it. They'd be satisfied doping themselves up on drugs. But they keep coming back and bringing more and more people in who are so sick. So many are tired of playing their doctor's drug games that cause adverse side effects and still doesn't fix their health problems.

> "Most doctors are unable to recognize wellness, simply because they're not trained in wellness but in disease."
> Robert Mendelsohn, M.D.

The committed doctor, who truly wants his patients to be healthy, attends alternative health seminars and begins studying what other complimentary health clinics around the world are doing do get effective results. He looks into the cancer clinics down in Mexico that have success in reversing disease, by using nontoxic therapies. He is intrigued and hungry to learn healing secrets that were never taught in medical school. He begins researching herbs, homeopathy, nutrition etc., and begins incorporating them into his practice. Patients get well as they use natural remedies to correct the cause and only use drugs as a last resort.

The AMA, FDA and other MDs harass him for not following along blindly and he is forced to stop accepting insurance. In extreme cases, he may even relocate to some foreign country so he can help people heal and practice medicine to the best of his ability without persecution from the big boys. He is likely to work with a naturopath or chiropractor.

> **"It is difficult to get a man to understand something when his salary depends upon his not understanding it."** Upton Sinclair

Do you pay a close-minded know-it-all to dull your God-given senses with drugs? And how does he or she know how much to prescribe for you? Or do you go to someone who really listens to your concerns and does all in his or her power to assist your body to heal so you can live the life you love, free of being a drug addict for the rest of your life? Is your doctor committed to healing the cause, or is he a symptom-suppressor with drugs that contributes to the 225,000 death figure each year? It's your health, your life, and your choice. May God bless you with wisdom to do what is best for you.

Courage to Wield the Sword of Truth

Former U.S. Air Force flight surgeon Dr. Fuller Royal shares his experience of being a drug dealer. *"I got tired of doling out pills and never having anyone get well."* He is a doctor of integrity, because he does what he believes is best for his patients and his track record proves his success.

Many doctors are persecuted in the name of truth. These doctors are the courageous ones who have the guts to step out of the medical box and do something different than administer poisonous drugs and unnecessary surgery, despite the lucrative profits that one can make. It's time doctors stand up to the current medical system and start addressing the cause so healing can occur. Sick people deserve to heal and they trust their doctor to teach them how. What type of physician do you trust with your health?

> **"A truth's initial commotion is directly proportional to how deeply the lie was believed…When a well-packaged web of lies has been sold gradually to the masses over generations, the truth will seem utterly preposterous and its speaker a raving lunatic."**
> Dresden James

Not all doctors are created equal. They understand the corruption in keeping sick people on drugs with no intention of really allowing the body to heal. After years of playing the prescription drug game with their patient's health they come to understand the insanity and protest it. At the AMA annual convention in New York City, Rick Kunnes, M.D., declared,

> **"Let's get one thing straight - The American Medical Association is really the American Murder Association."**
> Rick Kunnes, M.D. - American Medical News (Jan. 17, 1978, p. 11)

Another outspoken doctor is Robert S. Mendelsohn, M.D. At a convention in Long Beach, California in late January of 1980 he said, *"Modern medicine is now better geared for killing people than it is for healing them."* He went on to explain, *"The greatest threat to one's health is the physician who practices modern medicine. The treatments doctors use are often more harmful to their patients than the diseases themselves might be."*

Confessions of a Medical Heretic

After over thirty years of practice and serving as National Director of Project Head Start's Medical Consultation Service and Chairman of the Medical Licensing Committee for the State of Illinois, Dr. Mendelsohn concludes the following about modern medicine.

Robert S. Mendelsohn, M.D. – Says…

- I believe that the greatest danger to your health is the doctor who practices Modern Medicine.

- I believe that Modern Medicine's treatments for disease are seldom effective and often more dangerous than the ailments they're employed to treat.

- I believe that the dangers are compounded by the widespread use of dangerous procedures to treat non-diseases, procedures that produce real diseases that the doctor will then address with even more dangerous procedures in his efforts to repair the damage he has done.

- I believe that Modern Medicine endangers its victims by attacking minor ailments with hazardous treatments that should only be used when the patient's life is at stake.

- I believe that most doctors are the willing, if unwitting, tools of pharmaceutical manufacturers. Their patients become human guinea pigs for mass testing of drugs with dubious benefits and potentially lethal side effects that are unknown.

- I believe that more than 90 percent of Modern Medicine could disappear from the face of the earth—doctors, hospitals, drugs, and equipment—and the health of the nation would immediately and dramatically improve.

- I do not believe in modern medicine. I am a Medical Heretic …I haven't always been a Medical Heretic; I once believed in Modern Medicine.

Toxic Metals

> "It is interesting to note that cardiovascular disease has become widespread only since the 1920's, about the time of increased use of heavy metals in dental therapy but long after humans began consuming eggs, meat, milk, butter, and cheese, commonly thought to contribute to heart disease."
> Daniel F. Royal, D.O. - Medical Director of the Nevada Clinic and the Royal Center of Advanced Medicine, Las Vegas, Nevada

In 1840, dentists here in the U.S. formed the American Society of Dental Surgeons. Members of this association were required to sign pledges promising not to use mercury in dental fillings. Some dentists were even suspended from the dental society for using silver mercury fillings in 1848.

Mercury was referred to as "quicksilver" or "quacksalver." A "quack" is someone who pretends to cure disease and obviously a "salve" is medicine for a wound. It is interesting to note that the name "quack" was first given to anyone using mercury preparations on the skin to "cure" disease. Ironically, dentists not too long ago labeled you a quack if you claimed mercury fillings harmful and a possible cause of disease.

Most everyone knows mercury is a deadly poison. Researchers inform that mercury falls right underneath arsenic in terms of toxicity. It is so toxic that if a thermometer breaks in an elementary school, by law the children are required to evacuate and the fire department is called.

If mercury from a thermometer is toxic, then how could mercury in your silver fillings, in your mouth be safe? They are not. We have been lied to about the safety of silver dental fillings. Amalgam silver dental fillings are toxic. Mercury comprises over 50 percent of the silver dental fillings in your mouth. The five metals used in amalgam fillings are approximately: mercury (50%), silver (15-30%), tin (10%), copper (3-30%), and a trace amount of zinc (1%). The ADA and most dentists are under the impression that mercury and other metals are tightly bound and do not leak out, however research proves otherwise.

In 1979, Dr. Hal Huggins began measuring electrical currents coming off of metal fillings in the mouth. These electrical currents increase mercury release from the amalgams. Metals in a filling act as a standard battery. When two different metals are in an electrolyte (salt solution in your saliva), they generate electrical currents or a flow of electrons. These minute electrical currents can wreak havoc on your health because of their impact on the nervous system. The renowned German physician, Dr. Reinhard Voll, estimated, after more than forty years of research and observation, that nearly 80 percent of all illnesses are related to problems in the mouth.

R.P. Sharma and E.J. Obersteiner at Utah State University discovered mercury to be the single most toxic metal that they have investigated (even in such minute concentrations as 3.74×10^{-7} moles). Their research has proven that just a few micrograms disrupt normal cellular function. They inform that, *"Mercury is a strong protoplasmic poison that penetrates all living cells of the human body."*

Douglas Swartzendruber, Ph.D., experimental pathologist at the University of Colorado, explains that the accumulation of mercury from dental fillings in the central nervous system is an important connection to understanding neurological disorders such as multiple sclerosis. It has also been identified as a major contributor to ALS (Lou Gehrig's disease). The brain and the central nervous system tends to be a magnet for the accumulation of mercury and other heavy metals. Autopsy studies show that the level of mercury in brain tissue correlated to the number of metal fillings in their mouths (New England Journal of Medicine, vol. 349, Oct 30, 2003, pp. 1731).

Your immune system has a group of marine-like soldiers who roam around looking for enemies and these marines are called white blood cells. When they identify a cell that doesn't have proper identification to be in your body, their job is to destroy them. Each cell carries an I.D. card like a driver's license or passport. Healthy cells carry a five-protein I.D. card that allows them to exist in your body and escape harassment from white blood cells. Cells that have an altered code such as ones with an atom of mercury attached to them are ordered to be destroyed by the marines or white blood cells. When doctors see these internal wars, where the immune system is attacking itself, they call it an autoimmune disease not understanding the heavy metal toxicity issue as one of the causes. The only way to truly stop the war is to remove the mercury so cells can reveal themselves as "good guys" and the body's military-like immune system stops attacking what it thinks is the enemy. ALS is an example of this self-destructing internal battle occurring.

> **"Mercury kills cells by interfering with their ability to exchange oxygen, nutrients, and waste products through the cell membrane. Inside the cell, mercury destroys our genetic code, DNA, leaving us without the ability to reproduce that cell ever again."**
> Hal A. Huggins, D.D.S. - Founder of the Huggins Diagnostic Center and Author of *It's All In Your Head*

According to Mark A. Breiner, D.D.S., author of *Whole-Body Dentistry*, encourages you to ask your dentist why is it that before a silver (amalgam) filling goes into the mouth, it is considered a hazardous toxin? Then when it is removed, why must it be stored in a hazardous waste container and taken away by a licensed hazardous waste company? The answer is obvious.

Silver dental fillings are hazardous waste and according to the ADA the only safe place to put it is in your mouth! Now doesn't that make you feel good? Your mouth has become a toxic waste dump, and we pay to have the poison put in our teeth.

OSHA mandates that a Materials Safety Data Sheet for mercury be present in every dental office. Here are the rules for handling scrap amalgam dental fillings:
1. Store in unbreakable, tightly sealed containers, away from heat.
2. Use a no touch technique for handling amalgam.
3. Store under liquid, preferably glycerin or photographic fixer solution.

> "I don't feel comfortable using a substance (silver dental fillings) designated by the EPA to be a waste disposal hazard. I can't throw it in the trash, bury it in the ground, or put it in a landfill, but they say it's okay to put it in people's mouths. That doesn't make sense."
>
> Richard D. Fischer, D.D.S.

Mercury Facts

- If dentists are not careful when removing amalgams and one ends up on the floor, they could be fined a sizeable amount.

- Every time you eat food, chew gum, brush your teeth etc., mercury vapors come off the fillings. Drinking hot drinks and heated food accelerates the release of mercury vapors.

- A four-foot fluorescent light bulb contains approximately 22 milligrams of mercury and should be disposed of as hazardous waste. The average dental silver filling in your mouth contains about 1,000 milligrams of mercury.

- Multiple Sclerosis patients have been found to have 8 times higher levels of mercury in the cerebrospinal fluid compared to neurologically healthy controls (Eggleston, D.W., and M. Nylander, "Correlation of Dental Amalgam With Mercury in Brain Tissue." Journal of Prosthetic Dentistry, 58 (1987).

- Research has indicated that placement of amalgam fillings in monkeys has impaired kidney function by 60% in sixty days.

- Dr. Boyd Haley at the University of Kentucky has discovered that patients with Alzheimer's disease have higher than average levels of mercury in the tissue of their brains. When exposing rats to mercury vapors similar to what would typically be found in people with silver fillings, the rats developed changes in the brain that are similar to changes that occur in Alzheimer patients.

- Pregnant women who have amalgam fillings run the risk of passing heavy metals to their unborn. In Canada a study was done by Drs. Fritz Lorscheider and Murray Vimy where they placed amalgam fillings in pregnant sheep. The mercury in the fillings was radioactively labeled so that the scientists could definitively trace the mercury to the fillings. After a few days the sheep were examined and the findings were shocking. The amalgam-related mercury had spread to all the tissues of both the mother sheep and the unborn fetuses. Higher concentrations of mercury had accumulated in the kidneys, thyroid, intestines and jawbone.

- Every mother's worse nightmare is SIDS (Sudden Infant Death Syndrome). A German research team studied babies who died from SIDS. Upon close examination, the research team found that mercury in the babies' brains was directly proportional to the number of fillings in their mothers' mouths. It is currently illegal to use amalgam dental fillings in Germany.

> "Why is the ADA highly concerned about scrap amalgam while it preaches the safety of the amalgam in your mouth? It's the same stuff."
> Hal A. Huggins, D.D.S.

Is it coincidence that dentists who handle mercury fillings have the highest suicide and divorce rate among professionals? Dentists, according to insurance agencies, have one of the highest utilization rates of medical insurance. According to Joel Butler, Ph.D., professor of psychology at the University of North Texas, neuropsychological dysfunction was reported in ninety percent of dentists tested. These findings were reported at the ICBM conference November, 1988. Could it be more than just coincidence that female dental personnel have a higher spontaneous abortion rate, a raised incidence of premature labor and an elevated perinatal mortality than any other profession?

The bottom line is, your work environment affects your health. When you are around toxic metals all day, it has adverse effects. And for those who believe there is no harm in handling metals, try putting a piece of garlic in your shoe and walking around. In less than ten minutes you'll taste the garlic in your mouth. Anything you touch has the ability to pass through the skin and be absorbed into your blood.

> "Mercury may well be one of the biggest culprits in damaging DNA and setting the body up for various types of diseases."
> — Stephen B. Edelson, M.D.

At the Huggins Diagnostic Center for patients in treatment or consultation for heavy metal toxicity, 1,320 patients reported the following symptoms.

Heavy Metal Toxicity Symptoms

Symptom	%	Symptom	%
1. Unexplained irritability	73%	16. Shortness of breath	43%
2. Depression	72%	17. Heartburn	43%
3. Numbness and tingling	67%	18. Itching	41%
4. Frequent urination at night	65%	19. Rashes, skin irritations	40%
5. Chronic fatigue	63%	20. Metallic taste in mouth	39%
6. Cold hands and feet	63%	21. Jumpy, jittery, nervous	38%
7. Bloated feeling often	61%	22. Death wish or suicidal	37%
8. Loss of memory	58%	23. Insomnia	36%
9. Sudden anger	56%	24. Chest pains	36%
10. Constipation	55%	25. Joint pains	36%
11. Difficulty making decisions	54%	26. Tachycardia	32%
12. Tremors/shakes	52%	27. Fluid retention	28%
13. Twitching of muscles	52%	28. Burning tongue	21%
14. Leg cramps	49%	29. Headaches after eating	20%
15. Ringing in ears	49%	30. Diarrhea	15%

> "You should never put a gold crown in a mouth with amalgam (silver) fillings. The gold will speed up the release of mercury from the amalgams, so that your body burden of mercury will increase faster than it would with just amalgams alone."
> — Mark A. Breiner, D.D.S.

Root Canals

Root canals can be a contributor to disease because of the simple fact that it is very difficult to eliminate all bacteria from the roots during a procedure. Pockets of infection can exist in teeth with the estimated three miles of microcanals that are undetectable on X-rays. Once bacteria is trapped in and lives without oxygen, major health problems may occur. Infection can short circuit the meridians (energy pathways) and cause major health problems.

> "One third of all disease in this country can be either directly or indirectly traced to dental infections."
> George E. Meinig, D.D.S. - Author of Root Canal Cover-Up

Many health problems will simply not clear up if there is an infected tooth as the cause. Extraction of the root canaled tooth for some is the best solution, along with proper cleansing of the infected area (jaw). To demonstrate how toxic root canaled teeth can be, Dr. Weston Price implanted one under the skin of a rabbit. Within three days the rabbit died. It died from the same condition that the owner of the tooth had. Dr. Price continued repeating the experiment with the same tooth on twenty-seven different rabbits. Every rabbit died, even after autoclaving the tooth at high temperatures for twenty-four hours. To prove that these experiments with root canaled teeth could be the culprits for disease and death he performed other experiments to eliminate the possibility of coincidence. He took healthy teeth, non-decayed (wisdom teeth), and other sterile objects such as coins, pieces of glass and metal and sewed them under the skin of rabbits. No symptoms were reported and all rabbits appeared to be unaffected.

In conclusion, Dr. Price explains that bacteria from infected teeth can remain in the three miles of tubules, growing and multiplying and changing forms. These microbes produce toxic chemicals that, many times cause illness.

Autism – A Symptom of Heavy Metal Poisoning

We are bombarded with heavy metals without the help of doctors injecting them into our bodies through vaccinations and dentists filling our teeth with them. Most autistic children lack the capability to detoxify mercury from the brain. When mercury accumulates and begins to interfere with neurological behavior, the results are autistic behavior.

> "There is NO CONTROVERSY! The failure of others to recognize facts does not change the truth." Rashid A. Buttar, D.O. (Referring to Mercury Poisoning Causing Autism)

The Material Safety Data Sheet from Eli Lilly June 13, 1991 (Section 5 – Health Hazard Information) clearly warns that thimerosal, (an ingredient in vaccines) which contains mercury, is a chemical known to cause; birth defects, nervous system disorders, numbness in the extremities and even mental retardation. Why are we still allowing them to put this poison in our children's bodies?

> "Mercury is the "spark" that causes the "fires" of autism as well as Alzheimer's. Autism is the result of high mercury exposure early in life versus Alzheimer's is a chronic accumulation of mercury over a life time. A doctor can treat ALL the "fires" but until the "spark" is removed, there is minimal hope of complete recovery with most improvements being transient at best. However, once the process of mercury removal has been effectively started, the damage is curtailed and full recovery becomes possible and enhanced by utilizing various additional therapies including nutrition, hyperbarics, etc."
> Rashid A. Buttar, D.O., FAAPM, FACAM, FAAIM (Vice chairman, American Board of Clinical Metal Toxicology, Visiting Scientist, North Carolina State University)

Rashid A. Buttar, D.O., is the medical director of Advanced Concepts in Medicine located in Charlotte, North Carolina, where he has treated over 500 autistic children. By utilizing the best of conventional, traditional and alternative medical treatments his practice is highly successful in treating autism. He teaches that in order to heal autism, heavy metals, especially mercury must come out of the body. To learn more about his clinic and how he successfully treats autism as well as cancer, heart disease and other chronic conditions you can order his DVDs online at www.TheMedicalSeries.com. For additional information look him up at www.drbuttar.com or call his office at 704 895-9355.

> "I think that the biological case against thimerosal is so dramatically overwhelming anymore that only a very foolish or a very dishonest person with the credentials to understand this research would say that thimerosal wasn't most likely the cause of autism." Boyd Haley, Ph.D. - Department of Chemistry, University of Kentucky

Chapter 7
VACCINATIONS – WOLVES IN SHEEP'S CLOTHING

> **"Truth will ultimately prevail where there are pains taken to bring it to light."** George Washington

Michael Belkin was the proud father of a beautiful new daughter. Like most good parents, he wanted the best for his daughter so he trusted his doctors to give her vaccinations to make her healthy. When she was five weeks old, he took her in to get a second hepatitis B shot. That night she began having tremors and was extremely agitated. Within fifteen hours his precious beautiful baby girl was dead. The autopsy report revealed a swollen brain, typical of vaccination toxicity.

Hepatitis B is a blood-transmitted or sexually transmitted disease spread by drug users and sexually active homosexuals and heterosexuals. So why are we vaccinating our children who don't use drugs and have multiple sex partners with Hepatitis B?

> **"There is a great deal of evidence to prove that immunization of children does more harm than good."** Dr. J. Anthony Morris - Research Virologist & Former Chief Vaccine Control Officer at the U.S. Federal Drug Administration

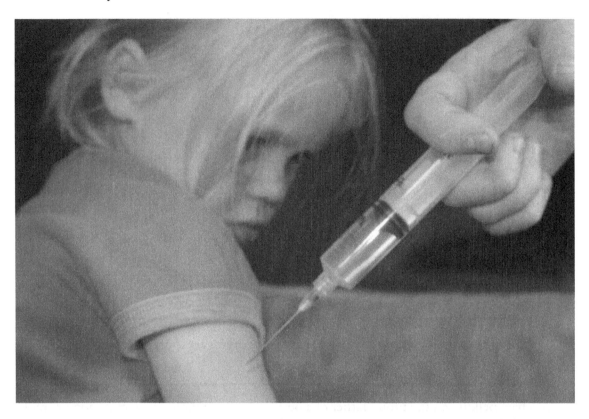

Tina took her beautiful, healthy three-month-old son, Evan, in to get a DPT shot. His body responded with a swollen leg, loss of head control, high pitched screaming and then he collapsed and died in a seizure. SIDS (Sudden Infant Death Syndrome) was the diagnosis.

In 1994 Tina gave birth to another beautiful baby, this time a daughter she named Miranda. When Miranda was nine months old, she took her in for her second DPT shot. She trusted her doctor when he reassured her that vaccines were safe and Evan's death had nothing to do with the DPT shot. The nightmare began all over again with little Miranda. She reacted with high-pitched screaming that could not be quieted, just as it happened with Evan. Within forty-eight hours little Miranda died. This time the pathologist concluded and the coroner agreed that the cause of death was the DPT shot.

> **"Can you inject a foreign substance of any kind into a little baby and believe that in any way it will improve its health?"** Wm. Howard Hay, M.D. – The Congressional Record (Founder & Medical Director, Sun-Diet Sanatorium, New York)

Unfortunately, it took two dead babies for the truth to be told. If you were Tina, what would you do about your two dead babies that were killed from the shot your doctor gave them? The truth is no one knows how these vaccines are going to react in a child's body. No tests are performed to screen out high-risk children. The CDC and most pediatricians say vaccinations are safe, but do they really know? Children acting strangely and then dying after receiving their shots is more than just "purely coincidence," like the CDC and other so-called professional groups try to claim.

> "The evidence for indicting immunizations for SIDS is circumstantial, but compelling. However, the keepers of the keys to medical-research funds are not interested in researching this very important lead to the cause of an ongoing, and possibly preventable, tragedy. Anything that implies that immunizations are not the greatest medical advance in the history of public health is ignored or ridiculed. Can you imagine the economic and political import of discovering that immunizations are killing thousands of babies?" William C. Douglass, M.D. (Honored twice as America's 'Doctor of the Year')

It is absolutely appalling that the CDC muscles their way around to get vaccines approved and made mandatory and then weasels their way out of any responsibility for death and injury when it occurs. Does it make sense to you that God created babies in such a way that they would need foreign toxic matter injected into them to make them healthy? Do you believe that God blundered when He created our children and forgot to create them with immune systems capable of keeping them healthy? For every doctor that says vaccines are safe and necessary, there is another one cautioning against them from what they have seen. Unfortunately, one side is much more widely reported than the other.

> "No batch of vaccine can be proved safe before it is given to children." Leonard Scheele - Surgeon General of the United States

Barbara Loe Fisher believed medical science was never wrong. She grew up in a family of doctors and nurses and trusted that vaccines were safe and effective. Her pediatrician never told her that her son was at high risk to receive another vaccine because he was recovering from the flu. The hot, red lump that developed at the sight of injection from his third DPT shot was a warning sign that Barbara shamefully admits she ignored.

Four hours after taking her two-year-old son in for his fourth DPT shot and oral polio vaccine, his face went pale and he sat lifeless in a chair for hours. She thought he had fallen asleep but in actuality he was unconscious and having a seizure. High-pitched screaming followed by bizarre behavioral patterns were an unexpected side effect from the shot. He was unable to recognize the alphabet that he knew before that shot. Vaccinations left her son with multiple learning disabilities, delayed motor skills, attention deficit and subsequently a life-long struggle with low self-esteem because he couldn't do what his peers could. *"I wish I could go back as so many parents do, and instead of holding my child down on the table like a sacrificial lamb, I could take him in my arms and walk out of that doctor's office, and give him back the future that was his birthright,"* pleads Barbara. But she can't. What's done is done. Now she helps educate others on the dangers of vaccinations.

> "I have been a regular practitioner of medicine in Boston for 33 years. I have studied the question of vaccination conscientiously for 45 years. As for vaccination as a preventative for disease, there is not a scrap of evidence in its favor. The injection of virus into the pure bloodstream of the people does not prevent smallpox; rather, it tends to increase its epidemics, and it makes the disease more deadly. Of this we have indisputable proof. In our country (U.S.) cancer mortality has increased from 9 per 100,000 to 80 per 100,000 or fully 900 percent increase within the past 50 years, and no conceivable thing could have caused this increase but the universal blood poisoning now existing." Charles E. Page, M.D.

The subject of vaccinations is a can of worms that has been deliberately lied about through erroneous statistics and faulty studies that have been marketed to persuade Americans to believe that vaccinations are necessary to eradicate disease. The CDC (Center for Disease Control) has disguised this wolf in sheep's clothing to be a harmless and safe blessing to the world. Nothing could be further from the truth.

> "Our children face the possibility of death or serious long-term adverse effects from mandated vaccines that aren't necessary or that have very limited benefits." Jane M. Orient, M.D. - Executive Director - Association of American Physicians and Surgeons

In order to solve the vaccination puzzle, we need to look at some facts. Most diseases such as smallpox, polio, measles, pertussis (whooping cough) were already rapidly declining around the world before vaccines were ever used. Experts conclude that better sanitation, hygiene, living quarters, healthcare, education, cleaner drinking water etc., are responsible for ending most disease epidemics. However, the vaccine manufactures who make between seven to ten billion dollars a year off of their concoctions of filth, want you to believe the vaccines are responsible for ending epidemics worldwide. This is simply not true.

> **"Every year, 35,000 children suffer neurological damage because of the DTP vaccine."** Edward Grant Jr. - Former Assistant Secretary of Health testified before the U.S. Senate Committee on May 3, 1985

The masses are being reeled in at record highs and the vaccine business is good. Vaccines are a business no different than selling satellite dishes and insurance policies. The problem is, when your pro-vaccination marketing plan has been sold to the masses like ice cream cones at a county fair and is making your company billions of dollars, how are you going to stop the train going down the tracks? What would the doctors tell their patients? It's not very professional in the business world to admit you were wrong. But an even greater incentive to keep on rolling down the tracks is the fact that this hoax is a multibillion-dollar moneymaker. What kind of business would cut their own throat when that kind of income is rolling in? If there were no money to be made at vaccinations, the whole ridiculous hoax would be abandoned like rats leaving a sinking ship.

> **"Take all the profit out of manufacturing and administration of serums and vaccines and they would soon be condemned, even by those who are now using them."** George Starr White, M.D.

Polio

Vaccination myths are touted as civilization savers. The truth is that vaccines cause far more disease than they ever prevent. Polio is a great example of how Americans have been brainwashed to believe that vaccinations are the reason polio has virtually disappeared.

The facts about the polio vaccine have been twisted like dough in a German pretzel shop. For example, are you aware that the polio epidemic was on the decline before the vaccine was ever introduced? In 1953, before the polio vaccine was ever introduced the death rate in the U.S. had already declined forty-seven percent. As a matter of fact, once the vaccinations began, the number of polio cases increased. For example, Rhode Island had a 450 percent increase and Massachusetts reported a 650 percent increase in polio after vaccines were given. In some countries, the polio epidemic ended without ever receiving the polio vaccine. In other countries, polio didn't even exist until people began receiving vaccinations. The developer of the polio vaccine himself, Dr. Albert Sabin, publicly admitted that the vaccine failed!

Dr. Bernard Greenberg, from North Carolina School of Public Health testified in May 1962, in the U.S. Congressional Hearings that polio increased substantially following mass immunization campaigns. He reports that from 1957-1958 there was a fifty percent increase in polio and from 1958-1959 there was and eighty percent increase. He testified that through manipulation of statistics that we have been lied to about vaccination facts.

> "Official data shows that large scale vaccination has failed to obtain any significant improvement of the diseases against which they were supposed to provide protection."
> Dr. Albert Sabin, (Developer of the Polio vaccine)

In 1976, Dr. Jonas Salk, creator of the killed-virus vaccine for polio, testified that the live-virus vaccine had been the principal, if not the sole cause, of all reported polio cases in the U.S. since 1961. What more evidence do you need than for the creators of the polio vaccine to publicly admit their concoctions are worthless and actually caused polio to increase? It doesn't get much simpler than this. Did your doctor forget to inform you of these facts?

Many years ago pharmaceutical companies, Cutter and Wyeth were sued by Americans who took their children in to receive polio vaccinations and were then later diagnosed with polio. Some 200,000 accidentally received the live polio virus and over 70,000 became ill. Further investigation revealed that two lots of the vaccine were contaminated with the live virus. Are you all right with an "Oops, sorry" when it comes to your health and someone messes up?

> "Many here voice a silent view that the Salk and Sabin polio vaccine, being made of monkey kidney tissue... has been directly responsible for the major increase in leukemia in this country."
> Frederick R. Klenner, M.D., F.C.C.P.

The law offices of Stanley Kops have proven that the oral polio vaccine has always been contaminated with SV-40 (simian virus #40), which has been linked by the FDA with cancers such as mesothelioma and meduloblastoma. Authorities have assured us that those polio vaccines which were grown on the kidney of the African Green monkey, did not contain this deadly contaminant . Stanley Kops has proven in the courtroom that not only is this not the case, but that the vaccine regulators who are responsible for keeping us healthy, have known all along that SV-40 virus was never removed from vaccines.

According to the Lancet 2002, SV40 viruses from the African green monkey have been detected in non-Hodgkin's lymphoma tumors. When toxic vaccine ingredients are showing up in cancerous tumors, it's time to put a stop to this genocide.

> **"The greatest lie ever told is that vaccines are safe and effective."**
> Dr. Len Horowitz

Measles

Measles was declining in the U.S. and England at a greater than ninety-five percent rate from 1915 through 1958. In 1920, 469,924 cases were reported. By 1955, less than three in ten million people had measles. The Measles vaccine was introduced in 1963, eight years after the epidemic had already ended naturally. Of course, most Americans have been spoon-fed the lie that the vaccine is responsible for ending measles outbreaks. However, the facts tell a different story. In the mid-1970's, after the measles vaccination had been administered to the masses, the death rate from measles remained exactly the same as it was prior to the introduction of the vaccine.

In a 1978 survey of thirty states, more than half of the children who contracted measles had been adequately vaccinated. The simple fact is, if vaccines worked, then why would you contract the disease after receiving vaccinations?

To blow an even bigger hole in the vaccination scandal, the WHO (World Health Organization) informs that chances of you contracting measles are fourteen times greater if you have been vaccinated for measles versus those individuals who have not been vaccinated! Come on now! In 1985, our federal government reported that eighty percent of the 1,984 cases of reported measles occurred in vaccinated individuals! Any reasonable scientist would look at this data and conclude that vaccinations are failing us, right?

> **"The only safe vaccine is one that is never used."** Dr. James R. Shannon – Former director of the National Institutes of Health

In a letter to Governor Edmund G. Brown of California, Eleanor McBean, Ph.D. states, *"I have uncovered some shocking data, showing that our government, medical and military authorities know that vaccination has killed and crippled thousands of innocent people; but the facts have been suppressed. The vaccine business has continued to thrive in spite of its disastrous failure, for the mere reason that it nets millions of dollars for the promoters, and this buys power with governments and propaganda control over the masses who don't know how to think for themselves."*

You were warned at the beginning of this book that some of this information may cause you to feel angry for what's happening in the name of healthcare. How does it make you feel to know that some of our so-called authorities label you as "someone who doesn't know how to think for yourself?" Are you ready to think or do you just go with the flow because everyone's doing it?

> "There is just overwhelming data that there's an association between the pertussis vaccine and seizures. I know it has influenced many pediatric neurologists not to have their own children immunized with pertussis." Jerome Murphy, M.D. - Former head of Pediatric Neurology at Milwaukee Children's Hospital

Vaccination Facts That Every Parent, Doctor and Nurse Should Know

- Infectious diseases were over 90 percent resolved by the time vaccines came onto the market.
- The risk from the pertussis vaccine is greater than the risk from the infection.
- The Hepatitis B vaccine was outlawed in France in 1983, after 15,000 citizens filed a class action suit against the government.
- After ten years of incorporating a mass vaccination program in the Philippines, where 25 million vaccines were given against smallpox, over 170,000 got smallpox, and 75,000 deaths were recorded from 1911 through 1920. (Townsend Letter for Doctors, Feb/Mar 1994)
- The incidence of asthma has been found to be five times more common in vaccinated children. (The Lancet, 1994)
- In 1976, more than 500 people were paralyzed with Guillain-Barre syndrome after receiving the flu shot and thirty of them died.
- The CDC has never done one study to see if it is a safe practice to inject nine vaccines into a newborn baby in the same day.
- Autism was unheard of until childhood vaccinations were introduced.
- *"...the combined death rate of diphtheria, measles, scarlet fever, and whooping cough declined 95% among children ages 1 to 14 from 1911 to 1945, before the mass immunization programs started in the United States."* (Bublin L, Health Progress, 1935-1945, Metropolitan Life Insurance Company, 1948, page 12)
- Mercury in vaccines exceeds the EPA levels of safety.
- In order to travel throughout the world no vaccines are required. They are only recommended, with the exception of Yellow Fever vaccine in certain areas of Africa.

The Origin of Vaccinations

> "I now have very little faith in vaccination, even as to modifying the disease, and none at all as a protective in virulent epidemics. Personally, I contracted smallpox less than six months after a most severe vaccination." R. Hall Bakewell, M.D. - Vaccinator General of Trinidad

In 1798, Edward Jenner inoculated an eight-year-old boy with pus from cowpox, a disease that milkmaids occasionally caught from cows. The boy never came down with smallpox when he was deliberately exposed to it later on. From this experiment, vaccinations were launched into the world and the masses have been receiving vaccines ever since.

> "I was working in one of the oldest lung illness treatment centers in Germany, and just by chance, I looked at the files of those people who had fallen ill during the first German epidemic of smallpox, in 1947…We had always been told that the smallpox vaccination would protect against smallpox. And now I could verify, thanks to the files and papers, that all of those who had fallen ill had been vaccinated. This was very upsetting for me."
>
> Gerhard Buchwald, M.D.

Everyone knows, that in order to perform legitimate studies to test the safety and effectiveness of a product, there must be a control group. Scientific studies require controlled, double blind placebo trials. It is ridiculous for the vaccine manufactures to think for one moment that they are above having to prove their products. The only studies done on vaccines compare new vaccines to old vaccines. So, if the question is, "Is drinking diesel fuel safer than drinking unleaded gasoline?" Well, that's not a very effective study is it? The question has to be "Is taking this vaccine more effective than doing nothing at all?"

Even our prescription drugs must be proven somewhat effective, despite all the possible adverse side effects. But when it comes to vaccines, they somehow miraculously end up above the law and are placed on the market when they have not been proven effective or safe.

Just as the IRS has a secret language they use to con Americans into paying income taxes on compensation for labor (which is not income and therefore not taxable), so does the CDC use words such as efficacy to confuse the public. They make the claim that vaccines effectively induce the production of antibodies and they are correct, however, that is only half of the equation. What they fail to honestly admit is that vaccines have not been proven to be clinically effective in protecting against disease.

> **"Confuse the meaning of words and you confuse the mind."**
> Vladimir Lenin 1870-1924

Could you imagine if you were perfectly healthy and your doctor convinced you to get vaccinated for polio so that you'd supposedly never contract it? So, being a good patient, you decide to follow your all-knowing doctor's advice and receive the vaccination. After receiving the polio vaccine, you suddenly begin having symptoms and eventually are diagnosed with polio. Come on Americans, wake up! When something isn't doing what it is supposed to do and healthy people are being harmed and killed, then something is wrong. Would loving and responsible parents subject their children to such risky and insane practices? It simply is not worth the risk.

> **"I am, and have been for years, a confirmed anti-vaccinationist...I have not the least doubt in my mind that vaccination is a filthy process that is harmful in the end."**
> Mahatma Gandhi 1869 - 1948 (Political & Spiritual Leader of India)

What happens when children are killed or severely damaged from vaccinations? Who is responsible? The CDC claims that:

1. The vaccine is not responsible.
2. The doctor who gave the shot is not responsible.
3. The vaccine manufacturer is not responsible.
4. The government who mandates mass vaccinations is not responsible.

WHO IS RESPONSIBLE?

According to the CDC, when children are harmed or killed from vaccines, the genetically defective child is to blame. Who are these people that blame vaccine damage and death on the child? The CDC, in their devious tactics and feeble attempts to cover up their harmful vaccine recommendations, has even warned that the DPT shot will look like it causes seizures, SIDS, autism etc., but states that it is not the vaccine. If it's not the vaccine, then what in the heck is it? It's time that these corrupt and dishonest officials pull their heads out of the sand and take some responsibility for their actions. Quit blaming innocent children as being genetically defective! It's time Americans demand a stop to this ridiculous nonsense.

To demonstrate how powerful these elite groups (CDC, vaccine manufacturers, government and doctors) are, it is interesting to note that each of them is legally exempt and in no way held accountable for adverse vaccine reactions. In other words, if you choose to vaccinate and disaster occurs (SIDS, seizures, autism etc.), then legal action against these groups is essentially impossible. You are just "out." Sadly, this may mean you are taking care of a disabled child for the rest of your life or attending their funeral.

Here is an example to help you understand the point being made. If you are charged with murder, it doesn't matter in this country whether or not you did it. What matters is whether or not your slick attorney can convince the jury you are innocent or guilty. If the jury agrees you are innocent, then you walk free. If they say you are guilty, then by all means don't drop the soap in the shower. It really has nothing to do with what you actually did.

Money is power and with it you can buy people off. Wealthy people who are guilty walk free all the time. Oh, they may be out thirty million or so, but they can buy their freedom. Just ask Michael Jackson how the system operates as he moonwalks his way to freedom yelling "Woo! Woo!" with one white-gloved hand over his crotch. Or ask O.J. how much it takes to make a glove not fit.

Just as wealthy criminals buy freedom through their money and power, so do vaccine manufacturers buy innocence with their harmful and sometimes deadly vaccinations. They are above the law because they are the law. The CDC can say and do what they want.

> "I did not find it difficult to conclude that there is no evidence whatsoever that vaccines of any kind – but especially those against childhood diseases – are effective in preventing the infectious diseases they are supposed to prevent. Further, adverse effects are amply documented and are far more significant to public health than any adverse effects of infectious diseases. Immunizations, including those practiced on babies, not only did not prevent any infectious diseases, they caused more suffering and more deaths than has any other human activity in the entire history of medical intervention. It will be decades before the mopping-up after the disasters caused by childhood vaccination will be completed. All vaccination should cease forthwith and all victims of their side effects should be appropriately compensated."
> Viera Scheibner, Ph.D. (Principal Research Scientist, Author of 3 books, some 90 scientific papers & co-developer of Cotwatch (a breathing monitor to prevent SIDS)

Many people have received vaccinations and their effects go unnoticed. Maybe your child will be one that is okay. However, I have personally worked with vaccine-damaged children and their parents. Watching parents break down and cry out of frustration and desperation because their most prized possession in life, their child, has been permanently damaged or killed from vaccinations is disheartening. And what makes matters worse is that the parent took the child in and held them still to be injected with harmful toxins that affected the child for the rest of their life.

In natural healing, it is possible to detoxify the child and help improve the quality of life, but we cannot push rewind. The effects of vaccinations are many times permanent. So, maybe it will kill or hurt your baby and maybe it won't. Are you willing to risk it?

Vaccinations Weaken Your Immune System

> "Only after realizing that routine immunizations were dangerous did I achieve a substantial drop in infant death rates. The worst vaccine of all is the whooping cough vaccine… it is responsible for a lot of deaths and for a lot of infants suffering irreversible brain damage. In susceptible infants, it knocks their immune systems about, leading to irreparable brain damage, or severe attacks or even deaths from diseases like pneumonia or gastro-enteritis and so on."
>
> Archie Kalokerinos, M.D., Ph.D.

Many allergies and respiratory illnesses are caused by increased levels of antibodies. Science has identified five classes of antibodies, which include; IgG, IgA, IgM, IgE and IgD. Vaccines can be a major cause for the development of IgE antibodies. Vaccines containing mercury (thimerosal), aluminum, Acellular Pertussis, Rubella, DT vaccine and gelatin in chickenpox vaccine have been reported to elevate IgE concentrations in the body, thus being a factor in many cases of allergies and asthma.

All vaccines with the exception of the oral polio vaccine (OPV) are injected directly into the bloodstream. When God created you, He put in your body a mucosal immune system also known as the secretory IgA. The secretory IgA is like a guard at a gate that prevents enemies from coming in and taking over. It filters microbes out so that, by the time an invading organism does get in the bloodstream, it is greatly reduced. So how does your body get rid of the microbes that do make it in? They are captured and taken right back out the gate through the mucosal barrier by sneezing, coughing and sweating. That is why it is dangerous to take drugs that suppress your sneezing, coughing and sweating. The guards in your immune system are trying to take the illegal alien microbes back out and you interfere with their work by suppressing your symptoms with cough syrup, Sudafed, antiperspirant deodorants etc.

> "Every day new parents are ringing us. They all have the same tragic story. Healthy baby, child, teenager, usually a boy, given the DPT, MMR booster followed by a sudden fall or slow, but steady decline into autism or other spectrums disorder."
>
> The Hope Project (Ireland)

Vaccines that are injected straight into the bloodstream, cross through your body's first line of defense, the mucosal barrier, with no warning. The guards in your immune system have no chance to sound the warning siren, no chance to recognize, duplicate or defend itself against future attacks from enemy microbes.

The body is sabotaged with these toxic vaccines like a thief in the night whose victim never sees him coming. When these foreign substances, including antibiotics, preservatives, and chemicals, that are designed to irritate the immune system, thereby strengthening its protective ability, come into the body bypassing all of your God-given natural barriers, then common sense cautions us to rethink what we are doing. Let's wake up to the fact that some people and animals cannot withstand such an assault without sustaining damage and sometimes even death.

Many of our children suffer from autism, seizures, mental retardation, dyslexia, hyperactivity and other development disabilities and we wonder why. Our overeducated and indoctrinated physicians do not have sense enough to stop this harmful experiment on humans. The problem is when your salary depends upon you not thinking for yourself, but just merely following routine procedures blindly, you keep your mouth shut in order to keep a paycheck every week.

> "Autism may be a disorder linked to the disruption of the G-alpha protein, affecting retinoid receptors in the brain. A study of sixty autistic children suggests that autism may be caused by inserting a G-alpha protein defect, the pertussis toxin found in the DPT vaccine, into genetically at-risk children." Mary N. Megson, M.D.

The immune system of healthy individuals is capable of dealing with the invasion of a single infectious disease. How else could we have survived for all the centuries before man created vaccines? The fact that you are reading this sentence says that you are the best of the best, survival of the fittest. Your ancestors survived the disease epidemics of the past without artificial vaccinations and now you are here. Those who were weak didn't make it. That says a lot about your immune system. Congratulations, you are a winner.

> "What we forget is that millions of years of evolution have taken place on this planet, and up until the last 100 years, humans have lived in relative harmony with microbes. Yes, there have been epidemic infectious diseases in history, but they have always resolved themselves. I don't think there is any real appreciation for what we may be doing by using so many vaccines to try to eradicate so many organisms. If we stay the present course, will mankind be free from infectious disease but crippled by chronic disease? Will eradication of feared diseases, such as AIDS, through mass vaccination be one of man's greatest triumphs or will we live in fear of deadly mutations of microbes that have outsmarted man's attempt to eradicate them? We may look back at the crossroads we are at today and wish we had decided to make peace with nature instead of trying to dominate it." Richard Moskowitz, M.D.

When we inject many different strains of vaccines through the skin directly into the blood, it is overwhelming for some and their systems cannot tolerate it. It does not happen that way in nature and the body was never meant to deal with such an exposure as the onslaught of vaccines present. Instead of strengthening Americans, we are weakening our immune systems by this artificial fraud and creating generations of new disease.

> "I've been practicing for 40 years, and in the past 10 years the children have been sicker than ever." Doris Rapp, M.D. - Founder of the Practical allergy foundation in Buffalo and Author of Is This Your Child

Possible Health Risks From Vaccinations

Allergies	Arthritis	Asthma	Autoimmune Disorder
Autism	Blindness	Cancer	Cataracts
Cerebral Palsy	Epilepsy	Diabetes	Ear Infections
Hyperactivity	Hypothyroidism	Lupus	ADD/ADHD
Leukemia	Meningitis	M.S.	Paralysis
SIDS	Death	Mental Retardation	

> **"The greatest threat of childhood diseases lies in the dangerous and ineffectual efforts made to prevent them through mass immunization."** Robert Mendelsohn, M.D.

Thimerosal, which is approximately fifty percent mercury by weight, has been one of the most widely used preservatives in vaccines. Research indicates that mercury is one of the most toxic metals known to man as previously mentioned. Mercury can interfere with the immune system by altering the cytokine status triggering autoimmune diseases and allergies.

The MSDS (Material Safety Data Sheet) on thimerosal from Eli Lilly states on their own letterheads that thimerosal is a "product containing a chemical known to the state of California to cause birth defects or other reproductive harm." Despite this blatant warning, Lilly still continues using thimerosal in the manufacturing of vaccines. Look up www.MomsAgainstMercury.com.

According to an article in JAMA (Journal of the American Medical Association) 1999, by Dr. Halsey (282) p 1763 entitled "Limiting Infant Exposure to Thimerosal in Vaccines, the EPA sets the limit at **.1mcg/kg/day** as a maximum "safe" level of exposure to mercury. Then they turn around and tell us to vaccinate our children with vaccines containing mercury levels that supersede way beyond the "safe" level. Let's take a look.

American Academy of Pediatrics Vaccine Schedule (www.aap.org)

Date To Administer	Vaccine	Amount of Mercury in Vaccine
Birth	Hepatitis B	12 mcg
4 months old	DPT & HiB	50 mcg
6 months old	Hepatitis B & Polio	62.5 mcg

Did our so-called health experts flunk their mathematics courses in school? We are injecting a known poison (mercury) into our children and to make matters worse, we ignore the safe level amount. Is it a mystery that childhood autism, ADD, cancer, asthma, diabetes etc., are skyrocketing each year?

> **"A single vaccine given to a six-pound newborn is the equivalent of giving a 180-pound adult 30 vaccinations on the same day."**
> Dr. Boyd Haley - Professor & Chair, Department of Chemistry, University of Kentucky

<u>Aluminum</u> is another toxic adjuvant used in vaccines. Itching nodules have been reported in 645 children out of 76,000 vaccines. The American Academy of Pediatrics admits, *"Aluminum is being implicated as interfering with a variety of cellular and metabolic processes in the nervous system and in other tissues."* The Hepatitis B vaccine given at birth contains aluminum hydroxide.

Official regulations state that aluminum should not exceed 1.250 mg levels in order for an individual to be safe, however the CDC ignores this just like they do with mercury by demanding that we bring our children in to receive DPT, Hepatitis B, HiB and Prevnar shots all in the same day. Each of these vaccines contains aluminum, which adds up to 1.475 mg of aluminum. This exceeds the recommended safety levels of aluminum.

> **"If you had five consecutive flu shots in any decade your chance of getting Alzheimer's Disease is ten times higher. This is partially due to the mercury and aluminum that is in every flu shot and most childhood shots."** Dr. Richard Schulze

Aluminum is eliminated from the body through the kidneys. However, infant kidney function is low at birth and doesn't reach full capacity until 1-2 years of age. According to medical literature, infants can't handle heavy metals, and yet we turn right around and inject them with aluminum in the hepatitis B shot at birth! Are we crazy or stupid? Why are we experimenting with our children's health? Perhaps it is all part of the plan to keep the disease maintenance business going strong. Maybe vaccination is the vehicle used to keep people coming in with symptoms and taking more drugs?

> **"... with measles vaccination, they went through Africa, South America and elsewhere, and vaccinated sick and starving children... They thought they were wiping out measles, but most of those susceptible to measles died from some other disease that they developed as a result of being vaccinated. The vaccination reduced their immune levels and acted like an infection. Many got septicemia, gastro-enteritis, etcetertera, or made their nutritional status worse and they died from malnutrition. So there were very few susceptible infants left alive to get measles. It's one way to get good statistics, kill all those that are susceptible, which is what they literally did."**
> Archie Kalokerinos, M.D., Ph.D.

Formaldehyde, which is used to embalm bodies, is used as an additive in vaccines. It has been proven to disrupt the nervous system, immune function and according to NCI reports may contribute to the cause of leukemia.

> "There is no evidence that any influenza vaccine, thus far developed, is effective in preventing or mitigating any attack of influenza. The producers of these vaccines know that they are worthless, but they go on selling them, anyway."
> Dr. J. Anthony Morris Research Virologist & Former Chief Vaccine Control Officer at the U.S. Federal Drug Administration

Vaccinations Are Crippling Our Immune Systems

- Since 1980 asthma has gone from 6.7 million cases to 17.3 million. Twelve percent of children under eighteen (approximately 9 million) have asthma now.
- Allergies and autism are dramatically increasing each year.
- Juvenile rheumatoid arthritis affects approximately 100,000 children under the age of sixteen.
- The cases of diabetes being reported are breaking records each week.
- Dr. Michael Odent reports his figures (JAMA 1994) that show a five times higher rate of asthma in pertussis vaccinated children compared to non-immunized children.
- Barthelow Classen, M.D., reported that juvenile diabetes increased 60 percent following a massive hepatitis B vaccination campaign for babies six weeks or older in New Zealand. He went on to further show that Finland's incidence of diabetes increased 147 percent in children under five after receiving three new vaccines in the 1970's, and that diabetes increased 40 percent in children from ages five to nine after receiving the MMR and Hib vaccines from 1988-1991.
- The New England Journal of Medicine concludes that the MMR vaccine is responsible for 35 percent of juvenile rheumatoid arthritis cases.
- AERS (Adverse Event Reporting System) reports that from 1991 to 1998 the rubella vaccine caused 55 percent of females to develop rheumatoid arthritis.

> "If an individual had 5 consecutive flu shots between 1970 and 1980, the chances of Alzheimer's Disease was 10 times greater than for those getting...no shots." Hugh Fudenburg, M.D. - Leading Immunogeneticist & author of some 850 peer-reviewed papers

Scientific research has shown that when Bacillus Pertussis (whooping cough germ) is injected into animals it leads to the secretion of insulin. In 1979, at the Fourth International Symposium on Pertussis, held in Bethseda, Maryland, it was shown that this same result occurs in those who have received pertussis vaccine. Drs. W. Hennessen and U. Quast reported in their publication "Adverse Reactions after Pertussis Vaccination," that the reactions after receiving the pertussis vaccine and the hypoglycemia syndrome have a close relationship.

> "The rise in IDDM (Juvenile onset diabetes) in the different age groups correlated with the number of vaccines given." Barthelow Classen, M.D. - Former researcher at the US National Institutes of Health and founder of Classen Immunotherapies in Baltimore

If your child has juvenile diabetes, it may be a result of the pertussis (whooping cough) vaccine. As Robert Mendelsohn, M.D. said, *"Maybe it's time to investigate whether the pertussis vaccine has anything to do with the rapidly rising number of people with juvenile diabetes, adult diabetes, hypoglycemia and all disorders of insulin metabolism."*

The pertussis vaccine is not the only one causing researchers to scratch their heads about the rise in juvenile diabetes. There is considerable evidence that shows that the hepatitis B vaccine is causing blood sugar imbalances as well. Go online to http://www.vaccines.net/toppage1.htm for a closer look at this ridiculous paradox.

> "My suspicion, which is shared by others in my profession, is that nearly 10,000 SIDS deaths that occur in the United States each year are related to one or more of the vaccines that are routinely given to children. The Pertussis vaccine is the most likely villain, but it could also be one or more of the others." Robert Mendelsohn, M.D.

Autoimmune diseases are becoming extremely popular. Just as cell phones and internet access twenty years ago were a rarity, now they are everywhere. So it is with the autoimmune diseases. Molecular mimicacy is when antibodies from vaccines began attacking your own body's organs and tissue. When we inject vaccines like Hepatitis B into the body and there is nothing for it to work against, then it is possible for it to start attacking our own organs, glands and tissue. Rheumatoid arthritis, type I diabetes, Kawasaki disease and lupus are examples of this inward attack taking place.

> "Immunization programs against flu, measles, mumps and polio may actually be seeding humans with RNA to form proviruses which will then become latent cells throughout the body...they can then become activated as a variety of diseases including lupus, cancer, rheumatism and arthritis."
> Dr. Robert W. Simpson - Rutgers University

The ticking time bombs called vaccinations that we have been injecting into humans are creating diseases to keep the doctor's office full. Doctors have even linked AIDS to the live oral polio vaccine. This vaccine is grown on the kidney tissue from the African Green monkey. Research has identified this monkey as the original source of the AIDS virus.

What man thinks he understands, we call science. Every fifty years that science changes drastically as new things are proven and old things are proven to be false. What do we really know? Mother Nature operating under God's intelligence has been producing life for a long time. Man has basically been living in harmony with microbes since the beginning of time until the last several decades. In man's blunderous attempt to fix things, sometimes we create a monster worse than the original one. When bacteria and viruses begin mutating and new strains are created because of our vaccination experiments, then the Frankenstein we have created may be stronger than what we can handle. Autoimmune diseases and cancer is skyrocketing, but it is just the beginning of the havoc that has been unleashed upon vaccinated Americans.

> "Studies have shown that while the oral polio vaccine contains three strains of polio virus, a fourth strain can be cultured from the feces of vaccine recipients. This indicates that viruses have recombined and formed a new strain in the process of vaccination."
> Virology, 1993

Doctors use a term called trancession, which means a virus can lay dormant in your body and then marry another virus to become something different. This is hardcore, scary science that we are creating through our vaccination experiments. What is even more frightening is that Americans are so brainwashed about this that if the news announces there is a shortage of vaccines then people will panic, push, and shove to claim their place in line to get their flu shot.

> "He who doesn't take the time to learn the truth someday will suffer the consequences." J. Rueben Clark

Chickenpox and Shingles

Most of us remember being kids and getting chickenpox. My mom wanted us to get it when we were young because all that happens is you break out with red itchy bumps on your skin and in about a week it clears up. You are then immune to it from then on as long as you are re-exposed to it every so often, as if to give your immune system a reminder quiz. The older you are, the worse the symptoms seem to be. Now we have a vaccine for chickenpox. Not as many children are coming down with chicken pox, but now we have adults who have never had chickenpox. Chickenpox in adults is called shingles and it is very painful and quite serious. Shingles is rare in adults who have had the chicken pox as a youngster. So, with all the shingles outbreaks you can guess what comes next.

The CDC is expecting large outbreaks of Shingles in the future and is in the process of creating a vaccine for it. Wouldn't it be best to stop vaccinating children for chickenpox, just let children get it naturally so they become immune and not have to worry about shingles in the future and a vaccine for it? Medical science fails to use logic when the opportunity to produce a drug or vaccine to treat disease comes to town. If there were no incentive to make a few dollars from vaccines, do you think they would still vaccinate for chicken pox?

What Doctors Have to Say About Mass Vaccinations

> "Vaccines are principally responsible for the increase of those two really dangerous diseases, cancer and heart disease." Dr. Benchetrit
>
> "Abolish vaccination, and you will cut the cancer death rate in half." Dr. F.P. Millard
>
> "My honest opinion is that vaccine is the cause of more disease and suffering than anything I could name. I believe that such diseases as cancer, syphilis, cold sores, and many other disease conditions are the direct results of vaccination. Yet, parents are compelled to submit their children to this procedure while the medical profession not only receives its pay for this service, but also makes sledded and prospective patients for the future." Dr. Henry R. Bybee

> "It is my firm conviction that vaccination has been a curse instead of a blessing to the race. Every physician knows that cutaneous diseases (including cancer) have increased in frequency, severity, and variety to an alarming extent. To no medium of transmission is the widespread dissemination of the class of diseases so largely related as to vaccination." B. F. Cornell, M.D.
>
> "I have removed cancers from vaccinated arms exactly where the poison was injected." E.J. Post, M.D.
>
> "Have we traded mumps and measles for cancer and leukemia?" Robert Mendelsohn, M.D.
>
> "Cancer was practically unknown until compulsory vaccination with cowpox vaccine began to be introduced. I have had to deal with at least two hundred cases of cancer, and I never saw a case of cancer in an unvaccinated person." W.B. Clarke, M.D.
>
> "The chief, if not sole, cause of the monstrous increase in cancer has been vaccination." Dr. Robert Bell
>
> "Immunized children have more ear infections and spend more days in hospitals." Dr. Michael Odent

Remember Dr. Alexis Carrel who kept the chicken heart alive for twenty-nine years? He has done his own scientific research into the vaccination hoax. He took highly diluted poisons, similar to formaldehyde in the Salk vaccine, which was at 1:4000 concentration. Dr. Carrel wanted to see what would happen if he injected these carcinogens at an even greater dilution, 1:5000 to 1:250000 in chickens. The results produced cancer in the inoculated chickens.

If we can produce cancer in animals with smaller dilutions of vaccine ingredients than the amount we give our own children, then why are we still vaccinating? Oh yes, that information isn't given out at the county health department or doctors offices. So, if the masses are unaware, they'll just follow blindly like hogs in the shoot at the slaughterhouse.

> "I am thoroughly convinced that the recent great increase in cancer is directly due to vaccination. I have written my report to several members of Parliament and invited them to the hospital to witness the dismal results of the Vaccination Act for themselves."
> William Forbes, M.D. - Medical Director, St. Saviours Cancer Hospital Regents Park, London, England

When my wife was pregnant with our first child, I was compelled to find the truth out about vaccinations. I had to know for certain what to do with my own children. After years of studying the pros and cons, I am thoroughly convinced that a child is better off to not be vaccinated. That is what I have done with my own three.

It's disturbing to see beautiful healthy children go in to receive vaccinations and then be diagnosed with autism and other disorders. I have worked with many vaccine-damaged children and it's sickening to see the adverse reactions firsthand.

> "Several of my personal friends now have cancer, some of them have died from it. I have inquired into the probable cause of the serious increase of this horrible disease. I believe, as do many other physicians, that cancer is due to impregnating the blood with impure matter and it is obvious that the largest method by which this is done is vaccinations and revaccinations." J.S. Preston, M.D.

Sherri Tenpenny, M.D., is the medical director of OsteoMed II, an integrative medical clinic in Middleburg Heights, Ohio. She had been an emergency room physician for twelve years when she started looking into the question of vaccinations. She has put in over 7,000 hours of research on vaccinations. Her conclusion is that vaccines are not safe or effective in preventing disease. The risks of adverse side effects are actually worse than the actual diseases themselves. She summarizes these findings on her very informative DVDs. They will answer your questions about vaccinations. For more information on her DVDs, books and vaccination seminars call (440) 239-1878 or go online to www.DrTenpenny.com or www.osteomed2.com.

> "...This...forced me to look into the question of vaccination further, and the further I looked the more shocked I became. I found that the whole vaccine business was indeed a gigantic hoax. Most doctors are convinced that they are useful, but if you look at the proper statistics and study the instances of these diseases you will realize that this is not so...My final conclusion after forty years or more in this business (medicine) is that the unofficial policy of the World Health Organization and the unofficial policy of the 'Save the Children's Fund'... (other vaccine promoting) organizations is one of murder and genocide.... I cannot see any other possible explanation...You cannot immunize sick children, malnourished children, and expect to get away with it. You'll kill far more children than would have died from natural infection."
>
> Archie Kalokerinos, M.D., Ph.D.

The pharmaceutical industry has done a tremendous marketing job in selling their, "Everyone needs to be vaccinated" campaign to the masses. Most gullible Americans reveal their ignorance by arguing how important it is to vaccinate when they know very little about vaccination history, disease epidemics and facts. What does the doctor know about the poisons he or she injects, other than what was taught in medical school with a corrupt twist to convince young doctors that if every child does not get vaccinated then the whole human race will be susceptible to disease epidemics that could annihilate the whole world? Be not deceived, when your drug and vaccine manufactures donate millions of dollars to medical universities, it influences the curriculum taught.

> Congressman Dan Burton testified to other members of congress the following:
>
> "How confident can we be in the recommendations with the Food and Drug Administration when the chairman (of Vaccines and Related Biological Products Advisory Committee) and other individuals on their advisory committee own stock in major manufacturers of vaccines? ...It almost appears that there is an "old boys' network" of vaccine advisors that rotate between the CDC and FDA—at times serving both simultaneously..."

The fear of not being vaccinated has been marketed and advertised with such efficiency that every college student studying marketing ought to use it as one of the finest examples in the world. They have literally made billions off of a junk product. The ingenious marketing ability of those who have pulled this off commands respect. On the other hand, it is frightening to know that many Americans don't care enough to look at the facts while cancer, allergies, fibromyalgia, lupus, autism etc., soar to new levels each year and our doctors shrug their white-coated shoulders as to why.

> "You can fool some of the people all of the time, and all of the people some of the time, but you cannot fool all of the people all of the time." Abraham Lincoln

Vaccination Ingredients

*Decayed animals	*Diseased blood	*MSG	*Bacteria
*Viruses	*Fungi	*Pus	*Urine
*Feces	*Formaldehyde	*Antibiotics	*Mercury
*Acetone	*Aluminum	*Carbolic acid	*Formalin
*Inactivated virus from infected cattle tongue epithelium			
*Virus strains prepared in chick embryo cell culture			
*Rabies from duck embryo origin			
*Live virus prepared from duck embryo or human diploid cell culture			
*Calf lymph			
*Formaldehyde suspension of Rickettsia Prowazekii grown in embryonate eggs			
*Dried mouse brain infected with French neurotropic strain of yellow fever virus			
*Rotten horse blood (diphtheria toxin and antitoxin)			
*Macerated cancerous breasts			
*Pus from sores on diseased animals			
*Mucus from the throats of children with colds and whooping cough			
*Decomposed fecal matter from typhoid patients			
*HiB saccarides cultured on cow's brains			
*Live measles virus			
*Live mumps virus			
*Live rubella virus			
*Monkey kidney cell cultures			
*Hepatitis-A vaccine contains MRC-5. Obtained from **aborted fetal cell cultures**			
*Rubella MMR-II vaccine contains WI-38 created from tissue of an **aborted fetus**			
*Pig blood			
*Mouse serum protein			
*Chicken pox (Varicella) is cultured on **aborted human fetus** (2002 PDR p. 2201)			
*Ethylene glycol (Antifreeze)			

> "Belief in immunization is a form of delusional insanity."
> Dr. Herbert Shelton

How barbaric and ridiculous can we get? To inject this toxic filth into the human body is most likely going to have harmful consequences. How many people will continue vaccinating their children when they know that some vaccine ingredients come from aborted fetuses? If I was ever introduced to something dark and evil, the ingredients in vaccines and the harmful effects they have had on our innocent children tops the list. To put this filth into a brand new healthy baby sounds like witchcraft, insanity, sorcery or an outright sin against a beautiful child of God that has been given as a gift to us to nurture, care for and raise. Vaccinating their little bodies with these toxins in an attempt to make them healthier is a sheer mockery to God who just created them. The intelligence within just created a mind-boggling heart, lungs, kidneys, brain, nervous system and a self-healing immune system and then we take that miracle and poison it in an attempt to make it healthier, as if it doesn't have enough sense to make it on its own and live? Children come into this world with an immune system far superior to anything arrogant scientists can conjure up in their labs to generate billions of dollars.

Are you like the hog at the slaughterhouse following blindly down the shoot because everyone else is doing it? Are you too busy watching "American Idol" at nights to educate yourself and family on the facts of vaccinations so you can make wise, informed decisions for the things that are most important in life, like your children's health? Your innocent children don't have a choice, they depend upon you to LOVE and care for them. Every choice has a consequence. It has been estimated that 1 out of 200 children suffer severe reactions from the DPT shot. It has been reported that approximately 4,000 children die each year from the DPT vaccine. Like Barbara Fisher said, "When it happens to your child then the risks are 100 percent."

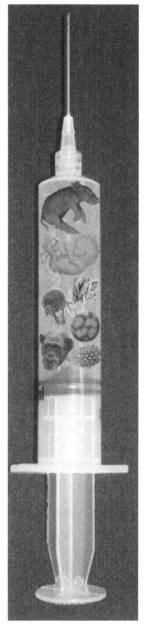

> "Fear can only prevail when victims are ignorant of the facts."
> Thomas Jefferson

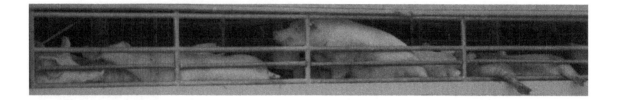

> "The dissenter is every human being at those moments of his life when he resigns momentarily from the herd and thinks for himself."
> Archibald MacLeish

Homeopathy – An Alternative to Vaccinations

Homeopathy has been used for over 200 years. Homeopathy is a safe, effective and inexpensive medicine that the pharmaceutical companies violently oppose because of the threat it poses to their billion-dollar monopoly.

> "You medical people will have more lives to answer for in the other world than even we generals." Napoleon Bonaparte

Just because the school your child attends says you have to have your child vaccinated does not mean there are not exemptions. You have the right to have a medical, religious, philosophical or proof of immunity exemption from vaccinations. For healthcare workers who do not want the Hepatitis B vaccine there is a federal exemption form online that you can download and give to your employer. Go to www.osha.gov and fill it out.

> "If you believe a law is immoral you have a duty to disobey it."
> Pat McKay – Author of Natural Immunity Why You Should NOT Vaccinate

Know your constitutional rights. Freedom of religion is guaranteed to Americans. It is against my religion to violate the trust God has granted me when He sent my wife and me our beautiful healthy children. To risk putting foreign toxic materials into their blood stream violates that trust that has been given to me when I became a father. I am their guardian and I have an obligation to give them the very best. Anything short of the best, I feel is totally unacceptable and irresponsible on my part.

> "When we give government the power to make medical decisions for us, we, in essence, accept that the state owns our bodies."
> U.S. Representative Ron Paul, M.D.

To say it simply, I love my children too much to risk giving them something that has been proven in the past to harm and kill other children. I feel God has trusted me with these choice spirits and I will not put toxic substances into their bodies. It is against my religion to do so.

> "Vaccination is not necessary, not useful, does not protect. There are twice as many casualties from vaccinations as from AIDS.
> Gerhard Buchwald, M.D. (West Germany)

Some doctors, school nurses, county health department workers etc., can get very pushy when you do not comply with what they have been instructed to do. You can request a religious exemption form from your county health department. When they ask why you choose to not vaccinate your child, a simple and firm, "It is against my religion" will suffice. Any other questions or harassment will usually cease if you simply respond by asking, "Do I need to have my attorney contact you?" Be kind, courteous, but firm and understand that they are simply doing their job. Here is a sample vaccine exemption form that may be used. Simply fill in the blanks, have it notarized and present it to the county health department, if you choose to not vaccinate your child and want them to attend public school. Obviously, this sample form is for an Alabama resident. It can be altered for the state where you reside.

Vaccine Exemption Affidavit

I (*Parent or guardian's name*) citizen of the State of Alabama and the United States of America affirm: Be it known to all courts, governments, and other parties that:

Being a person of strong Christian Morals, it is against my religious convictions to accept the injection of any foreign substance into my body or the body of my child. This includes, but is not limited to, any and all vaccinations, shots, tests for diseases, oral vaccines, epidermal patches, and in any other way that live or killed bacterium, viruses, pathogens, germs, or any other microorganisms, that may be introduced into or upon my body or any of my children's bodies.

This written statement to exempt my child from any immunizations, TB testing, and other shots/injections, because I hold genuine and sincere personal religious beliefs which are inconsistent with these medical procedures and experimentation. The practice of vaccination and the injection of any foreign substance is contrary to my conscientiously held religious beliefs and practices, and violates the free exercise of my religious principles.

I (*Parent's name*), as the parent of (*Child's name*) am exercising my rights under the **First Amendment of the U.S. Constitution** and **C.R.S. 25-4-1704 (4) (b)** and (Alabama Government Code Section 16-30-3 and Alabama Code 22-20-3 Section 22-20-3) to receive religious exemption from vaccinations & testing.

Applicable law has been interpreted to mean that a religious belief is subject to protection even though no religious group espouses such beliefs or the fact that the religious group to which the individual professes to belong may not advocate or require such belief. Title VII of the Civil Rights Act of 1964 as amended Nov. 1, 1980; Part 1605.1-Guidelines on Discrimination Because of Religion.

SENATE BILL #942 SECTION 1 CHAPTER 7

3380 – IN ENACTING THIS CHAPTER, IT IS THE INTENT OF THE LEGISLATTURE TO PROVIDE: EXEMPTION FROM IMMUNIZATION FOR MEDICAL REASONS OR FOR PERSONAL BELIEFS.

3385 – IMMUNIZATIONS OF A PERSON SHALL NOT BE REQUIRED FOR ADMISSIONS TO A SCHOOL OR OTHER INSTITUTION ... IF THE GUARDIAN, PARENT, OR ADULT WHO HAS ASSUMED RESPONSIBILITY FOR HIS OR HER CUSTODY AND CARE IN THE CASE OF A MINOR, OR THE PERSON SEEKING ADMISSION FILES WITH GOVERNING AUTHORITY, A LETTER OR AFFIDAVIT STATING THAT SUCH VACCINATIONS ARE CONTRARY TO HIS/HER BELIEFS.

I affirm that vaccination & injections of any foreign substances and proteins conflict with my religious beliefs as stated above. Therefore, I would request that you accommodate my religious beliefs & practices by exempting my child from any vaccinations, injections, and testing of any kind.

Subscribed and sworn, without prejudice, and with all rights reserved, (Print Name Below)
_____,
Principal, by Special Appearance, in Propria Persona, proceeding Sui Juris.

_____
Signature of Affiant

Acknowledgement

State of Alabama

County of_____:

On this_____ day of _____, 200____, before me

Personally appeared _____, to me known to be the person described in and who executed the foregoing instrument and acknowledged that he executed the same as his free act and deed, for the purposes therein set forth.

_____
(Notary Public)

My Commission Expires _____, 200_____

For more vaccine exemption forms and specific information regarding each state's law go to www.vaclib.org/exemption.htm or www.thinktwice.com/laws.htm.

> **"Any action that is dictated by fear or by coercion of any kind ceases to be moral."** Mahatma Gandhi

If you do choose to vaccinate, remember that antibiotics and cortisone suppress the immune system. So, if you have or are taking these, you don't want to vaccinate at that time. Be wise, be informed and be smart so that you can be healthy.

> **"The price of freedom is eternal vigilance…Never trust your government. You need a revolution every twenty years, just to keep the government honest!"** Thomas Jefferson - 3rd President of USA & author of the Declaration of Independence (1743-1826)

Barbara Fisher explains that Mandatory vaccination is the only law in this country that requires an American citizen to risk his or her life for their country. In times of war, when the draft was in effect, the young men being asked to take that risk were 18 years old and could consciously object if they chose too, they were not one day old infants.

If you choose to vaccinate your child, simply ask your doctor what the health risks are. Most will reassure you that vaccines are safe and necessary for health. After they promise you how safe and effective they are, pull out a form such as the one below, and simply ask your physician to sign it since he or she is so confident that vaccines are safe.

Physician Vaccination Signature Form

> **"I certify that the** (*Name of Vaccine*)_____**vaccine being administered to** (*Name of Child*)_____ **is free from all known and yet unknown zoonotic or human viruses or viral fragments and will not cause acute or chronic illness in the recipient due to viral contamination or as a reaction to the components of this vaccine.** (*Signature of Physician*)_____ **Date** _____.

Most physicians will refuse to sign such a form because they know that the vaccines are not safe and that there are risks. If your physician refuses to sign such a form, then that is evidence enough to convict vaccines guilty of harmful side effects and possibly murder in some cases. Don't let your child be the next statistic.

For doctors, concerned parents and other intellectuals who still don't believe that vaccinations can do no wrong, there are some books you my want to look at, if you are not afraid. If you want hard core scientific research on vaccinations, here is a list of books that will allow you to discern the facts from the myths. Do your own research if you want to know the truth.

> "If you want the truth on vaccination you must go to those who are not making anything off of it. If doctors shot at the moon every time it was full as a preventive of measles and got a shilling for it, they would bring statistics to prove it was a most efficient practice, and that the population would be decimated if it were stopped."
> Dr. Allinson

Books Your Doctor Never Read About Vaccinations

1. Vaccinations and Immune Malfunction by Harold E. Buttram, M.D.
2. Vaccinations Do Not Protect by Eleanor McBean, Ph.D.
3. How To Raise A Healthy Child …In Spite Of Your Doctor by Robert Mendelsohn, M.D.
4. But Doctor, About That Shot… The Risks of Immunizations and How to Avoid Them by Robert Mendelsohn, M.D.
5. Immunizations: The Terrible Risks Your Children Face That Your Doctor Won't Reveal by Robert Mendelsohn, M.D.
6. Vaccination? A Review of Risks and Alternatives by Isaac Golden, Ph.D.
7. Vaccines: Are They Really Safe and Effective? By Neil Z. Miller
8. Natural Immunity Why You Should Not Vaccinate! By Pat McKay
9. Don't Get Stuck: The Case Against Vaccinations by Hannah Allen
10. The Case Against Vaccination by M. Beddow Bayly
11. Homeopathy In Epidemic Diseases by Dorothy Shepherd
12. Vaccination, Social Violence, and Criminality: The Medical Assault on the American Brain by Harris L. Coulter
13. Immunization: The Reality Behind the Myth by James Walene
14. The Case Against Immunizations by Richard Moskowitz, M.D.
15. The Poisoned Needle by Eleanor McBean
16. The Dangers Of Immunization by Harold E. Buttram, M.D.
17. Dangers Of Compulsory Immunizations – How to Avoid Them Legally by Tom Finn (Attorney)
18. Murder By Injection by Eustace Mullins

19. What Every Parent Should Know About Childhood Immunization by Jamie Murphy
20. Vaccination: 100 years of Orthodox Research Shows that Vaccines Represent a Medical Assault on the Immune System by Viera Scheibner, Ph.D.
21. A Shot In The Dark by Harris L. Coulter and Barbara Loe Fisher
22. What About Immunizations? Exposing the Vaccine Philosophy by Cynthia Cournoyer
23. The Immunization Decision by Randall Neustaedter
24. Vaccination and Immunization: Dangers Delusions and Alternatives by Leon Chaitow
25. The Sanctity Of Human Blood: Vaccination Is Not Immunization by Tim O'Shea

> **"As well consult a butcher on the value of vegetarianism as a doctor on the worth of vaccination."** Bernard Shaw

Chapter 8
NEVER SURRENDER

Chiropractic Adjustments Allow Me to Compete

Growing up with three older brothers who thought it was fun to pick on their younger sibling, made me feel somewhat like Johnny Cash's song, "A boy named Sue." I had to get tough or die. Somehow I managed to survive all of our front yard tackle football games and living room wrestling matches. I followed in my brothers' footsteps and competed in football, wrestling and lifted weights intensely. I have always enjoyed a good fight. To find out who is the toughest, meanest, strongest, fastest athlete around has always caught my attention. Whether I was the man in the pit doing battle or a fan cheering for my brother, I love competition. My philosophy has been, "Talk is cheap, put your money where your mouth is."

Barely escaping my brother's death grip holds, I somehow managed to live long enough to make it to kindergarten. Experience is the greatest teacher and I was well prepared when it came time for me to go to school. I was always considered the toughest, strongest kid in my grade. In elementary school we would play tackle football when the teachers weren't looking. It wasn't fair when I played, because no one could tackle me and I would score every time I got the ball.

As I grew bigger, so did my intensity for the game. I was feared for being the hardest hitter on the team and many friends didn't enjoy lining up across from me in hitting drills. I loved it. In fact, I lived for it. My bent facemask and battered helmet proudly bore the honor of devastating collisions I dished out every chance I had.

Practice days would find me screaming intensely, as blood dripped from my charred fists that jackhammered through offensive lines. The adrenaline rush that surged through me from flying down the field as fast as I could and exploding into someone like a freight train surpassed the high of any drug stimulus. It was a time I could hit someone as hard as I could and not get in trouble for it. I loved to hit and I loved practice, but when the lights lit up Lion's field on Friday nights, I unchained the beast. I was a football playing maniac, a loose cannon, flying down the field trying to knock someone's head off.

I practiced with such intensity that my coach made me sit out on the kick off team, because too many players were getting hurt trying to block me. In my opinion, that's when we found out who was honest all summer long in the weight room and who played the game just so their girlfriend could wear their letterman's jacket.

> **"Get knowledge of the spine, for this is the requisite for many diseases."** Hippocrates 460-377 B.C.

I considered myself to be tough, but without chiropractic adjustments my football and wrestling days would have come to an abrupt halt. Excruciating pain shooting through my back as I shot in for a double leg take down was more than I could bear. I knew something was seriously wrong with my back. My coach told me to go see my doctor. So my Mom and I went in to see Dr. Halpin. He knew me well from my broken wrists I had in previous years of athletics and was considered the best in town. He X-rayed me from every direction possible and then came in and we studied my back. There were no fractures and he diagnosed me with a sprained back. He told me to sit out for six weeks and to take a prescription for painkillers he was writing. To tell me I was going to have to sit out for six weeks was as bad as telling me that I was going to have to wear a dress, march in the band and play the flute.

Not being able to bend down and tie my shoes, I knew something was wrong and just because my doctor couldn't see a broken bone in the X-rays didn't mean I was okay. This ordeal taught me that doctors only find what they are looking for, not necessarily what is causing the pain or disease.

> **"Chiropractors adjust subluxations, relieving pressure from the nerves so that they can perform their functions in a normal manner. The Innate can and will do the rest."**
> B.J. Palmer, D.C. – Developer of Chiropractic

Not satisfied with taking a painkiller to dull my God-given senses, I went to see a chiropractor. Dr. Roger Fairbanks had me stand and while keeping my right leg straight, I put my heel on his adjusting table. He then told me to stretch my arm out and try to touch my toe. I did great, I could reach about sixteen inches past my toe (good hamstring stretch). Then he had me switch legs. As I attempted to touch my toe, there came the pain and tightness. I couldn't even make it past my knee. "That's how far you are out of balance," he explained. My neck was no different. I could turn my neck and look to the right pain free, with fair flexibility, but when I turned to the left it was jammed. It was as if someone had a door stop embedded in my neck preventing my range of motion.

Dr. Fairbanks adjusted me twice a week and as the days went by I loosened up and felt better. He encouraged me to ice my back and neck to remove inflammation and within a short time, I was pain free. For the rest of my football and wrestling days, I continued to receive chiropractic adjustments to keep me aligned and pain free.

> **"Why search the world over for an exterminator or an antidote for dis-ease? Why not look for the cause of the ailments in the person affected and then correct it?"** B.J. Palmer, D.C.

If you are going to play brutal sports with physical contact, you would be wise to get adjusted periodically. The collisions in football and the brute force of wrestling can easily jerk you out of alignment. When the neck, vertebrae and hips are out of alignment, a tremendous amount of stress is placed on the body, especially the nerves. If not corrected, serious injury can occur.

Pinched nerves can cause excruciating pain. I remember after playing fullback on offense and nosetackle on defense for the entire game my neck was so far out of alignment that I couldn't move it. I was hurting so badly, that when the bus finally arrived home that night, I couldn't sleep. I sat the whole night on the couch wishing the night was over because I was in so much pain. Aspirin didn't faze me. I knew what I needed, and the remedy was not a pill. I needed to be adjusted, to unlock the jammed vertebrae in my neck. I know it is absolutely insane to beat your body up like that in sports, but when you are seventeen years old it means the world to you. As soon as I got adjusted, the pain subsided and my neck unjammed like gears in a transmission. Within a short time I was healthy again, pain free, and running down the field punishing opponents with my facemask, as I exploded into them with every ounce of energy my body could muster.

> **"It is useless to administer a powder, potion, or pill to the stomach when the body needs an adjustment."** B.J. Palmer, D.C.

Motorcycle Accident Crushes My Football Dreams

After high school, I pursued my goal of playing college football for a short time until I got my butt kicked. No, it wasn't from a 300-pound offensive guard, it was a 3,000 pound Ford Escort that sent me flying twenty-five torturous feet.

One beautiful spring day I was riding my motorcycle to Gold's gym. A Ford Escort pulled out right in front of me. Before I had a second to hit my brakes, I smacked him going 40 mph with no helmet. My football dreams were crushed like a ripe tomato on a cobblestone street in a Spanish bull-run. I lost that battle and it hurt on all levels; physical, mental and emotional.

I don't remember much, except waking up in the emergency room. I looked down at my pillow to see it saturated in blood from my poor battered melon. It was no surprise that my head took quite a lick.

Doctors said I was a miracle. I was told I was very lucky to be alive. The doctor looked at me and said, "Most people who take a shot like you did die, the impact snaps their spine." Surprisingly, the X-rays they took revealed no fractures. However, I felt like every tendon, ligament and muscle in my hips and shoulders had been sent through a meat grinder and made into bratwurst sausage links. I was in so much pain, that I couldn't bend down to sit on the toilet. Talk about being down and out, embarrassed, frustrated and down right miserable. I couldn't sleep at nights because the slightest movement would wake me up in excruciating pain. I felt like the coyote on the Bugs Bunny Roadrunner show-whipped.

Controversy in the Doctor's Office

I had a bubble of fluid on my lower back the size of a baseball. My doctor wanted to stick a needle in the pocket of fluid and drain it. A second emergency room physician looked at it and said he would leave it alone. I decided I'd get a third opinion. I called my cousin, Steve Pincock, who was a sports medicine trainer for the university's football team. Steve took me in to see Dr. Kimball who was considered the best. He looked at me and reasoned, "If we lance that pocket of fluid and try to manually drain it, you run the risk of infection. Why not just let the body heal naturally? The body is smart and when it is ready it will eventually drain on its own." That made perfect sense to me and so that was my decision. It took some time, but eventually my body healed itself. Was that a miracle? Yes and no. Yes, in the sense that the whole way our human body functions and heals is a miracle. On the flip side, it's no miracle because that is how God engineered our bodies. He made us SELF-HEALING.

> "Miracles happen, not in opposition to Nature, but in opposition to what we know of Nature." St. Augustine

I continued going in for painful physical therapy sessions all summer long. The fall football season kicked off without me and instead of putting on a helmet and shoulder pads, I was strapping on ice packs trying to get the baseball-size pocket of fluid on my lower back to go down. If there was ever a time for an antidepressant drug to magically turn my hell into a heaven, I needed it then. I was tempted, but never took a "happy pill."

My Struggle

That was a very depressing summer for me. Many negative thoughts went through my mind. I was mad. I was mad at the guy who pulled out in front of me. I was mad at the pain I was experiencing. I was mad about my future. I wanted my shot to play football and within a second it had been robbed. What I didn't realize at the time was that I was giving away all of my power by allowing an experience to control me. I was feeling like a poor victim.

I didn't want to change directions in life. I wanted to play football and now I couldn't. I was resisting "what was." Have you ever spent thousands of hours preparing for something and then at the last minute, the roof caves in and you can't do what you have been anticipating doing for the last fifteen years? That is where I was. I was wishing for something different and didn't want to accept my new direction.

One night I walked outside and thought about ending my life. I looked up at the stars in the blackness of the night and prayed to God for help. I thought about the sadness that killing myself would bring to my family, especially my dear, sweet mother and I knew deep down that that wasn't the answer. But I was so mad, frustrated and confused. I didn't know what I was going to do.

> **"Blame is a smoke screen that hides reality by focusing in the wrong direction."** Valerie Seeman Moreton, N.D.

As I starred at the stars in a rage of anger, something magic happened. I caught a glimpse of something that I can't explain. The anger slowly disappeared and a sense of reverence overtook me. A type of peace and quietness came over me. I felt a loving presence reassuring me that everything would be fine and that this would soon pass. I understood that I would heal up and be fine, but for some reason I wasn't supposed to go and try to be a football hero. I decided to accept that and I made the decision that I would not fight it any longer.

I was taught that night that all things work for our greatest good. I knew that our loving Father in Heaven was the creator of all, and that things happen in life so that we can learn and grow. God doesn't just allow the good things to happen, he allows it all so that we get our money's worth here.

Looking back, that accident was a blessing in disguise because it taught me some valuable, but painfully humbling lessons. I was too proud and cocky to listen to any other way, so the Lord knocked me off my high-horse to get my attention. It wasn't long afterwards, that I met my sweet wife, who has been my best friend ever since.

> "I am the Lord… and there is none else, there is no God beside me… I form the light, and create darkness; I make peace, and create evil; I the Lord do all these things." Isaiah 45:5

True peace and happiness in life comes when we stop resisting what is and accept it, as part of God's divine plan for each of us. I learned that the only way to have peace in our lives is to flow with the process of life and accept things for what they are. I am grateful for the experiences God blesses me with; they have been great teachers in disguise.

Back to Gold's Gym

After months of excruciating physical therapy, I found myself lifting weights in the gym with just the bare bar, trying to get my range of motion back. It was painful, frustrating and depressing, but I could not suppress my passion to lift heavy weights and be strong. I was determined to regain my strength. I am a fighter and to get up one more time after being knocked down was the only way I knew. Nothing could or would stop me and I was willing to prove this to myself and the world.

I went back to the gym and worked mainly on range of motion and flexibility, lifting bars with no weight on them. It hurt to bench press a bare 45-pound Olympic bar. As the weeks trudged on, my weakling exercises progressed and I put a 2 1/2-pound plate on each side of that bar. Later I moved up to the 5's and then the 10's. I slowly inched my way up until I could put the 45's on. Once my range of motion came back to normal, I made good progress.

> "If children gave up when they fell for the first time, they would never learn to walk." Louise L. Hay

From a corner of the gym through a cloud of chalk and groans of pain is where I first met Misi Inoke and Tui Filiaga. They are two of the strongest men I have ever met. These modern-day Samsons toiled with 100-pound plates on each side of the bar like kids do inner-tubes at a beach party. Coaching them every step of the way was their trainer, Ray Weber, an Italian boxer from Pittsburgh. Ray trained just as hard as they did, but didn't compete in powerlifting due to some old injuries.

When I saw Misi and Tui warm up on the bench press with 315 pounds for ten reps and then 405 for ten more reps and then 495 (that's five 45's on each end) for eight reps, my mouth dropped open like an Italian opera singer on a Saturday night. I was in awe of their strength. I once saw Tui bench press 315 pounds 43 times at the end of a workout! Needless to say, people got out of their way when they walked into the gym to slam the iron. They were all brute strength, no show, unlike so many pretty-boy bodybuilders, with their massive physiques, but no power behind it.

I had met Tui and Misi at the gym earlier in the Spring when I was training for football and they took me under their wings. They would occasionally coach (spot me) on my lifts and encouraged me to get stronger for football. So, after the accident, they invited me to join their powerlifting team and start competing. Since I wasn't playing football, I decided to give powerlifting a shot.

Powerlifting

In late November, 1997, I went to the Idaho State Powerlifting meet with Tui, Misi and Ray. I was nervous and intimidated, but at the same time, honored to compete with modern day Samsons. Being weak from the accident, I felt way out of my league, but I went anyway and took fifth place in the 220-pound weight class. I was proud of myself for squatting 500 pounds, bench pressing 315 and deadlifting 520, but I was in no way satisfied with a measly fifth place. My desire to be crowned champion was kindled like a stack of wooden crates burning at a bonfire.

Misi won, "Lifter of the Meet" and was awarded a huge trophy as he smoked his competition in the 275-pound weight class. He squatted a bar-bending 800 pounds, benched 600 pounds and heaved up 685 on the deadlift! We took third place as a team and I was highly honored to be a part of it.

With a raging desire to win, I went back to the gym and heaved the iron until total exhaustion. Training with Misi, Tui and Ray was motivating, fun and intense. I caught on fire. I couldn't wait to go to the gym and slam the iron. When you have a 600 pound bench presser and a 800 pound squatter as a training partner, it's very inspiring.

Before bed I would train mentally as I envisioned myself crushing records with mind-boggling strength. This is a very important part of achieving your goals. If you can't see, feel and believe in something it will probably never happen physically.

Seven months later, we went to see how hard I had really worked in the gym. We competed in the Rocky Mountain States Powerlifting Championships. I moved up to the 242-pound weight class and squatted 650 pounds, slammed 400 on the bench press and groaned up a 585 deadlift. I earned that first place trophy and it felt great. This made me feel as if I had redeemed myself from being crushed by a white Ford Escort that had my forehead signature on its side.

What does any of this have to do with health? A lot actually, I want you to understand that in order to be healthy we need something to do, something to work towards. We need goals. We need a reason to get out of bed in the morning. We need something that gets us excited. For me, it's the ability to go to the gym and workout like a crazy lunatic. An intense workout releases endorphins that make us feel good. It's also a great stress-releaser. Lifting weights makes me feel good and sleep well at nights.

Just last night, I had an awesome upper body workout in my gym in our basement. It may sound ridiculous but it gives me something to look forward to after work. This enthusiasm for life is what keeps us healthy. Get out and get involved with something that motivates you. There are millions of possibilities out there and lifting weights is one of mine. Find something to do and do it. Do something that brings fulfillment into your life. Turn the TV off, it doesn't count as a hobby.

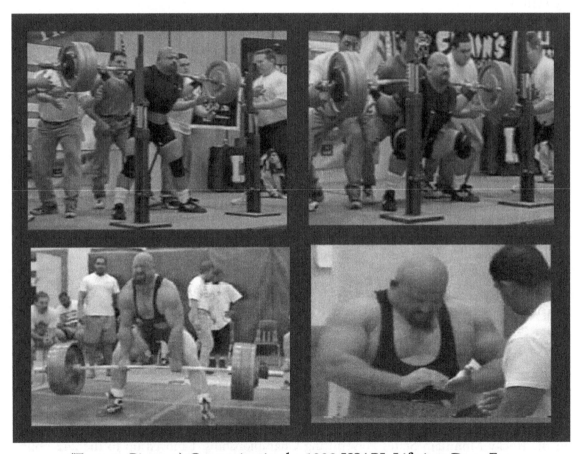

(Top two Pictures) Competing in the 1998 USAPL Lifetime Drug Free National Powerlifting Championships in St. Louis, Missouri - 650 lb. Squat (Bottom two pictures) Winning 1st place at The Rocky Mountain States Powerlifting Championships – 1998, Pocatello, Idaho

Chapter 9
MASTER OF PUPPETS

How Much Do Your Drugs Actually Cost?

> "I use to have a drug problem but now I make enough money."
> David Lee Roth (Van Halen)

Considering that spending on prescription drugs has tripled between 1990 and 2001 to over $140.6 billion according to Kaiser Family Foundation, it would be accurate to say that prescription drugs are a profitable business.

Who finances the medical schools in this country? Cynthia Crossen, from the Wall Street Journal, in 1996 published a book called, *Tainted Truth: The Manipulation of Fact in America*. Her book exposes the corruption of lying with statistics. She goes on to reveal that, in 1981, the drug industry gave $292 million to colleges and universities for research to ensure that every medical university around promotes disease maintenance through the use of pharmaceuticals. In 1991 the drug lords rubbed the backs of universities by giving them $2.1 billion.

If a homeopathic or herb company were to give $2 billion to colleges, do you think they would be promoting the benefits of these natural healers? Like the old German proverb says, *"Who eats my bread dances to my tune."*

The pharmaceutical industry, with its generous financial contributions, has a monopoly on health care in this country. Very little research is done by the big boys on anything natural because if they cannot patent something and make millions they are not interested.

> "Researchers are like prostitutes. They work for grant money. If there is no money for the projects they are personally interested in they go where there is money." Dr. Sydney Singer

The following drug cost statistics are from Federal Budget Analysts in Washington, D.C. According to Sharon Davis and Mary Palmer of the U.S. Department of Commerce and the Bureau of Economic Analyst this is what they report:

DRUG	RETAIL COST	ACTUAL COST OF INGREDIENTS	% OF MARKUP
Xanax	$136 – 100 tabs	.24 cents	569,958 %
Celebrex	$130 – 100 tabs	.60 cents	21,712 %
Claritin	$215 – 100 tabs	.71 cents	30, 306 %
Keflex	$157 – 100 tabs	$ 1.88	8,372 %
Lipitor	$272 – 100 tabs	$ 5.80	4,696 %
Norvasec	$188 – 100 tabs	.14 cents	134,493 %
Paxil	$220 – 100 tabs	$ 7.60	2,898 %
Prevacid	$ 44 – 100 tabs	$ 1.01	34,136 %
Prilosec	$360 – 100 tabs	.52 cents	69,417 %
Prozac	$247 – 100 tabs	.11 cents	224,973 %
Tenormin	$104 – 100 tabs	.13 cents	80,362 %
Vasotec	$102 – 100 tabs	.20 cents	51,185 %
Zestril	$ 89 – 100 tabs	$ 3.20	2,809 %
Zithromax	$1,482–100 tabs	$ 18.78	7,892 %
Zocor	$350 – 100 tabs	$ 8.63	4,059 %
Zoloft	$206 – 100 tabs	$ 1.75	11,821 %

Should this be considered price gouging? When Hurricane Katrina hit New Orleans, people were arrested for selling gas, water, generators etc., for double the price. If someone tries to sell gasoline for six dollars a gallon and the government fines them for price gouging, then surely our government would intervene on this prescription drug scandal, right? Selling Xanax for $136 bucks when the actual ingredients only cost about .24 cents is a first class rip-off.

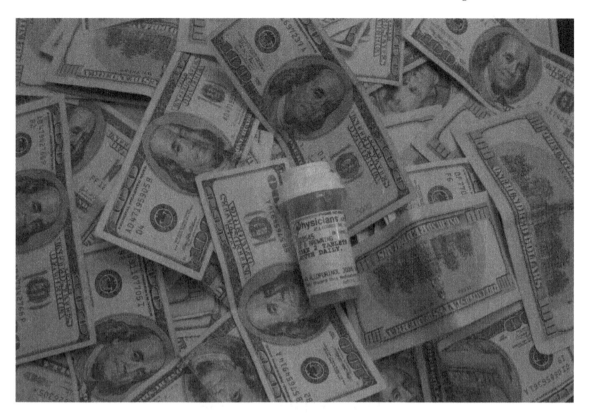

Do you know what is even smarter than making a fortune off your drug concoctions? Get your medical doctors to legally prescribe the drugs to about ninety-million Americans and get them hooked. This produces a generation of addicts. Then influence insurance companies, the government, AMA, FDA and everyone else who needs to be on your team in order for you to win the game to jump on the "Do Drugs" campaign and oppose any natural remedy that cannot be controlled by the pharmaceutical industry.

> **"I am quite confident that if gravity had to be approved by the FDA it would clearly meet strong resistance from the multi-national drug corporations."** Joseph Mercola, D.O.

Every car salesman in this country has the goal of learning how to buy cheap and sell for the highest price possible. Thank goodness other car dealerships offer competition that keeps the prices somewhat affordable. Could you imagine how much a Honda Accord would cost if there was a monopoly on selling automobiles? Instead of paying around $24,000 perhaps you would pay over $100,000?

The stock market is built upon this whole game of buying cheap and selling high. But the pharmaceutical industry commands respect for their ingenious monopoly they have created to legalize, patent and distribute the goods. They have mastered the art of dealing drugs. Al Capone and his band of henchmen wouldn't hold a candle to what Eli Lilly and his co-partners run. They have done it with such elegance and grace to the point of suckering the masses, doctors and other government leaders into believing that drugs are all we need for health. What we have in this country is the biggest scam ever perpetrated against the American people. Drug sales have soared to over 500 billion dollars per year.

This industry is so big and powerful that when a deadly drug harms and kills people to the point that the FDA recalls it, they can easily afford to throw millions out left and right to whoever has been harmed. The attorneys are stumbling over each other trying to get in on the action so they can rub their mitts on forty percent.

> "There is no room in the Hall of Fame for the founder of a cure that involves eating certain foods and giving up others. Dis-ease is so easily prevented and so easily cured, it warrants no 'heroes'."
> Giraud Campbell, D. O.

If We Could Patent the Sun

If something can't be patented and marketed to make millions, then mainstream medicine has no interest in it. No one has figured out how to sell the sun to Exxon. Therefore, we do not see the majority of houses equipped with solar panels being used to heat and supply electricity to our homes and power our cars. Gas, oil and electricity are what our cars and homes are powered with and it generates trillions of dollars. It is residual income, meaning everyone will need to pay their gas, oil and electric bill next month in order to drive a car and enjoy the comforts of electricity in their homes. The petroleum industry and power companies know that money will come in next month and next year because people need their products and services to live. That is smart business. What is their enemy? An inventor who could mass-produce an electrical device that could capture the energy from the sun and store it to be used to generate enough energy to power your car and home. This would threaten their business. If an inventor could offer the public this, then Americans would no longer need them. Could you imagine what would happen if you could buy such a device for a one-time fee of maybe $5,000 and never have to pay another electric or gas bill for your home or car again? The device would pay for itself within the first year of use. It would revolutionize the world.

> "I have no doubt that we will be successful in harnessing the sun's energy.... If sunbeams were weapons of war, we would have had solar energy centuries ago." Sir George Porter

Money is the great motivator. Money buys and controls, and many times enslaves, people. Would you get up and go to work tomorrow if you weren't going to receive a check? How many fathers would love to come home early from work to spend time with their children, but can't because of work? Money is why no one has mass-produced electrical devices to capture the sun's power.

The Drug Business

As mentioned earlier, many prescription drugs originate from herbs. Chemists take molecular structures and rearrange them, thus forming a man-made imitation of the natural substance. The rearranging of the molecules is like a combination lock. If someone else doesn't know the combination, they can't open it or duplicate it. This way they can patent their drug and market it for whatever price they choose.

In 2004, Pfizer, the largest drug company, made a whopping fifty-three billion dollars! Ensuring that every consumer and doctor is aware of their drugs, they spent thirty-two percent of those sales on marketing and administration and only fifteen percent on research and development.

Money Equals Power

> "To achieve world government, it is necessary to remove from the minds of men, their individualism, loyalty to family traditions, national patriotism and religious dogmas." Brock Chisolm (Director of the U.N. World Health Organization - SCP Journal 1991)

After reading the above quote, hopefully, every American who cherishes their family traditions, national patriotism and religion will realize that some of our so-called leaders apparently have a different agenda for us.

It is interesting to know that President Bush and his administration's push for medical liability reform is legislation to protect the pharmaceutical industry from liability lawsuits filed by injured patients who trusted their chemical drugs to make them healthy. Why would President Bush be so in favor of such a law? Once again, if we look at the cause, the symptom makes sense. The pharmaceutical industry was the largest corporate sponsor for the Bush election campaign. Ah ha! Now the pieces of the puzzle start to make sense. When someone donates millions of dollars in your behalf, most people feel obligated not to turn around and bite the hand that just fed them. Always remember, those who pay the piper get to call the tune.

Rockefeller Oil Interests and I.G. Farben

John D. Rockefeller, Sr. (1839-1937) was a wealthy businessman who founded Standard Oil of New Jersey, and later, OPEC (Organization of Petroleum Exporting Countries). OPEC functions as a cartel by maximizing profits from crude oil. An elite group of very wealthy oil/business men pool their resources together for the strict purpose of limiting competition by price-fixing the market. By selling your product for the highest possible price and squashing out all competition, you can create a monopoly and thus set any price you want on your products. So if you like to complain about high gas prices, you can thank Rockefeller oil interests.

Venezuela has its own oil refineries. Do you think it costs them $3.85 a gallon to pump their gas tanks full? No way. They pay seventeen cents a gallon for gasoline. Under the Rockefeller oil cartel here in the U.S., we pay what they tell us to pay.

By the 1860's, Rockefeller owned the world's largest refinery and was consolidating most of all oil refining into one giant corporation. By 1879 he owned ninety percent of America's oil refining capacity and owned stock in forty-one other corporations. Who cares, right? What in the world does Rockefeller's oil have to do with your health? If you want to unwind the noose and trace it back to its roots to understand why medicine is the way it is, then we find it goes way back to a deal Rockefeller made with a German chemical/drug company called I. G. Farben.

I.G. Farben (Interessen Gemeinschaft) means, "Community of Interests." This German-based company controlled nearly the entire German drug and chemical industries during the 1930's. They gained ownership of the technology for producing synthetic fuels from coal, a process called hydrogenation.

In the late 1920's, I.G. Farben became a threat to Rockefeller's oil empire by offering a less expensive synthetic substitute. Rockefeller was too smart of a business man to allow this to happen, so he came up with a solution.

The Big Drug Deal

If you can't beat them, join them. Money-driven businessmen don't fight one another. They make deals with their competition to keep business up to par, so both can benefit the most from the masses paying high prices for their goods.

In 1929 I.G. Farben met with John Rockefeller and made possibly the biggest drug deal in the world. They shook hands on a deal that would allow Rockefeller to sell oil but not drugs and have the hydrogenation patent for use outside of Germany, while I.G. Farben would sell only chemicals. In 1930 these two super-powers established a joint company to develop the oil-chemical field. By 1940 I. G. Farben's operations were in ninety three countries and were the world's largest chemical manufacturer. They controlled 380 companies, many of them pharmaceuticals, such as Bayer, Proctor and Gamble, Monsanto, Dow chemical and Hoffman-LaRoche Laboratories. The Rockefeller/I.G. Farben cartel was well on its way to being in control of most of the world's manufactured chemicals, including drugs that require coal tar or crude oil as a component in the manufacturing process. Obviously a medical system that didn't involve their drug use would be competition and a threat to their empire, so with their money and power they helped shape what America's disease maintenance system is what it is today.

> **"Power tends to corrupt, and absolute power corrupts absolutely."**
> First Baron Acton

Restructuring Medicine in the USA

In 1900 there were more than 15,000 homeopathic practitioners here in the U.S., one sixth of the entire medical profession! We also had twenty-two homeopathic medical colleges training doctors. By 1923 only two homeopathic schools remained. What happened?

At the turn of the century the AMA had established a council on Medical Education in the U.S. Their objective was to reform U.S. medical schools. In 1910 Abraham Flexner, a layman, produced "The Flexner Report" while being employed by Andrew Carnegie, John D. Rockefeller and Simon Flexner. He was paid to produce a report that would discredit homeopathy, naturopathy and other natural healing modalities so that the drug/oil cartels could control the future medical market.

Our medical schools here in the U.S. were restructured by a nonphysician, Abraham Flexner, while being financed by Rockefeller oil interests. They began reforming medical schools and for obvious reasons would not license hundreds of schools teaching natural healing modalities. Fourteen of America's homeopathic colleges all of a sudden didn't meet "criteria." So after our homeopathic/naturopathic colleges were denied licensing, the only medical schools left were those schools that favored drug-oriented medicine. You can bet your bottom dollar this was no coincidence.

> **"No one should approach the temple of science with the soul of a money changer."** Dr. Thomas Browne - English Physician

Over one hundred years, later many people are enslaved into America's disease maintenance system by being hooked on the prescription drugs Rockefeller and I.G. Farben set out to manufacture and control long ago. We pump $3.75 a gallon gas in our cars and many can't even afford the co-pay on their prescription drugs. Whether you believe it or not, you are a slave to the drug and oil business unless you don't do drugs and don't drive a car.

These unseen powers are why we have a disease maintenance system, not a health care system. It's time for gullible Americans to wake up and quit being deceived, no different than our high spirited founding forefathers did when they finally mustered up enough courage to revolt against foreign governments controlling them and taxing them unfairly. They wrote the Declaration of Independence and won our freedom. Americans deserve health care, not disease maintenance.

> "The reality, therefore, is that government becomes the tool of the very forces that, supposedly, it is regulating."
> G. Edward Griffin – Medical Historian

Who Owns Insurance Companies?

To understand why insurance does not cover natural healing, we need to look at the cause. By 1974, Rockefeller owned a large portion of stock in the first and third largest insurance companies in the U.S. Within time the Rockefeller/I.G. Farben monopoly muscled their way around, buying many other insurance agencies. Owning and controlling drugs, oil and insurance companies could ensure residual income and cinch the knot for eliminating competition in the future.

For financial business purposes, alternative medicine was conveniently ridiculed and unfairly represented in clinical trials and still is to this day. You don't have to have a Ph.D. to figure out why. Creating a health care system that would only allow a licensed medical doctor (no homeopaths or naturopaths in most states) to treat and diagnose disease using the I.G. Farben/Rockefeller expensive, addictive, patented drugs to being covered by mainstream insurance would ensure a lucrative financial pay off. Some medical doctors haven't a clue for whom they really work. They are pawns in the game, legalized drug dealers for I.G. Farben/Rockefeller business.

> "In the specialized field of drugs and pharmaceuticals, the Rockefeller influence is substantial, if not dominant." Edward Griffin

Dr. Ralph Moss was fired from Memorial Sloan-Kettering in the 1970's for refusing to play ball with these drug dealers. Laetrile, which comes from apricot pits, was then and still is effective for healing cancer. When he refused to cover up the research, he found himself without a job. Since so many of our insurance and government agencies are intertwined and controlled through this cartel, they hold tight reins on the market. The field of U.S. cancer care is organized around a medical monopoly that ensures a continuous flow of money to the pharmaceutical companies, medical technology firms, research institutes, and government agencies such as the Food and Drug Administration (FDA) and the National Cancer Institute (NCI), and quasi-public organizations such as the American Cancer Society (ACS). This is "the cancer industry," exhorts Ralph Moss, Ph.D.

> "...For the truth is that the medical industry is far less than optimal. It is basically controlled by those who support the drug companies. The drug companies are owned by those who control the banking industries. They manipulate nations and war. Enough said. If anyone does not believe me, I say: Seek truth with an open mind and you will find all the proof of that which I have said. We all need to know the truth and the sooner the better, if we want to save the freedom and health we still have." Richard Anderson, N.M.D.

The FDA - A Pawn in the Game

Is it coincidence that about half of our high-ranking FDA officials have previously been employed by major pharmaceutical companies immediately before coming on board with the FDA? Studies show that another half of those employees take executive jobs in pharmaceutical companies when they leave the FDA. An article in USA Today in September 2000, showed that fifty-four percent of the experts on advisory committees had a direct financial interest in the drug or topic they were asked to evaluate.

> "The FDA is supposed to regulate the pharmaceutical industry, but instead they are teaming up to work on an antifraud campaign against an industry that some could construe to be an economic competitor."
> Mark Blumenthal – Executive Director, American Botanical Council

Years ago in the days of prohibition, Al Capone bought off many law enforcement agents to make sure his alcohol was taken care of. He ran a business. In order to run a large successful business, you must have employees. Pay them enough money and people will make sure the ball rolls in your direction. The current medical establishment in this country is the way it is because of the money being paid to keep the pharmaceutical industry in charge.

> "The FDA and the drug companies are doing everything they can to prevent you from learning about these safer, gentler (yes, and much cheaper) ways to heal and help yourself."
> Earl L. Mindell, Ph.D. – Author of the Vitamin Bible

In 1974, FDA scientists testified before congress that the FDA is nothing more than a pawn for the pharmaceutical company. Of course things of this nature never receive much media attention and soon it is hushed up and swept under the carpet. However, it is interesting to note that during that same fraud/conspiracy ordeal, Congress identified 150 FDA employees who owned stock in twenty-seven of the companies they were supposed to regulate.

Money Handlers

> "Permit me to control the currency of a nation and I care not who makes its laws!"
> Baron de Rothschild - Rothschild Banks of London and Berlin

The Rothschilds and their seven business partners control the currency in this country and although most Americans think that they live in a free society, it is highly controlled by an elite group. Presidents and leaders of countries are merely puppets whose strings are pulled to keep them dancing to their tune. When a president like Abraham Lincoln refuses to borrow money at a high interest rate from these international bankers to finance the Civil War they have him assassinated. Years later when another president like John F. Kennedy started talking about how he was going to do away with the Federal Reserve and take back our country then he became a threat to "the big bankers." When he didn't conform and play ball with them, they bumped him off, end of story. To cover their tracks they had, Jack Ruby (who was in bad health and knew he would soon die) murder Lee Harvey Oswell, the original assassin suspect. They are smart enough to know that, if you don't want a murder trial with an investigation, you destroy the suspect and evidence and that is what they did to avoid the truth behind John F. Kennedy's assassination.

The following is a list of very wealthy people who have enough money and power to, "care not who makes the laws."

> 1. Rothschild - Banks of London and Berlin
> 2. Lazares Brothers - Bank of Paris
> 3. Israel Moses – Sieff Banks of Italy
> 4. Warburg – Bank of Hamburg, Germany and Amsterdam
> 5. Lehman Brothers – Bank of New York
> 6. Kuhn, Loeb and Co. of Germany and New York
> 7. Chase Manhattan (Rockefeller) – Bank of New York
> 8. Goldman Sachs – Bank of New York

These eight international bankers are the owners of the phony Federal Reserve System set up by Paul Warburg of Kuhn – Lobe and Co., who used President Woodrow Wilson as a puppet to sign this corporation into existence in 1913. The privately owned Federal Reserve is no more federal than Federal Express.

> **"Because the Federal Reserve Bank of New York sets interest rates and controls the daily supply and price of currency throughout America, the owners of that bank are the real directors of the entire system. These shareholders have controlled our political and economic destinies since 1913."**
> Eustace Mullins - Secrets of the Federal Reserve

If I started the Bank of Sainsbury today and bought my own printing press and began to print money without it being backed by gold and silver and then loaned the money out to people at a high interest rate, it wouldn't take long before I became very wealthy. This money would be created from nothing, since I have no gold or silver to back it. That is what the Federal Reserve has been doing since 1913. They make a fortune off the interest paid from phony currency and we Americans are slaves to this debt. It is such a debt that we can't even pay the interest.

> **"If the people understood the rank injustice of our money and banking system there would be a revolution before morning!"**
> Andrew Jackson 7th U.S. President (1767-1845)

The hard working American middle class has been paying for it dearly ever since, as we struggle to make ends meet. Now many families have both spouses working to make a living while we pay high taxes. The IRS is the collection agency that most Americans pay for these super wealthy bankers to keep us in bondage.

> **"Whoever controls the volume of money in any country is absolute master of all industry and commerce."** President James Garfield

Medical Ghost Writing

What do you do when you manufacture a proven harmful product that has the potential to make billions, if you can sneak it past the authorities and get it out on the market for your drug dealers (doctors) to pedal for you? According to Erica Johnson of CBC news, medical ghostwriting is the practice of hiring Ph.D.'s to come up with clever drug reports, purposely leaving out negative side effects, for drug companies to get their poisons on the market. Next, they recruit doctors to put their name on the report as the authors. Once they have dishonestly manufactured their golden goose, they submit it to be published in prestigious medical journals, such as the Lancet and British Medical Journal, etc. It is reported that these devious ghostwriters can receive up to $20,000 for every report they swindle.

More and more of these frauds are being exposed in our disease maintenance system. It is appalling that the New England Journal of Medicine has admitted that deceitful ghostwriters have written fifty percent of the drug reviews in their journal! Dr. Jeffrey Drazen, the New England Journal's editor, explains that pharmaceutical money muscles its way in and around everything to the point that he simply can't find experts to write for him that do not have pharmaceutical connections. So what does this mean? Your doctor is reading falsified drug reports that leave negative side effects out that make the drug look better than it actually is.

> **"The relationship between medical journals and the drug industry is somewhere between symbiotic and parasitic."**
> Richard Horton - Editor of the Lancet

Dr. M. Michael Wolfe, a medical expert, received an unpublished drug review on Celebrex from the editors of JAMA. He read it and was impressed because it was made to appear to be superior to two other arthritis drugs, not causing as many ulcers. Dr. Wolfe and colleagues promoted the product by submitting a highly favorable editorial of their own to accompany the newly released findings in JAMA. Consequently, doctors began prescribing Celebrex to millions of arthritis sufferers.

Over time most drugs show their true face riddled with harmful side effects. Celebrex was no exception. Dr. Wolfe continued to investigate why Celebrex was not as the report he had endorsed said it to be. As more and more data was located on Celebrex, he quickly came to realize the initial report he had received was a product of ghostwriting. Numerous discrepancies were found between the first report and his newly found data such as reports of ulcers after six months deliberately being left out of the first report. Once all the pieces of the puzzle lined up, Celebrex was no better then the other two drugs but once again the drug companies hoodwinked the masses, including the FDA and doctors, and made millions on their poison before the "experts" could uncover their conniving ways.

Digging a little deeper into the rat's nest, Dr. Wolfe came across some more interesting dot-connecting information. He found that the initial report he was given included sixteen authors who were faculty members of eight medical schools and every single author was either an employee of Pharmacia (Manufacturer of Celebrex) or a paid consultant of the company. As a matter of fact, between 1990 and 1997, nearly all clinical trials performed on non-steroidal anti-inflammatory drugs (NSAIDS) such as Vioxx, aspirin, Motrin, Aleve, Bextra etc., were sponsored by your pharmaceutical lords who buy and pay for whatever they want.

> **"Robert Mendelsohn, M.D. had a rule: You never hear about the dangers of a drug unless another drug to replace it is available."**
> Ted Koren, D.C.

To punch another hole in the already flat tire, when all of these NSAIDS were researched between 1990 and 1997, the results showed the sponsored drug to have equal or superior efficacy when compared to all other NSAID products. For more information look at (JAMA July 27, 1998, p.31S and USA Today. McLean, Va.: Aug 1, 2002. Page A11).

> **"We are being hoodwinked by the drug companies. The articles come in with doctors' names on them and we often find some of them have little or no idea about what they have written."**
> Editor of the British Journal of Medicine

For those of you who trust the drug industry to be honest in helping us achieve optimum health, good luck. Any researcher or detective can look at their information and laugh at the ridiculousness of the whole rotten sack of corruption. As long as there is money to be made at someone else's expense, lies will be told.

> **"Scientists should always state the opinions upon which their facts are based."** Author unknown

Paying to Squash Competition

Mark Fisherman in his book, *Manufacturing the News*, brings to light that under the current system of journalistic reporting, a favorable support will always be given to the status quo and those who control the big money, power and political scenes, regardless of what the true facts might. Money can buy almost any report to show virtually anything you want. One example of this appeared in a national newspaper with a study entitled, "Saint John's Wort Not Effective for Treating Depression." This one-sided, deceiving article failed to tell the whole truth about what was found. The actual study was kept from the public. It was done on both Prozac and Saint John's Wort but the article led you to believe that it was only about Saint John's Wort.

The results, after giving depressed patients Prozac and Saint John's Wort, revealed that neither the drug nor the herb had any effect on the patients. Of course the headline news was claiming Saint John's Wort to be ineffective for treating depression, while they conveniently left out even mentioning that Prozac failed to show any improvement in this study either.

> **"The deception going on in the media is appalling."** Bill O'Reilly

Something else the article failed to mention is the fact that there are lots of other scientific studies that have proven Saint John's Wort to be extremely effective for depression. The media will twist, distort, cut-and-paste whatever they want you to hear as they take orders from their bosses to manufacture the news. It is doctored up to meet expectations of the big boys with money who pull puppet strings to get what they want. So next time you are reading or watching the news, remember what you are hearing is what they want you to know. There is a good chance that the money spent to put that information in front of you will go towards you absorbing it like a sponge and adhering to it like glue. You will then defend it with your life as "THE TRUTH." Why? You heard about it and read about it and suddenly think that you have become an expert on the subject.

> **"It appears that money can't buy you love but it can buy you any 'scientific' result you want."** Carolyn Dean, M.D., N.D.

No Honest Opinions in the Media

Former chief of staff for the New York Times, John Swinton, was asked to give a toast to the independent press before the New York Press Club. Exposing the corruption in journalism, he said the following.

> "There is no such thing, at this date of the world's history, in America, as an independent press. You know it and I know it. There is not one of you who dares to write your honest opinions, and if you did, you know beforehand that it would never appear in print. I am paid weekly for keeping my honest opinion out of the paper. Others of you are paid similar salaries for similar things, and any of you who would be so foolish as to write honest opinions would be out on the streets looking for another job. If I allowed my honest opinions to appear in one issue of the paper, before twenty-four hours my occupation would be gone.
>
> The business of journalists is to destroy the truth; to lie outright; to pervert; to vilify; to fawn at the feet of mammon, and to sell his country and his race for his daily bread. You know it and I know it.
>
> What folly is this, toasting to an independent press? We are the tools and vassal of rich men behind the scenes. We are the jumping jacks; they pull the strings and we dance. Our talents, our possibilities and our lives are all the property of other men. We are intellectual prostitutes."
>
> John Swinton (Former Chief of Staff for the New York Times)

How are Doctors Educated About Drugs?

> "To pass our examinations and get qualified, we must accept what our teachers tell us. In other words, we must cultivate what Josh Billings called a well-balanced mind---one that will balance in any direction required." Major R. Austin M.R.C.S., L.R.C.P

Many medical doctors will admit that the only knowledge they have about the drugs they prescribe is what pharmaceutical representatives tell them and give them to read. How does this make them professionals? For example, take a magic drug to get rid of acid reflux. Most will say it works like a charm, taking no thought as to what they are setting themselves up for in the future. Sure it works because it shuts down the secretion of digestive juices which stops the acid from coming up the esophagus, but now the person doesn't break down and digest his food properly. What's the effect of that? Arthritis, osteoporosis and hundreds of other malnutrition diseases because now the poor person has an imbalance in the digestive system where he is not breaking down food, so bones become brittle and weak. Two years later "the doc" is writing him a prescription for arthritis medication. Within ten years the poor guy is on a long list of prescriptions to address problems caused from previous medications. He goes in for Cortisone and Prednisone shots and other steroids, which temporally kill pain but further deplete the body of its already nutrient-deficient state. This is the sad and vicious disease maintenance program most medical doctors employ in this country. It's time for a change, Americans deserve a whole lot more, a whole lot better.

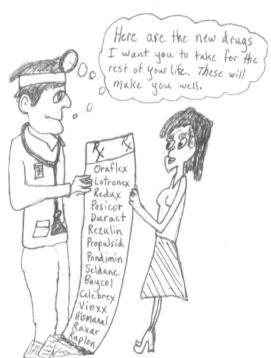

Several months ago a woman came to see me with some health problems. We performed a CEDSA exam on her to identify the cause of her imbalances. We found her liver and kidneys to be inflamed and toxic. We suggested two products for her which were a combination of herbs that flush, drain and supports the liver. She took the bottles to her medical doctor to get his approval and he told her not to take them because they could damage her liver. Obviously, this doctor was ignorant to the fact that the drugs he had her on were causing liver damage and that these herbs have been proven scientifically as remedies that will help heal her. Of course what can you expect, he hasn't been trained in nutrition or any other natural, cost affective modality. All he knows is what was taught to him in medical school, which is drugs and surgery. So why should we expect anything different than that?

> "The most dangerous untruths are truths moderately distorted."
> Georg Christoph Lichtenberg - Physicist

Your Doctor is Not God

Similar to finding a good auto mechanic to fix your car, you would be wise to find a good doctor who studies health and understands how the body heals. When your doctor tells you, "There is nothing more we can do to help you. You will just have to learn to live with your disease and maintain it with drugs for the rest of your life," then that is your wake up call. If the drugs you have been on haven't dulled your God-given senses too much, then common sense should awaken you to realize that you don't have the right doctor. Obviously his attempt to make you well with man made drugs has failed. It's time to address the cause of your disease and quit playing the symptom cover-up game. Let's find a solution to the problem and stop being a guinea pig for the pharmaceutical industry's guessing game that kills 225,000 Americans every year.

> "Call a doctor's strike and the death rate goes down!"
> Robert Mendelsohn, M.D.

Cancer patients hear death sentences from their doctors such as, "There is no hope, get your affairs in order, you have six months left to live." What your doctor is really saying is, "Well, I've tried to cut, burn, and poison the cancer and it's not working, so I have nothing else in my bag of tricks. I guess you'll just have to give up and die."

> "I believe that it is second-degree murder, if a patient dies after a doctor sends him home telling him that he will die because there is no cure. What the doctor should say is that he (the doctor) does not know what to do, therefore the patient should go to someone who does know. Or, the doctor could say, 'based upon what I know about your disease and what I know about my treatments, you will die in xx months, if you follow my program.'"
> Richard Anderson, N.M.D.

Just because your doctor's education involved drug treatment and surgery, but failed to study what promotes the phenomenon of cellular healing, does not mean that you and others around the world have to suffer and die. Your doctor is not God, only you and your Creator know when your time to depart this mortal existence is, and you do not leave until you are ready. If you are fed up with not feeling well, then you are ready to stop playing the disease maintenance game and start healing.

> "Every creative act in science, art, or religion involves a new innocence of perception liberated from the cataract of accepted beliefs."
> Arthur Koestler – Author of The Thirteenth Tribe

What is a drug anyway? Webster's Dictionary defines a drug as "A substance other than food intended to affect the structure or function of the body." In the Bible there is mention of sorcery. The word sorcery comes from the Greek word phar-ma-kia which translates into the English language as drugs.

> "Thy merchants were the great men of the earth; for by thy sorceries (phar-ma-kia) were all nations deceived." Revelation 18:23

Americans are being deceived when it comes to health. There is no money in curing disease in comparison to treating symptoms with drugs and surgery. No one can argue against this fact. When people come into our clinic and we correct the cause of disease with natural remedies, then they no longer need our services. A wise person might take some natural things to occasionally prevent, but for the most part they do their recommended program and then go on about their lives. This is how healthcare should be.

> "If our scientists and medical colleges would put forth the same effort in finding the virtues in the "true remedies" as found in nature for the use of the human race, then poisonous drugs and chemicals would be eliminated and sickness would be rare indeed."
> Jethro Kloss

Hypocrites

We have been led down a dark, shady path to believe in drugs. Yet, we shout to our young school children at the top of our lungs, "Just say no to drugs," while we take Prozac to be happy and pop Tylenol for our headaches and Prilosec for heartburn.

If a child watches mom take Tylenol for a headache and Prozac for depression, is that reasonable? Most Americans think it is totally fine because these drugs are legal. Well, if we silently teach our children to take a drug to fix our problems, then it is absolutely logical to think it reasonable to have a drink, smoke marijuana and who knows what else to relax, de-stress and fix our problems.

What kind of message do we send to our children when we look externally to fix internal problems? If we are emotionally out of balance and never address the reason and simply dry up our tears with a "happy pill," we are teaching our children that dulling our senses with drugs is acceptable. We all want our children to grow up to be happy, healthy and an influence for good in the world. But are we silently saying to our children "DO AS I SAY, NOT AS I DO?" I believe the saying goes, "I cannot hear what you are saying because your actions scream so loudly."

> **"Ignorance is not knowing but knowing what isn't so."**
> Mark Twain 1835-1910

It's time to change. Let's teach this next generation to fix problems instead of hiding them. Let's teach them to take care of themselves by paying attention to their minds and bodies. When issues come up, as they always will, let's teach our children to find the source of the problem and correct it at its root. Let's do this ourselves and lead by example, if we love our children who will eventually take care of us.

The unspoken language of example is one that's never erased from a child's mind who is searching for direction and purpose in life. Nothing ever needs to be said. Your example does all the talking for you on what's right and wrong, good and bad. Talk is cheap. Walk the walk and make a difference.

> **"Wherefore by their fruits ye shall know them."** Matthew 7:20

In the book, *Magnet Therapy* by Ron Lawrence, M.D., Paul Rosch, M.D., and Judith Plowden the following history of medicine is given.

A Short History of Medicine	
2000 BC	Here, eat this root.
AD 1000	That root is heathen. Here, say this prayer.
AD 1850	That prayer is superstition. Here, drink this potion.
AD 1940	That potion is snake oil. Here, swallow this pill.
AD 1985	That pill is ineffective. Here, take this antibiotic.
AD 2000	That antibiotic is artificial. Here, eat this root!"

Chapter 10
YOUR HEALTH UNDER ATTACK

Balancing the Body

1. **Circulatory System** - Consists of veins, arteries and the heart. A fresh supply of nutrient rich, oxygenated blood feeds your 100 trillion living cells that make up you.

    Ginkgo biloba, ginseng, butcher's broom, cayenne, ginger and flaxseed increase circulation.

    Hawthorne, magnesium, potassium, L-carnitine, L-taurine, and Coenzyme Q-10 support the heart.

Our best products for circulation are Circu Plus & Gota Plus.

2. **Lymphatic System/Immune System** - Includes the spleen, tonsils, appendix, thymus, adenoids, lymphocytes, lymph nodes, lymph vessels and lymph fluid. Any swelling (edema), fluid retention, usually indicates insufficient drainage or infection. The lymphatic system drains toxic waste from the body similar to a septic tank and drain field that allows waste material to be flushed from the toilet out of your house.

    Swelling occurs when your immune system is working and fighting infection or when there is insufficient drainage. Removing any of these organs is simply throwing part of your immune system in the trash, as if God made a mistake when He created you. Why would you want to get rid of your own soldiers who are fighting to get you healthy?

The immune system fights off invading organisms such as bacteria, viruses, fungus and other environmental toxins. Lymphocytes are white blood cells that clean up garbage. Each person has about one trillion of them working like little "Pac-Man" garbage eaters. From the time you began reading this sentence, over 800,000 of them have been created and destroyed! The thymus gland is the training camp that sends out special forces like navy seals we call B and T cells to sound the alarm of danger and fight. After the war, all the dead soldiers (cells) are taken to be disposed of in the spleen.

To drain the lymphatic system we have found echinacea, nettles, solidago, dandelion, elderberry, Oregon grape, red root and yellow dock to work well. *My best lymphatic drainage products are lymphatic drainer, Alpha E Spleen & Trifolo Plus.*

To build up the immune system and charge our infection fighters we use; echinacea, goldenseal, cat's claw (una de gato), elderberry, astragalus, myrrh and pau d'arco.

My favorite immune boosting formulas are Echinacea Plus, Immu Boost, Arcozon, Immu Plus and Thymo Plus.

3. **Digestive System** – Includes the stomach, liver, gallbladder, pancreas, small intestine and large intestine. The stomach needs potassium and zinc in order to manufacture hydrochloric acid to mix with your food. Once the food is mixed properly, it goes into the small intestines where enzymes are called in for the chemical break down that changes food into the nutrients that enter the blood. The left over wastes are then passed into the large intestine or colon and then released through bowel movements. Healthy individuals have a bowel movement after every meal. If you have fewer, you are constipated. Two or three bowel movements a day is normal.

The liver is a filtering station that performs over 500 different functions. No one can be healthy without a properly functioning LIVE-ER. Bile is made in the liver and then stored in the gallbladder. Every time we eat something with fats, bile is secreted to help us break down the fats, just like you squirting dish detergent in hot sink water to cut the grease and wash the dishes.

The pancreas secretes insulin to regulate blood sugar levels. Sodium bicarbonates from the pancreas helps neutralize stomach acids. The pancreas also manufactures enzymes to break down foods.

Nettles, dandelion, milk thistle, barberry and hydrangea support the liver and gallbladder. Black Radish, betaine, pepsin and chlorophyll are good stomach supporters. *For liver support I suggest Dandi Plus and Hepachol. To support the gallbladder and break up gallstones we use Hydrangea, LGB – AP (for parasites) and Beta Plus.*

Chromium, vanadium, cinnamon, bitter melon, gymnema sylvestre, nopal cactus, American ginseng and fenugreek support the pancreas and blood sugar. To move the bowels we use aloe vera, senna leaf, cascara sagrada and psyllium husk.

*For digestive support I recommend Alpha Gest and Diadren Forte. *(Do not take Diadren Forte if you have an ulcer – the protease will irritate it).*

4. **Nervous System** – Major parts of the nervous system are the nerves, spinal cord, brain and sensory organs. Subluxations of the spine and emotions are common nervous system disrupters. Magnesium, potassium, ginkgo biloba, valerian root, passion flower, skullcap, kava, evening primrose oil and chamomile help restore balance to the nerves.

Manganese nourishes discs in the back and can help chiropractic adjustments hold.

I recommend Nerve Formula, MG/K Aspartate and Circu Plus.

5. **Endocrine System** -

Pituitary - This is the master gland that controls the activity of all the other glands. Headaches can be caused from an imbalance in the pituitary due to a manganese deficiency.

Manganese, yarrow, calcium and pituitary concentrate supports pituitary function. *Pitui Plus is our pituitary support formula.*

Pineal - The pineal produces melatonin which helps balance our sleep/wake cycles.

Botanical melatonin and magnesium can help you sleep. *Our Melatonin formula helps with insomnia and is a natural sleep aid.*

Thyroid - The thyroid controls body weight, metabolism and body temperature.

Iodine from kelp, bovine thyroid concentrates, magnesium, suma, maca, yarrow and amino acids support the thyroid. *Thyro Plus and Kelp Complex are our thyroid support remedies.*

Parathyroid - The parathyroid regulates calcium levels in the body. Arthritis, kidney stones and bone spurs can be caused from an imbalance in the parathyroid.

Detoxification for the sycosis miasm will help balance the parathyroid gland so that excessive calcium doesn't build up in the body causing kidney stones and spurs.

Thymus - The thymus is part of the immune system that trains B and T cells to fight infection and keep you healthy.

Vitamins C, B-complex, folic acid, chromium, natural tocopherols, calcium, pantothenic acid, echinacea and cat's claw support immune function. *Thymo Plus and Echinacea Plus are thymus support formulas.*

Adrenals - The adrenals help us deal with stress and give us energy. They control electrolyte (mineral levels) in the body and help regulate metabolism. Afternoon fatigue, blood sugar issues and dizziness when standing up too fast can be signs of sluggish adrenals. Most respiratory issues usually involve weak adrenals.

Pantothenic acid, royal jelly, bovine adrenal concentrates, ginger, licorice, vitamin C, suma and maca support the adrenal glands. *To support the adrenals we use Adrena Plus, Sumacazon and Licro Plus.*

Pancreas - The pancreas controls blood sugar levels and glucose metabolism.

Calcium, magnesium, digestive enzymes (amylase, lipase and protease), pancreatin, choline, inositol, chromium, L-lysine, hydrochloride, pepsin and ginger support the pancreas. *Diadren Forte, Ginger Plus and Cinnamon 6 are pancreas support formulas.*

Gonads – Females have ovaries and males have testicles. They secrete hormones responsible for the development and functioning of secondary sex characteristics.

<u>FEMALES</u> – Amino acid complex, zinc, bovine ovary and uterus concentrates, blue cohosh, black cohosh, dong quai, yarrow and natural progesterone cream support the female reproductive system.

I suggest Endo Glan F, Sumacazon, Ovary-Uterus Plus and Female Formula.

MALES – Ginseng, ginger, yarrow, eleuthero, sarsaparilla, kola nut, yohimbe, saw palmetto, flaxseed oil, calcium, magnesium, boron, zinc and amino acid complex supports the male reproductive system and prostate.
Endo Gland M & Male Formula are good. For prostate problems I suggest Prosta Plus and Juni Plus.

The Endocrine System

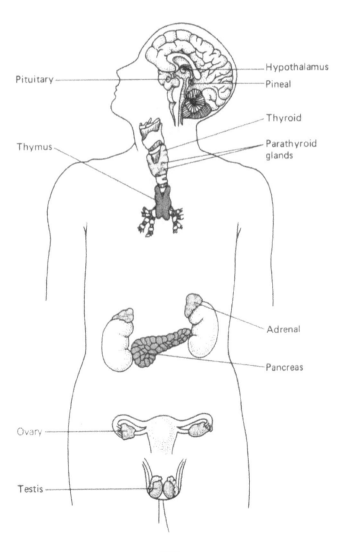

6. **Urinary System** – The kidneys, ureters, bladder and urethra process fluids in the body. The kidneys filter the blood to remove wastes (urea-protein metabolism waste) and maintain proper balance of water, salts and acids.

Solidago, juniper berries, echinacea, cat's claw, uva ursi, corn silk, parsley, horsetail and bovine kidney concentrate supports the urinary system.

I recommend Rena Plus, K/B Plus & Solidago.

7. **Respiratory System** - The respiratory system includes the nose, mouth, sinuses, pharynx, trachea, bronchial tree and lungs. Your cells need oxygen in order to live. The respiratory system brings oxygen into the body and expels the waste products better known as carbon dioxide.

Mullein and lobelia are good for the lungs. Myrrh, echinacea, bee pollen, royal jelly and eucalyptus help open the sinuses.

I suggest Mullein Plus, Pneumo Plus & Adrena Plus to support the lungs. To support the sinuses we use Myrrh Plus, Hista Plus and Adrena Plus.

8. **Reproductive System** – The male genitalia includes the penis, testicles and prostate. The female genitalia includes the ovaries, fallopian tubes, uterus, vagina and mammary glands.

*See male and female gonads above for nutritional support.

For females I recommend Endo Glan F, Sumacazon & Ovary Uterus Plus. For Male support take Endo Glan M, Male Formula, Prosta Plus & Sumacazon.

> "Tomorrow is the most important thing in life. It comes into us at midnight very clean. It's perfect when it arrives and it puts itself in our hands. It hopes we've learned something from yesterday."
>
> John Wayne

Circulation

Every organ and gland is nourished with oxygen and nutrients from the blood. If calcium begins plaquing in the body, then blood flow in the arteries can become sluggish and eventually blocked. Cholesterol and fat build up can also cause restriction of blood flow, which may lead to blockages. When circulation becomes sluggish, organs and glands begin to starve. Naturally, cells will become diseased and eventually die without proper nutrition and oxygen supply. The blood is your 100 trillion cell's lifeline.

High blood pressure is an emergency warning sign sent out by the cells when they are starving for oxygen and nutrition. When the troops are starving they send a message to increase the blood pressure so more nutrition and oxygen can squeeze through clogged arteries and reach cells far away from the heart. We take blood pressure medication that acts as a dictator to force the body to reduce the pressure. The cells that screamed for nutritional support were told to "shut up" as the new high blood pressure dictator drug is now running the show. Eventually, those deprived cells become diseased and then we ask for more drugs to deal with neuropathy, numbness, tingling, cold hands and feet, poor memory, etc. It's time we understand that the body is producing symptoms for a reason and the purpose is to get our attention so that we fix the problem.

Many Americans have poor circulation. Do you get cold hands and feet easily? Is your memory getting worse? These are common symptoms of poor circulation, because when too little blood makes it to the cells in the brain, they become malnourished and you have trouble remembering. When the blood flow to the hands and feet is sluggish, then they get cold easy. Another symptom of poor circulation can be erectile dysfunction in men. When blood flow is restricted to the muscles of the penis, then it has a difficult time rising to the occasion.

Cancer is a symptom of poor circulation. When the blood flow is healthy then oxygen nourishes the cells and brings along a team of white blood cells (cops) whose job is to destroy any cancer (criminals). Remember, Dr. Warburg proved that cancer thrives in a low oxygen environment. By increasing circulation you decrease your risks of cancer. If the cops can't get to the crime seen then criminals can get away with murder. Cancer patients almost always need circulation support.

Heart disease is the number one killer in the U.S. and coronary artery bypass surgery is a $3.3 billion a year industry. If you want to stay off of their operating table you would be wise to periodically support your blood vessels with some circulation support. There are approximately 70,000 miles of blood vessels in the average human. When a blockage occurs in the arteries near the heart, bypass surgery is usually performed. Doctors will cut a short section of vein from the leg and use it to replace the clogged vessels near the heart. There is no doubt that many times this can save a life and the doctor becomes a hero. But what has been done to remove blockages in all the rest of the blood vessels? Nothing. It will be a matter of time until you need another bypass surgery.

> **"Most modern heart disease is caused by magnesium deficiency."**
> Mildred S. Seelig, M.D.

The Circulatory System

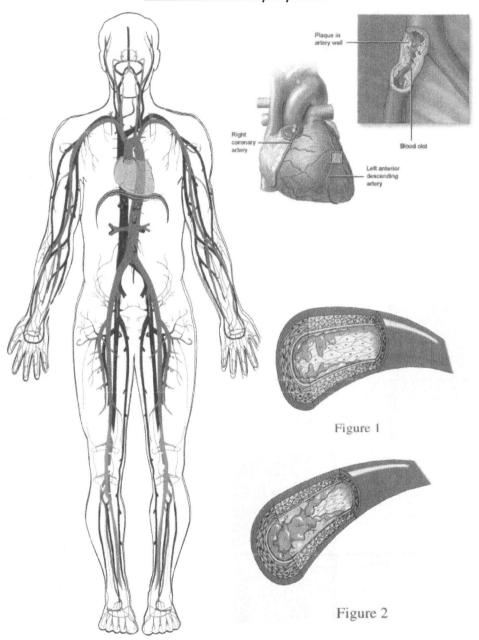

Figure 1

Figure 2

(Figure 1) shows an artery with plaque build-up beginning to restrict circulation. (Figure 2) shows plaque build up completely restricting circulation. Our best products to dissolve plaque build-up and increase circulation are Circu Plus and Ginkgo Complex.

Why Do Arteries Get Blockages but Veins Don't?

Medical doctors, who are committed to seeing their patients heal, address the causes for symptoms to manifest. A friend of mine, Johnnie Strickland, M.D., from Prattville, Alabama, focuses on healing the cause. He has found CEDSA to be an effective way of identifying what his patients need to get well. He has an interesting way of looking at what causes disease. As a medical doctor, he asks the question, "Why do arteries get cholesterol blockages but veins don't?" Dr. Strickland explains that arteries have muscles in the walls but veins don't. When the muscles contract, they produce lactic acid. If the body's pH is acidic, then it pulls calcium out of the bones to neutralize the acids. When this acid comes in contact with the calcium, it turns to stone. This combination leads to hardening of the arteries, which then causes the blood pressure to drop. When blood pressure drops below the 22mm of mercury in the capillary bed, then oxygen and nutrients are hindered from reaching cells. The cells then send out panic messages to increase blood pressure to get oxygen and nutrients to their starving cells throughout the body. Without food, cells cannot function and eventually die.

Most mainstream medical doctors will prescribe high blood pressure medication when the central pressure is elevated to bring the pressure to normal. By doing this, we get blood pressure too low in the capillary beds and over time shrinkage of tissues and cell death occurs that eventually leads to organ failure.

> "Animals don't get heart attacks, because – as opposed to humans – they produce their own vitamin C in their own bodies. Heart attacks and strokes are not diseases but the consequences of chronic vitamin deficiency and they are therefore preventable." Matthias Rath, M.D. – World-Renowned Physician & Scientist www.dr-rath-research.org

Enzymes for Health

Enzymes are the essence of life. Enzymes equal activity. Proteins, nor vitamins, nor minerals can be utilized without enzyme activity. Enzymes are the active ingredients that cure disease. How do you suppose your immune system destroys infectious microorganisms or harmful bacteria? The white blood cells release enzymes that attack and kill pathogens.

Each of us has a limited supply of enzymes at birth. The faster we use up our enzyme supply, the faster we die. The fewer enzymes we have, the weaker our immune system becomes and the more dis-ease we experience.

> "Both the habit of cooking our foods and eating them processed with chemicals, and the use of alcohol, drugs, and junk food, draw out tremendous quantities of enzymes from our limited supply."
> Dr. Edward Howell Author of Enzyme Nutrition

Raw fruits and vegetables are packed with healing elements and life giving energy. They are also filled with their own enzymes, which means they help digest themselves instead of taxing the body of its supply. Heating food over 118 degrees destroys all enzymes and most vitamins.

Enzymes help digest food, but when taken on an empty stomach, they act like the "Pac-Man" video game and eat cancer and digest garbage in the blood stream. Two German scientists, Drs. Max Wolf and Karl Ransberger, began using enzymes for health back in the 1930s. To this day, enzymes are used throughout the world to help improve health and reverse cancer.

> "The cancer cell shields itself from anticancer agents by forming a fibrin coating around each individual cell; this fibrous coating is made of protein. Proteolytic enzymes digest this protein coating, which allows the body's white cells to attack the cancer cells and destroy them." Dr. Harold W. Manner

Dr. Charles Hallquist, DCh, DD, founder of Enzyme Research operates the Oswego Center for Natural Health in Lake Oswego, Oregon. Go to www.enzymeres.com for more information. He uses enzymes to achieve optimum health with great success. Fungal forms, bacteria and parasites are all made up of protein. Viruses are protected by a protein-based shell coating. Protease is the enzyme that digests proteins.

Protease Has Been Used Effectively On The Following Symptoms

Infections	Parasites	Fungal infestations
Bacteria	Viruses	Weakened immunity
Skin eruptions	Abscess	Inflammation in ear
Hepatitis	Slow tissue repair	Hormonal imbalance
Osteoporosis	Hypoglycemia	Kidney dysfunction
Candidiasis	Canker sores	Water retention
Gout	Toxicity of the blood	Gum disorders
High blood pressure	Gingivitis	Hyperglycemia

Our protease formula used on an empty stomach helps clear up infections and clean up the bloodstream. Two capsules taken upon rising and two more before bed will help strengthen the body by cleaning up toxins in the bloodstream. This saves the immune system from extra work. When you are ready to make an investment in your health, try a couple of bottles of Protease to gobble up toxins in your blood. This is a valuable product you don't want to leave out of your arsenal. It may be wise for you to cleanse your bloodstream with Protease every six months if you want a strong immune system and vibrant health.

If you have an ulcer or gastritis, do not take Protease. It may cause a burning sensation. It's important to heal the gastritis first with our Gastro formula that does not contain protease.

Diabetes

> "To say diabetes is genetic is an evasion of the truth. The incredible rise in the incidence of diabetes does not indicate a sudden change in genes but points to an environmental cause."
> Carolyn Dean, M.D., N.D.

Diabetes is a favorite disease for mainstream medicine to maintain with drugs. Once you start their drugs, you become their life long customer. Instead of supporting the circulatory system, pancreas, liver and adrenal glands with nutrition, they monitor glucose levels and maintain it with drugs. If you are willing to make some changes in your diet and lifestyle, your body can heal.

Diabetes (type II) was unheard of before we started processing foods. Once these processed foods hit the market, diabetes began to skyrocket. Hydrogenated fats and oils are found in so many of our processed foods like crackers, chips, desserts and the fake butter substitute, margarine. Almost everything that comes in a box or package contains these highly toxic health-destroyers. This man made junk is like putting silicon sealer on the cells of your body. It seals cellular glucose receptor sites, keeping glucose out and insulin up. The result is diabetes, not to mention the clogging of arteries. Only a fool would eat silicone sealer, however, when we ingest these hydrogenated oils we are sealing glucose receptor sites and arteries no different then you sealing the outside of a window in your house. Why do you think diabetics always have poor circulation to their feet?

After watching his mother die from diabetes and cancer, James Chappell D.C., N.D., Ph.D., M.H., launched a crusade to find the cause and cure for diabetes. He reports his phenomenal findings in his book, *A Promise Made, A Promise Kept: One Son's Quest For The Cause and Cure of Diabetes*. Although the FTC and the FDA have barred him from being involved with the manufacturing of any products that help reverse diabetes, he continues to teach and write educational material under the Freedom of Speech clause in the United States Constitution.

> "I have found the ingredients that have been scientifically and historically proven to reverse (cure) diabetes."
> James Chappell, D.C., N.D., Ph.D., M.H.

The seven remedies Dr. Chappell has identified to reverse diabetes

1. Cinnamon 2. Bitter Melon 3. Gymnema Sylvestre 4. Nopal Cactus
5. Fenugreek 6. American Ginseng 7. Chromium Picolinate

Chromium

Sugar and starches break down into glucose. The pancreas secretes insulin which helps the body use glucose. Glucose is either burned as energy or stored as fat.

* Chromium is the mineral that supports proper blood sugar levels.
* Chromium helps with weight loss, high cholesterol, endurance, high triglycerides, depression, hypoglycemia and diabetes.
* *"Chromium is an essential trace mineral that helps the body maintain normal blood sugar levels. Chromium picolinate increases fat loss and promotes a gain in lean muscle tissue."* Yale New Haven Health

Cinnamon

* Dr. John Anderson of the United States Department of Agriculture (USDA) discovered a polyphenol compound called MHCP in cinnamon that mimics insulin. *"Cinnamon's medicinal properties demonstrate the most significant nutritional discovery I have seen in 25 years,"* says Dr. Anderson.

  Laboratory experiments show that cinnamon lowers glucose, blood fat and cholesterol levels along with neutralizing free radicals. If we consume too much sugar, glucose builds up in the blood and causes symptoms such as weight gain, blurred vision and fatigue. When cells begin to lose their ability to react with insulin, doctors diagnose you with diabetes. Cinnamon rejuvenates the ability of cells to react with insulin.
* Research indicates that the positive affects of cinnamon last for at least twenty days after people stop taking it. *"I don't know of any drug or product whose effects persist for 20 days, cinnamon must be an exception,"* reports Dr. Frank Sacks (professor of Nutrition at the Harvard School of Public Health).

* *"Cinnamon can improve glucose metabolism and the overall condition of individuals with diabetes; thereby improving cholesterol metabolism, removing artery damaging free radicals from the blood and improving function of small blood vessels."* Alam Khan, Ph.D. from the Agricultural University in Peshawar Pakistan

Bitter Melon

Bitter Melon is an excellent herb to help your body regulate blood sugar. When you inject yourself with insulin and take medication, your body becomes dependent upon these outside influences. Bitter Melon does not do the work for the body. It strengthens the body so it can do the work itself. Much testing has been done on this phenomenal herb and it has a promising future in the diabetic community.

* *"Pharmacological and clinical evaluations indicate that bitter melon had a significant blood glucose lowering effect and that the long term use may be advantageous over chemical drugs in alleviating some of the chronic diseases and complications caused by diabetes. The use of natural agents in conjunction with conventional drug treatments, such as insulin, permits the use of lower doses of the drug and/or decreased frequency of administration which decreases the side effects most commonly observed."* Journal of Phytotherapy, Dr. W Jia, W Gao and L Tang
* Memorial Sloan-Kettering Cancer Center acknowledges bitter melon as an important remedy for health issues. They claim, *"Bitter melon has been used to treat diabetes, cancer, viral infections and immune disorders. Data suggests it has a significant hypoglycemic effect."*
* *"Bitter melon appears to have multiple influences on glucose and lipid (fat) metabolism that strongly counteract the effects of a high-fat diet,"* says Dr Q. Chen and Li Et from the University of Hong Kong, The People's Republic of China.

Gymnema Sylvestre

Gymnema sylvestre in Hindi means, "sugar destroyer," because it actually blocks the sugar receptor sites. This plant has been used to treat diabetes in India for over 2,000 years. It has proven to be effective in enabling cells to take in glucose while preventing adrenaline from stimulating the liver to produce glucose thus reducing blood sugar levels. This plant is simply amazing.

* Harvard Medical School along with Natural Standard states, *"There is evidence to suggest that gymnema can lower blood sugar levels in people with Type I and Type II diabetes."*
* Yale New Haven Health from Yale University states, *"Gymnema sylvestre will often improve blood sugar control in diabetics. Although no interactions have been reported, gymnema may decrease the required dose of insulin."*

* *"Results confirm the stimulatory effects of gymnema sylvestre on insulin release indicate that this herb acts by increasing cell permeability,"* reports Drs. SJ Persaud and PM Jones (Journal of Endocrinology November, 1999 at the School of BioMedical sciences, King's College, London, England).
* From the Journal Ethnopharmacol, October 1990, Dr. ER Shanmugasundaram, et al, from the University of Madras, India, says, *"Gymnema sylvestre therapy appears to enhance endogenous insulin, possibly by regeneration and/or revitalization of the residual beta cells in insulin-dependent diabetes mellitus."*

Nopal Cactus

The ancient Aztecs in Mexico used this "prickly pear" to treat and cure diabetes and it is still being used in Latin America today. Nopal cactus blocks absorption of sugar in the intestinal tract, which results in lowered blood sugar levels. It is also good for lowering blood pressure, cholesterol and triglycerides. It helps curb the appetite and break down fat.

* In The Archives of Medicine as reported by the Department of Internal Medicine in Mexico, Drs. AC Frati, N Diaz Xiloti, et al., state, *"Diabetic patients had a significant decrease of serum glucose reaching from 41 to 46% when taking nopal cactus."*

American Ginseng

Ginseng is considered "The king of all herbs," in Asia. It is very effective for chronic fatigue, stress, mercury poisoning, circulation, memory, nervous system disorders and diabetes. It is also antibacterial and anti-viral. Ginseng lowers blood glucose levels.

* Pritzker School of Medicine, University of Chicago, Dr. Jing-tian Xie, states in the Pharmacology Res. 2004, *"American ginseng possesses significant anti-hyperglycemia and thermogenic activity and may prove to be beneficial in improving the management of Type 2 diabetes. American ginseng berry possesses significant antihyperglycemic and anti-obese effects."*
* The University of Toronto, Canada concludes that American ginseng produces a significant reduction in blood sugar for diabetics.

Fenugreek

* *"Fenugreek significantly reduced blood sugar and improved the glucose tolerance test with a 54% reduction in 24-hour urinary excretion,"* states Drs. R.D. Sharma, T.C. Raghuram and N.S. Rao from the National Institute of Nutrition, Council of

Medical Research, Hyderabad, India.
* Jaipur Diabetes and Research Center reported in the India Journal Association of Physicians by Drs. A. Gupta, R. Gupta and B. Lal, *"Use of fenugreek seeds improves glycemic control and decreases insulin resistance in mild Type 2 diabetes.*
* Sloan Kettering Cancer Center states, *"Fenugreek exhibits hypocholesterolemic, hypolipidemic, and hypoglycemic activity in healthy and diabetic humans and animals."*

Scientific research has been proving the benefits of herbs. If your doctor fails to acknowledge that research, then what does that say about him or her? It's time we give the body nutritional support that actually empowers the body to heal. Who wants to maintain disease with toxic, expensive drugs when Mother Nature has a far superior and less expensive product without the side effects?

Chiropractic Adjustments

"The body is controlled by the nervous system, which is made up of your brain and spinal cord. The brain sends signals to the rest of your body via the spinal cord. These signals go to every organ, muscle and tissue of the body. If at any time there is an interruption to these signals due to a misalignment of one or more vertebrae, then not only will the body not receive the proper communication from the brain, but it can not properly send messages back to the brain. This interruption of neurological signals is called a subluxation. The cause of the subluxation is stress. There are three kinds of stress; physical, chemical and mental/emotional.

The primary purpose of a chiropractor's profession should be the detection and removal of subluxations. The chiropractor does this with what is called an adjustment. An adjustment is a very specific force put into the body. This force may be applied by the chiropractor using their hands, an instrument or even a very light touch. The purpose of the adjustment is to re-establish the communication between the brain and the rest of the body, thereby allowing the body the opportunity to heal itself."

Dr. Jon Alan Smith

Let's suppose your car tires keep wearing unevenly. Within six months of buying new tires they are so worn on the inside that they blow out. Now you have a choice. You can buy new tires every six months when the inside tread wears away, or you can take your car in and get it aligned so that the tires wear evenly and last seven times as long. What makes sense to you? You can do the same thing with the bones and joints in your body.

If you are out of alignment, then it would be wise to have a chiropractor adjust you so that the vertebrae are aligned and the joints aren't wearing unevenly. Some people who "trust their doctor" will go in every three years for some type of back, neck, hip or joint surgery. Others get aligned so that their joints wear evenly similar to tires on a car. Headaches and pain subside once subluxations are corrected because the pressure is taken off the nerves. Your organs and glands can, once again, function properly with restored nerve function.

Chiropractic care has been proven to be very beneficial for promoting health and eliminating disease. Anything we do to balance your body is promoting health. Remember, balance is the key to life. Too much sunshine can burn and damage your skin and not enough, creates a vitamin A deficiency. Too much water will drown you, not enough and you will wither up like a prune and dehydrate to the point of death. Balancing your system through chiropractic adjustments is a necessary step in achieving optimum health.

Your nerves are like electrical wiring in a house. It's nice to flip the switch and have the lights come on. What happens when you flip the switch and the light fails to illuminate? An electrician has to trace the electrical line looking for a short. A short in your nervous system many times is caused by a subluxation, where pressure is placed on a nerve, thus short circuiting the energy flow to an organ or gland. No electricity flowing to your adrenal glands can cause a symptom known as chronic fatigue.

A kinked garden hose restricts the flow of water. A kinked (pinched) nerve in your body turns the energy off to that particular area, setting you up for pain and disease.

Which way makes the most sense to fix the problem?

1. Surgery: Cut a hole in the hose before the kink and insert a new hose to reroute the water around the kink and splice back into the main hose.
    #### Or...
2. Adjustment: Take the hose by the end and straighten it out, then adjust it by twisting it in a manner that takes the kink (pressure) out and allows the water to flow out smooth and unrestricted?

Healing Poisoned Medicine

Effects of Spinal Misalignments

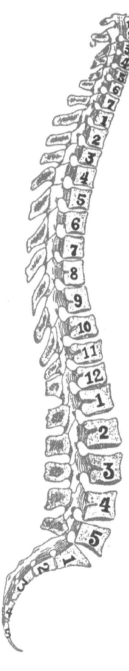

Vertebrae	Areas Affected		Common Effects of Subluxation	
Cervical 1	• Blood to the head • Pituitary gland • Facial bones • Scalp	• Brain • Inner & middle ear • Sympathetic nervous system	• Headaches • Nervousness • Insomnia • Head colds • High blood pressure	• Migraine headache • Nervous breakdown • Amnesia • Chronic tiredness • Dizziness
Cervical 2	• Eyes • Optic nerves • Auditory nerves • Sinuses	• Mastoid bones • Tongue • Forehead	• Sinus trouble • Allergies • Crossed eyes • Deafness	• Eye troubles • Earache • Fainting spells • Certain cases of blindness
Cervical 3	• Cheeks • Outer ear • Teeth	• Trifacial nerve • Face bones	• Neuralgia • Neuritis	• Acne or pimples • Eczema
Cervical 4	• Nose • Lips	• Mouth • Eustachian tube	• Hay fever • Catarrh	• Hearing loss • Adenoids
Cervical 5	• Vocal cords • Pharynx	• Neck glands	• Laryngitis • Hoarseness	• Throat conditions: coughing or croup
Cervical 6	• Shoulders • Tonsils	• Neck muscles	• Stiff neck • Pain in upper arm • Tonsillitis	• Whooping cough • Croup
Cervical 7	• Thyroid gland • Elbow	• Shoulder Bursae	• Bursitis • Colds	• Thyroid conditions
Thoracic 1	• Forearms to fingers • Esophagus • Trachea		• Asthma • Cough • Difficulty breathing	• Shortness of breath • Pain in the arms and hands
Thoracic 2	• Heart (valves and covering) • Coronary arteries		• Heart conditions • Certain chest conditions	
Thoracic 3	• Lungs • Breast • Pleura	• Chest • Bronchial tubes	• Bronchitis • Pleurisy • Pneumonia	• Congestion • Influenza
Thoracic 4	• Gall bladder	• Common duct	• Gall bladder conditions	• Shingles • Jaundice
Thoracic 5	• Liver • Solar plexus • Blood		• Arthritis • Fevers • Anemia	• Low blood pressure • Poor circulation • Liver conditions
Thoracic 6	• Stomach		• Dyspepsia • Indigestion	• Heartburn • Stomach troubles
Thoracic 7	• Pancreas	• Duodenum	• Ulcers	• Gastritis
Thoracic 8	• Spleen		• Lowered resistance	
Thoracic 9	• Adrenal and supra renal glands		• Allergies	• Hives
Thoracic 10	• Kidneys		• Kidney trouble • Nephritis	• Artery hardening • Chronic tiredness
Thoracic 11	• Kidneys	• Ureters	• Skin conditions	• Eczema, boils, acne
Thoracic 12	• Small intestines	• Lymph circulation	• Rheumatism • Gas pain	• Sterility
Lumbar 1	• Large intestines	• Inguinal rings	• Constipation • Colitis	• Diarrhea and dysentery • Hernias
Lumbar 2	• Appendix • Lower leg	• Abdomen	• Cramps • Acidosis	• Difficulty breathing • Varicose veins
Lumbar 3	• Sex organs • Knees	• Uterus • Bladder	• Bladder trouble • Menstrual trouble • Bed wetting	• Impotency • Change in life symptoms • Knee pains
Lumbar 4	• Prostate gland • Sciatic nerve	• Muscles of low back	• Sciatica • Lumbago	• Frequent or painful urination • Backaches
Lumbar 5	• Lower legs	• Ankles and feet	• Poor circulation • Cold feet	• Swollen or weak ankles • Leg weakness or cramps
Sacrum	• Hip bones	• Buttocks	• Sacroiliac conditions	• Spinal curvature
Coccyx	• Rectum	• Anus	• Hemorrhoids • Pruritus (itching)	• Pain while sitting

The example seems ridiculous, but so do the numerous real life experiences people have reported of doctors performing unnecessary surgeries that many times make the problem worse. It makes no sense to not try chiropractic adjustments first, before letting someone drill or cut into your body. If a few adjustments can correct the problem (as it usually does), you have saved yourself a huge ordeal. Do not be mistaken. Sometimes surgery is necessary for some individuals in certain situations, however, if we can correct a problem through simple noninvasive adjustments, then doesn't that make better sense?

The following case study is a great example of what an amazing healing capability the human body possesses. When Kelly Lee came to see me, she handed me the following list of what she had been diagnosed with and symptoms she was experiencing.

Symptoms Kelly Was Experiencing

Chronic Fatigue	Insomnia	Restlessness	Weight Gain
Sluggish Metabolism	Allergies	IBS	Acid Reflux
Indigestion	Halitosis	Gas	Poor Circulation
Muscle Pain	Joint Aches	Foggy Thoughts	Poor Memory
Headaches	Irritability	Yellowing of Eyes	
Depression	Oral Candida	Black under Eyes	

> **"If prescription drugs really worked-we would already be a disease-free society!"** James F. Balch, M.D. – Author of Prescription For Nutritional Healing

Case Study – Aug, 2007

For many years I felt that my health was coming to the end of the road. Luckily, I found that there was a light at the end of the tunnel. It started a long time ago when I was just a child. It seemed when I was young that I was always sick. I know now, in retrospect, that much of that was caused, at least in part by the fact that I was severely emotionally abused. My health got progressively worse with age.

When I was 29 years old I became very ill with extreme fatigue, and abdominal pains that rendered me unable to eat. I started having panic attacks, oral candida, and diarrhea. I went to the emergency room on numerous occasions because I was so sick. They would give me shots and a bag of glucose and send me home. On Christmas Eve in 1997, I was admitted to the hospital. They removed my gallbladder, diagnosed me with acid reflux and a hiatal hernia. After being released from the hospital, I still felt sick. I continued going in for test after test and the doctors couldn't find anything wrong. I was put on numerous drugs that never cured me. At this point in my life I felt so sick and hopeless that suicide was my only answer. Through the help of my family I went to see a mental health physician and she diagnosed me with IBS (Irritable Bowel Syndrome) due to depression. I was prescribed antidepressants. I was sick on and off for the next nine years. I took truckloads of antibiotics and pain pills.

In 2005 I began gaining weight like I was pregnant and fluid buildup was causing me to swell so badly that I couldn't see my ankles. My doctor prescribed fluid pills and then an extreme burning began in my legs and feet that made me feel as if I were on fire. From that point on, I was juggled back and forth from doctor to doctor who could never help me.

At this point in time I could hardly walk. It was then that I was introduced to a chiropractor by the name of Dr. Jon Alan Smith. He helped me tremendously. Soon I was able to walk again.

I was still experiencing some moderate pain in my legs when I heard about Dr. Sainsbury. On Aug 17, 2007 I went in for an appointment with Dr. Sainsbury and that is when my world changed. He did a CEDSA exam on me and what he found was overwhelming. I cried. My body was so toxic. My liver was especially weak. My blood sugar levels were out of balance and my body was extremely acidic.

I went home and cleaned out my medicine cabinet and threw away the drugs. I am now off of my prescriptions and doing well. I cleaned out my kitchen and bought healthy foods. I have been on the program over a month now and I feel great. I have lost 35 pounds and feel like I am ten years younger. I would give a million dollars for this program. It has been an amazing journey. I can't wait to see how far I can go.

I encourage anyone who feels like having good health is hopeless, not to give up. I thank God everyday that I was able to heal using chiropractic health care and naturopathic remedies. Thanks, Dr. Jon Alan Smith and Dr. Reed T. Sainsbury for giving me my life back.

Kelly Michelle Lee
Albertville, Alabama

The Healthiest People in the World

> "Those who now advocate eating natural foods as the only source of vitamins and minerals live in a dream world of yesterday. What was yesterday's law is today's folly. It really doesn't matter how well you balance your meals, or if you're a meat-eater, vegetarian, or a raw-foodist, you still run the risk of malnutrition if you try to get all your vitamins and minerals exclusively from the foods you eat."
> — Paavo Airola, N.D., Ph.D.

Where do the healthiest people in the world live? Researchers have identified five cultures whose people live on the average of our human genetic potential of 120 years of age with no major diseases as Americans know so well. In the January, 1973, issue of National Geographic Magazine these cultures were examined. They are all Third World countries with no modern day medicine.

Five Long-Lived Healthy Cultures

1. The Himalayan Tibetans of Northwestern China
2. The Hunzakut of Eastern Pakistan near Mount Rakaposhi
3. The Russian Georgians of the Caucasus Mountains in Western Russia
4. The Vilcabamba Indians in the Andes Mountains of Ecuador
5. The Titicaca Indians in the Andes Mountains of Southwestern Peru

What do all these cultures have in common? Dr. Wallach lists the following in his book, *Rare Earths Forbidden Cures*.

1. The communities are found at elevations ranging from 8,500 feet to 14,000 feet in sheltered mountain valleys.
2. The annual precipitation is less than two inches.
3. Their water source for drinking and irrigation comes from glacial melt and is known universally as "Glacial Milk" because the highly mineralized water is an opaque white or gray color from the presence of an enormous amount of suspended rock flour.
4. There is no heavy industry or modern agriculture to pollute their air, water, or food.
5. Only natural fertilizer including animal manure, plant debris, and "Glacial Milk" is applied to their fields.
6. Western allopathic medicine is not available to these cultures.

> "The difference between the child prodigy (i.e. - music, art, math, physics, athletics, etc.) and the high school dropout is not genetics or income level of the parents, but rather the nutritional (and especially the mineral intake) competency of the child during pre and postnatal development." Joel Wallach, D.V.M., N.D.

According to Dr. Wallach's research, millions of people are born each year with totally unnecessary physical defects. Allopathic medical doctors try to pin defects on genetics, but the research proves otherwise. For example, it is true that Down's Syndrome or Trisomy is a chromosomal defect in which there is an extra chromosome twenty-one. However, Dr. Wallach has proven that Down's Syndrome is not genetic. He explains, *"It in fact is the result of a preconception zinc deficiency which produces a chromosomal/DNA injury or defect similar in nature to the changes created by radiation."* He continues explaining that, *"Nutritional studies in animals and cell cultures have demonstrated that Trisomy 21 or Down's Syndrome can be created at will in the laboratory by preconception zinc deficiencies during the formation and development of the sperm and the egg – these facts underscore the critical nutritional needs for sexually active men and women. It has been clearly demonstrated in the laboratory animal, pet animal and agriculture experiments 98% of all birth defects are not "genetic" in nature, but in fact are nutritional deficiencies of the egg, embryo and fetus and can be prevented by preconception nutrition."* Dr. Wallach continues to explain that, in the animal industry, these tragic and expensive birth defects have been eliminated by giving correct nutrition to breeding animals.

"To understand how the developing embryo is so dependent upon a proper and adequate supply of vitamins, minerals, amino acids and fatty acids, we have to appreciate that embryonic tissues develop faster physically and biochemically than the most aggressive cancer cells; this rate of growth and development requires dizzying amounts of essential nutrients to complete certain biochemical and tissue maneuvers on time – the train only passes by once, if it is missed there is no going back and the child will be born with one or more biochemical, physical, mental or emotional defects." To say it simply, if we want to be healthy then we need to supplement our diets and make sure we have the necessary minerals for health. The research has been done which proves a great scientific breakthrough in preventing diseases yet the powers that be suppress it.

Mineral Functions and Deficiency Symptoms

ANTIMONY – effective against blood flukes
BISMUTH – ulcers & bacteria (Heliobacter Pylori)
BORON – bone metabolism, osteoporosis, proper endocrine function
CALCIUM – arthritis, back pains, Bell's Palsy, bone spurs, brittle fingernails, calcium deposits, depression, eczema, high blood pressure, hyperactivity, insomnia, irritability, kidney stones, limb numbness, muscle cramps/spasms/twitches, nervousness, osteoporosis, panic attacks, periodontal disease, PMS, pica, rickets, tooth decay
CESIUM – cancer aid: produces alkaline condition
CHROMIUM – ADD/ADHD, anxiety, aorta cholesterol plaque, coronary blood vessel disease, depression, diabetes, Dr. Jekyll/Mr. Hyde rages, elevated blood cholesterol, elevated blood triglycerides, fatigue, hyperactivity, hypoglycemia, infertility/decreased sperm count, learning disabilities, peripheral neuropathy, retarded growth
COBOLT – anemia, anorexia, growth and nerve system function
COPPER – hair loss, anemia, aneurysms, arthritis, cerebral palsy, criminal/violent behavior, depression, diarrhea, dry brittle hair, fatigue, hernias, high blood cholesterol, hypo/hyper thyroid, ptosis (sagging tissue), Kawasaki disease, learning disabilities, liver cirrhosis, ruptured discs, low blood sugar, respiratory disease, swachman's syndrome, varicose veins, white/gray hair
EUROPIUM – doubles the life span of laboratory animals
FLUORIDE – in plant based colloidal form will aid bone strength & no toxicity
GERMANIUM – oxygen utilization, enhances immune function. Deficiency may cause arthritis, cancer, low energy, osteoporosis
GOLD – reduces joint inflammation
IODINE – *Copper is needed to utilize iodine. Iodine is needed for proper thyroid function. Deficiency may cause* cold intolerance, brittle nails, bulging eyes, constipation, depression, dry skin & hair, elevated blood cholesterol, excessive sweating, fatigue, goiter, hair loss, hand tremors, heat intolerance, heavy periods or less than 28 day cycles, hypothyroidism, irritably, inability to concentrate, insomnia, low basal body temperature, low sex drive, muscle aches/pains/cramps/weakness, nervousness, poor memory, puffy face, rapid pulse, under-active thyroid, weight gains & weight loss.
IRON – anemia, anorexia, brittle nails, confusion, constipation, depression, dizziness, fatigue, fragile bones, GI upset, headaches, heart palpitations, irritability
LANTHANUM – chronic fatigue
LITHIUM – ADD, depression, infertility, manic depression, reproductive failure
MAGNESIUM – anxiety, asthma, anorexia, birth defects, calcification of small arteries, confusion, depression, hyperactivity, hypotension, insomnia, irritability, menstrual migraines, muscle pains/tremors/weakness, Nervousness, neuromuscular problems, restlessness, seizures, SIDS, tachycardia/palpitations, tetany/convulsions, tremors, vertigo
MANGANESE – asthma, arteriosclerosis, convulsions, dizziness, hearing loss, hypoglycemia, infertility, loss of sex drive, poor cartilage formation, still births, spontaneous miscarriages, tinnitus
MOLYBDENIUM – helps enzyme functions

NEODYMIUM – doubles life span of laboratory animals, enhances cell growth
NICKEL – anemia, dermatitis, poor growth, rough dry hair
PHOSPHORUS – anorexia, anxiety, bone pain, fatigue, irritability, numbness
POTASSIUM – acne, constipation, depression, edema, fatigue, glucose intolerance, insomnia, mental apathy, muscular weakness, nervousness, palpitations, salt retention, tachycardia
PRASEODYMIUM – doubles life span in lab animals, proper cell growth
SAMARIUM – doubles life span in lab animals, proper cell proliferation
SELENIUM – age spots, Lou Gehrig's disease, Alzheimer's, anemia, cardiomyopathy, cataracts, cystic fibrosis, cancer, fatigue, heart palpitations, HIV, infertility, keshan disease, liver cirrhosis, multiple sclerosis
SILICA – increases collagen in bones, brittle fingernails, dry brittle hair
SILVER – kills over 650 bacteria, viruses and fungals. systemic disinfectant
STRONTIUM – can replace calcium
SULFUR – collagen diseases, lupus, degeneration of cartilage, ligaments and tendons
THULIUM – doubles the life span of laboratory animals
VANADIUM – aids in glucose transport. Enhances insulin effectiveness. Deficiency may cause cardiovascular disease, diabetes, infertility, obesity
YTTRIUM – doubles life span of laboratory animals
ZINC – brain defects, clubbed limbs, Down's syndrome, hiatal hernia, spina bifida, webbed toes or fingers, acne, anemia, depression, enlarged prostate, eczema, fatigue, infertility, loss of sense of smell, poor memory, sterility, white spots on nails & weak immune function.

U.S. Senate Document #264

"The alarming fact is that foods – fruits and vegetables and grains, now being raised on millions of acres of land that no longer contains enough of certain needed minerals, are starving us – no matter how much of them we eat! No man of today can eat enough fruits and vegetables to supply his system with the minerals he requires for perfect health because his stomach isn't big enough to hold them."

"The truth is that our foods vary enormously in value, and some of them aren't worth eating as food....Our physical well-being is more directly dependent upon the minerals we take into our systems than upon calories or vitamins or upon the precise proportions of starch, protein or carbohydrates we consume."

"It is bad news to learn from our leading authorities that 99% of the American people are deficient in these minerals, and that a marked deficiency in any one of the more important minerals actually results in disease." U.S. Senate Document #264 published by the 2nd session of the 74th Congress (1936).

The fact that our soils are depleted of minerals and therefore our foods lack necessary minerals for health is one cause of disease. Farmers fertilize their fields with NPK (nitrogen, phosphorus and potassium). Why? Because these are the primary nutrients required by plants to give farmers a maximum yield for maximum profits. The other 57 minerals are many times lacking from the foods we eat. Supplementing your diet with minerals is a wise insurance policy to make sure your body is getting what it needs for optimum health.

So what do you do to make sure you are getting minerals into the body that are absorbable and utilized at the cellular level? We recommend a liquid product by Drucker Labs called intraMAX. It's a 100 percent organic microcomplexed ALL-IN-ONE "carbon-bond" living product. Dr. Richard A. Drucker, N.D., N.M.D., Ph.D. formulated the intraMAX product to be 100 percent vegetarian, drug free, ultra hypoallergenic, 100 percent natural with no additives. Go online to druckerlabs.com for more information.

The intraMAX formula contains over 415 organic minerals and nutrients.

70+, trace minerals	154 antioxidants	12 essential fatty acids
42 amino acids	stabilized oxygen	16 plant derived enzymes
49 super green foods	59 herbs	80 vitamins & nutrients
22 macrominerals	27 vegetables	65 electrolytes
11 optimum seeds/sprouts	36 fruits	Noni (organically bound)
13 probiotics	12 carotenoids	25 fibers (all natural)
119 bioflavonoids	aloe vera (organic)	8 essential sugars
38 essential oils	carbon (living)	silver (organically bond)
39 Bach flowers	fulvic acid	8 protein minerals
24 healing colors		

Water

> "When the well's dry, we know the worth of water."
> — Benjamin Franklin

Clean water is a scarcity. Every year eighteen billion pounds of new pollutants and chemicals are released by industry into the atmosphere, soil and groundwater. Think of all the prescription drugs taken by Americans and then being urinated out into the sewers. Some city water is reprocessed sewer water loaded with these cancer causing drugs. They then put more chemicals in it that supposedly makes it FDA approved and safe. Safe for what? Some agencies have a different language they use when it comes to health matters. I guess it depends upon the researcher's definition of what is safe. My mother-in-law once tested her drinking water with her swimming pool water testing kit. Her drinking water had more chlorine in it than what was safe to swim in.

> "Don't assume that just because the water coming out of your tap is tested that it is safe. The EPA has cataloged over a quarter million unsafe water violations affecting over 120 million people on public water systems."
> Lono Kahuna Kupua A'O - Author of Don't Drink The Water

Chlorine

There's no doubt that chlorine kills bacteria and helps make our water supply safer than it was a hundred years ago. However, now we have a new problem. If chlorine kills bacteria, what do you think it does to our "good" or "friendly" bacteria we need in the gut? We must have this friendly bacteria in order to be healthy and keep candida yeast from getting into our blood steam. When chlorine kills off our good bacteria, we face other health issues like fibromyalgia and Lupus which usually have candida yeast as toxic culprits producing the dis-ease.

Most scientists will admit that chlorinated acids MX and DCA are two of the most dangerous chemicals you may be exposed to in our society. Both of these are in chlorinated drinking water. Chlorine is a powerful killer that harms delicate cells and DNA strands in our bodies. As a matter of fact, it has been linked to elevated trihalomethane (THM) levels found in many cancer patients (Joseph G. Hattersley, Journal of Orthomolecular Medicine vol. 15, 2nd Quarter 2000). The Journal of the National Cancer Institute reported a study that showed that drinking chlorinated water increases one's risks of developing bladder cancer by eighty percent. A Norwegian study, published in the International Journal of Epidemiology in 1992, claims that drinking chlorinated water increases the incidence of colon and rectal cancer twenty to fourty percent.

Chlorine has been found to injure red blood cells, which can lead to anemia. Chlorine in our drinking water has been proven to cause scarring of the arteries. This may lead to heart attacks and strokes. Health care professionals recommend drinking lots of water. Make sure you are drinking a healthy water and not one loaded with harmful chemicals.

Reed T. Sainsbury

Poison in Our Drinking Water

> "Fluoride is toxic to bones and increases risk of fracture at all levels of exposure including fluoridation at 1 ppm. Regardless of any other consideration, this is reason enough to discontinue fluoridation immediately."
>
> John R. Lee, M.D. - Author of Natural Progesterone

Sodium fluoride (hydrofluosilicic acid) is an industrial pollutant, a waste byproduct of aluminum manufacturing and phosphate fertilizer companies. If you are a highly intelligent business owner, the best way to get rid of your trash (byproducts) is to convince someone else it is highly beneficial for them and you'll sell it to them at a bargain price.

Sodium fluoride is rated more toxic than lead in chemistry indexes and just a hair less toxic than arsenic. It's also a halogen that destroys enzyme function and a deadly toxin used in rat poisoning products. It kills rats by destroying their digestive system. Our taxes pay millions of dollars to put this deadly junk into our drinking water!

According to John R. Lee, M.D., there have been eight reliable scientific studies done (and no reliable contrary ones) showing that fluoridation is associated with increased hip fractures. Furthermore, there is a significant association of fluoride and osterosarcoma. Dr. Lee points out that the chance of osterosarcoma for males ten to nineteen years old was 6.9 times higher in fluoridated municipalities compared to nonfluoridated areas.

Does Austria, Belgium, Denmark, Egypt, Finland, France, Germany, Greece, Holland, India, Italy, Luxembourg, Norway, Spain, Sweden, and Switzerland know something we Americans don't? What do they all have in common different then the United States? They have researched the fluoride myth and have banned the trash from being put in their drinking water.

In 1977, Dr. John Yiamouyiannis and Dr. Dean Burk (Former head of cytochemistry at the National Cancer Institute) conducted a study on cancer rates in ten fluoridated American cities and ten non-fluoridated cities over a twenty-year period. Americans never heard about this study because the results were counterproductive to aluminum manufacturing companies selling their waste product to us to put in our drinking water. What the study revealed was an increased mortality rate from cancer in those living in cities with fluoridated water.

When we ingest fluoride at levels as low as 1ppm in drinking water, it causes chromosomal damage by interfering with the DNA's ability to repair itself. Hey, isn't that what cancer does? Sounds like some pretty bad stuff, doesn't it? In this day and age with one out of every three Americans coming down with cancer, isn't it about time we stay away from chemicals and practices that have shown any possibility of increasing disease and harming our body? Why in the world do we tolerate this poison being put in our drinking water?

The only difference between the fluoride in rat poison and your fluoridated toothpaste is the parts per million. In fact, it is documented that as little as one-tenth of an ounce of fluoride can cause death. You'll notice that on your tube of toothpaste the FDA has a warning label to contact poison control or a physician if you accidentally swallow the crap.

A can of fluoride sold over the counter comes in a can marked "poison" with skull and crossbones. Wouldn't it be wiser to use something natural that won't poison your body if accidentally swallowed? There is no way you can brush your teeth with fluoridated toothpaste without some of it being absorbed in your mouth's sensitive cells. How much toothpaste do our children accidentally swallow each time they brush?

> **Let me state clearly and loudly that fluoridation of the water is the biggest hoax in medical history perpetrated on innocent people in the name of science."** Paavo Airola, Ph.D., N.D.

Calcium fluoride is what helps strengthen teeth, not sodium fluoride. We have been bamboozled into believing that by disposing of this pollutant into our drinking water, we can help prevent cavities in teeth. What a bunch of utter nonsense. There is plenty of scientific proof if you're willing to investigate the matter instead of believing whatever ALCOA (Aluminum Company of America) tells you to believe.

It is completely absurd to think that putting sodium fluoride in our drinking water is no different then using calcium fluoride because they're both fluoride. Dr. Richard Anderson explains, *"It would be like saying that the air we breathe is a gas (which it is), so therefore breathing Mustard Gas must be good also. Mustard Gas is good for killing just like sodium fluoride is good for killing."*

In 1938, Gerald H. Cox, a biochemist for the Mellon Institute (The Mellons were owners of ALCOA), presented the plan for adding fluoride to our drinking water. A big shot attorney, Oscar Ewing, supported Cox's plan. Clever reports surfaced to persuade us to put this toxic waste in our drinking water while other reports that proved fluoride to actually increase tooth decay were buried.

> **"The great mass of people will more easily fall victim to a big lie than a small one."** Adolf Hitler - Mein Kampf (1925)

The fact is that there were no animal studies, nor any double blind, controlled studies done to prove fluoride to be safe. They just went ahead and subjected 40,000 humans to the left-over-trash from aluminum. Before they began the studies, there were no thorough dental examinations, no X-rays performed, on the people in the experimental area. How were they expecting to find out if fluoridation was harmful, safe or effective? No double-blind control studies were done, nor any measures taken to check for possible adverse effects from the fluoride on adults. Why would we just accept fluoride being put in our drinking water without proof that it was safe and effective?

The Grand Rapids-Muskegon, Michigan study is supposedly the one study that proved fluoride acceptable to be put in our drinking water. Muskegon was considered the non-fluoridated control city. This was to be a ten year study. However, five years into the study things weren't turning out how the fluoride pushers had hoped. Tooth decay in non-fluoridated Muskegon was decreasing at the same rate as the fluoridated Grand Rapids. So, what was their solution? They just decided to drop Muskegon from the study. What kind of scientific study can just drop their control group in the middle of a ten year study and then later come out with their conclusive report that tooth decay dropped in Grand Rapids after putting fluoride in the drinking water? From this, and other phony reports like it, most of the U.S. now drinks fluoridated water.

> **"For cartilage to repair, the system must be fluoride free. Fluoride in all forms, including toothpastes, should be avoided by everyone."**
> John R. Lee, M.D.

Another flaw in the fluoride hoax is that fluoride can't actually penetrate teeth because they both carry a negative charge. No study has ever been able to prove that fluoride prevents cavities. The U.S. public health service shows no difference in tooth decay statistics between fluoridated areas and low fluoridated areas.

The World Health Organization conveniently voted on fluoridation when only sixty out of 1000 delegates were present. It just so happened that it was a day when those sixty who were present were the ones who favored fluoridation. Do you think it was a coincidence?

In 1990, the National Cancer Institute publicly announced that fluoride was carcinogenic (cancer causing). Scientists at Seibersdorf Research Center in Austria have concluded that as little as 1 ppm of fluoride slows down the activity of the immune system. To hammer another nail in the fluoride coffin, U.S. geneticist have demonstrated that the degree of chromosomal damage increases proportionally in direct relationship to the amount of fluoride in the water. In fact, at the Nippon Dental College in Japan, studies show that putting the same amount of fluoride commonly found in U.S. water supplies into drinking water, causes normal cells to mutate into cancer cells. In 1982, researchers at the Japanese Association of Cancer Research in Osaka reported, *"Last year at this meeting, we showed that sodium fluoride, which is being used for the prevention of dental caries (cavities), induces chromosomal aberrations in the irregular synthesis of DNA. This year, we report findings that show malignant transformation of cells is induced by sodium fluoride."*

Statistics prove that in every city where fluoride is used in the drinking water, disease increases, tooth decay increases, births of mongoloid children increases, and crime rates are higher. Of course these reports are the ones that are kept behind the scenes. We are only given the reports they want us to hear in the news. Many doctors and scientists write books exposing these types of frauds and corruption, but sadly most of us are too busy to read their findings.

> **In point of fact, fluoride causes more human cancer death and causes it faster than any other chemical."** Dean Burk - Chief Chemist Emeritus of the National Cancer Institute

It's time to demand that we quit poisoning our water with this left over trash. Other educated countries do not allow fluoride to be put in their water supplies. We pay for the crap to be put in our water and then have health problems. Start drinking natural spring water or some form of purified water that does not contain chlorine and fluoride.

Antidepressant Drugs Cause Abnormal Behavior

> **"In my talks, I show how the molecules of emotion run every system in our body, and how this communication system is in effect a demonstration of the bodymind's intelligence, an intelligence wise enough to seek wellness, and one that can potentially keep us healthy and disease-free without the modern high-tech medical intervention we now rely on."** Candace B. Pert, Ph.D.

Doctors prescribe Prozac even with the FDA warnings of 575 side effects. As of October, 1993, there were 28,623 complaints of adverse side effects filed with the FDA, including 1,885 suicide attempts and 1,349 deaths.

> **"The modern medical system, officially known as allopathic medicine, is the most dangerous system in terms of the survival of the human race. In number of casualties (total U.S. casualties during all four years of WW 11 equal 234,874, as compared to 392,556 medical casualties in 1996 alone) it has outranked war by many times. Yet, the vast majority of people in the Western World adhere to it like glue, support it like it was their friend, trust in it like it was God, and like cattle walking to the slaughterhouse, become weaker, maimed and often, dead-long before their time."**
> Richard Anderson, N.M.D.

Many of the violent acts committed in our society and schools are committed by those who are on antidepressant or psychiatric drugs. These mood-altering drugs cause some people to do bizarre things. It's important to understand that we were meant to feel emotions. Hormones are released in tears. When we take a drug it dulls our God-given senses and suppresses our natural feelings, putting us in zombie-mode. Suppressing these emotions and tears may produce toxic grief hormones.

Dr. Joseph Glenmullen, a Harvard psychiatrist and author of *The Antidepressant Solution* explains that the reason Prozac causes behavioral disturbances is because it is similar to cocaine in its effects on serotonin. Since the 1950's it has been known that serotonin is a stress neurohormone. It is so disruptive it can cause docile animals like rabbits to become aggressive in laboratory experiments. Ann Blake Tracy, Ph.D., explains how serotonin drugs such as Prozac, Zoloft, Paxil and Effexor are extremely dangerous. We wonder why kids bring guns to school and go on a killing spree, after their doctor prescribes drugs to interfere with serotonin levels similar to cocaine.

> "In my mind, both kinds of user - the one who gets the drugs from a doctor and the one who buys them from a dealer - are doing the same thing: altering their chemistry with an exogenous substance that has widespread effects, many of which are not fully understood, in order to change feelings they don't want to have."
> Candace B. Pert, Ph.D.

Headaches

What causes headaches? Too many toxins in the body overwhelming the small blood vessels of the brain, which causes pressure against the vessel walls, can trigger headaches. Headaches can also be caused by subluxations (pinched nerves), stress, oxygen depravation, hormonal/endocrine imbalances, heavy metal/chemical poisoning, constipation and dehydration to name a few. So what do you do? If you're like most Americans, you take an aspirin or the like. Is your headache caused by a deficiency of aspirin? Of course headaches aren't caused from a lack of aspirin. Aspirin is a quick, but temporary fix.

The dangerous part of taking aspirin is that we have done nothing to fix the real problem. It is equivalent to you driving your car home and suddenly, the red engine oil light begins to flash a warning sign that something is wrong. Only a fool wouldn't stop their car and check the oil level and immediately fill it to the proper level, because he understands that continuing on without oil could result in disaster. God created your body with warning signs, called pain. The wise person heeds the warning signs and fixes the problem. Putting a bandage on a headache is like sticking duct tape over your check engine light.

Most Americans are taught to ignore their warning signals and take painkillers. The sad fact is that most people end up dealing with a much bigger problem than a headache later on. They end up in the emergency room with problems that could have been prevented. If Americans treated their health half as well as they did their automobiles, we'd be much better off.

> **"My general philosophy is the fewer drugs people take, the better off they are."** Jere Edwin Goyan - San Francisco Pharmacist, Former head of FDA

Aspirin

Americans consume more than thirty tons of aspirin per day. Since 1852, when the German chemist Gerhardt formulated it in a lab, aspirin has been no stranger in American households. Many people can't make it through a day without aspirin. Are you an aspirin addict? Do you bow down and worship the Tylenol and ibuprofen gods to make you feel good? Do you have faith and trust in these pills to work their pain-disappearing magic tricks? If not, then why do you take them? Are you aware that aspirin alone causes over 1600 people every year to go to the hospital and die from gastric bleeding? Did you know that aspirin poisons more children every year than any other toxic substance?

If you are an aspirin pill-popper, you might want to know that aspirin is a form of salicylic acid, which is also the basis for an anticoagulant used in rat poisons. How does it work to kill rats? The poison causes internal hemorrhaging and the rodent bleeds to death on the inside. You really didn't believe that little aspirin pill you've gulped down all these years was magic did you? It causes internal bleeding which eases the pressure off of your capillaries thus allowing pain to subside. So, you trade your headache in for gastric bleeding, what a bargain. In the process, it also destroys the natural mucous lining in the stomach which leads to bleeding ulcers while leaving you depleted of electrolytes.

Tylenol causes 50,000 cases of kidney failure each year. Five thousand of these are severe enough to require a kidney transplant, not to mention any liver damage that is done. Of course your doctor never tells you that the reason your liver and kidneys don't work anymore is caused from all the aspirin, painkillers and other drugs he prescribed for you to take for the last twenty years. But don't worry because once again they have you covered. Dialysis centers are being built all over to treat your drug-damaged kidneys.

Reed T. Sainsbury

Actions Speak Louder Than Words

Our children watch mom and dad pop pills to get rid of pain. Then, we sit around and wonder why they get mixed up with drugs. Being a teenager can sometimes be painful when you are trying to fit in and find out who you are and what you believe. For some, there may be times when they feel all alone and that mom and dad don't have a clue as to what they go through. They may feel pressured by friends to try drugs to fit in. Some may do it to relax and relieve stress or to just have a good time. If they have grown up their whole life watching mom and dad pop pills for headaches, heartburn, depression etc., then they may rationalize that they need more pain relief then mom and dad do in certain stressful situations.

A teenagers emotional, mental and social battles that they go through sometimes are brutal. Breaking up with boy/girl friends and trying to fit in and be accepted at school can be extremely stressful. If mom and dad's shining example of popping pills to feel good is what they've seen, then why shouldn't a teenager try drugs to "feel good?" Twenty years later, when they are addicted to crack cocaine or other substances, we tell our sob story about our child's drug abuse to others. We complain about all the money spent on rehab, battling to overcome the addiction. We just can't believe it happened to one of our babies. Perhaps our silent example to pop pills for headaches and pain spoke loud enough to tell our children that that is the solution for our pains in this world? What's the difference in popping a Tylenol for pain in the head versus some heroin when you are feeling a little down and overwhelmed by the stress of life?

Aspartame: The Poison in Our Food

> **"Aspartame (NutraSweet) is a neurotoxin and should be avoided like the plague. Aspartame has been shown to cause birth defects, brain tumors and seizures, and to contribute to diabetes and emotional disorders."** Carolyn Dean, M.D., N.D.

The U.S. has jumped on the bandwagon against sugar. Clever chemists have figured out how to manufacture a substance that tastes sweet like sugar, without calories. Are these artificial sweeteners like Aspartame the answer to our sweet tooth cravings? Doesn't it sound too good to be true? Popular artificial wonders such as NutraSweet, Equal and Splenda taste like sugar minus the calories. A dream come true for those who lack self-discipline when it comes to over indulgence in sweets. These artificial sweeteners have been incorporated into some 9,000 food products. So what's the big deal?

When Aspartame containing products such as NutraSweet and Equal are used as sweeteners and the product reaches a temperature higher than eighty-six degrees Fahrenheit (when ingested), then Aspartame breaks down into wood alcohol also known as methanol. As it breaks down further it converts into formaldehyde. Formaldehyde is made by the oxidation of methyl alcohol. This deadly neurotoxin is a common embalming fluid. It has proven to be a class A carcinogen that affects the respiratory, gastrointestinal and central nervous system. Formaldehyde is grouped in the same class of drugs as cyanide and arsenic, which are deadly poisons.

In 1969, the Searle Company approached Dr. Harry Waisman to study the effects of aspartame on primates. Seven infant monkeys were fed the artificial sweetener in milk. One died after 300 days, five others had gran mal seizures. Searle deleted these findings when they submitted this study to the FDA. Some researchers have gone as far as defining NutraSweet as nerve gas that eradicates brain and nerve functions.

Dr. H.J. Roberts, a specialist in Diabetes and world expert on Aspartame, has warned us of the dangers of using Aspartame in his book, *Defense Against Alzheimer's Disease.* He explains how Aspartame poisoning is escalating Alzheimer's Disease.

Contrary to popular belief, Aspartame in diet drinks and foods doesn't help you lose weight, it actually promotes weight gain. Dr. Roberts reports that when he got his patients off Aspartame, they lost an average of 19 ½ pounds. He says, "I now advise all patients with diabetes and hypoglycemia to avoid aspartame products." The Congressional record stated, "Aspartame makes you crave carbohydrates and will make you fat."

Most diet drinks contain high amounts of sodium. This causes people to retain water in their bodies and they become edemic. Examples of this epidemic are obvious in hospitals. Many obese nurses walk around with a diet drink in their hand at work, yet they fail to understand the principles of weight loss.

Not only do soft drinks cause weight gain through water retention, but they interfere with proper kidney and bladder function. The sugar destroys beneficial bacteria (flora) in the intestinal tract, which leads to constipation, another culprit in weight gain. Constipation, not having two or three bowel movements per day, locks toxins in the body so they can't be eliminated properly. As a result, your blood becomes toxic which feeds every cell.

In order to lose weight, fat must be flushed from the cell. The enzymes responsible for aiding the process of fat release are paralyzed when they are poisoned and cannot do their job. People defeat their purpose when they try to lose weight by drinking diet soft drinks.

Many American soldiers who served in Desert Storm returned home only to find their health deteriorating. Many complained of chronic fatigue and neurological problems. Our military consumed diet drinks that sat in the 120-degree sun for weeks while the Aspartame broke down into methanol and formaldehyde. After consuming these poisons many soldiers were diagnosed with serious health problems.

Dr. Luis Elsas, Pediatrics Professor of Genetics at Emory University, has testified before Congress stating that, in his lab tests, animals given Aspartame developed brain tumors. It is also interesting to note that when brain tumors in humans are removed and examined, many contain high levels of Aspartame residue.

Aspartame should be absolutely avoided by diabetics. It prevents stable blood sugar levels and can cause vision problems, comas, and even death. Betty Martini exposes ninety-two side effects from Aspartame poisoning that has been reported to the FDA.

Aspartame is a neurotoxin and is capable of going past the blood brain barrier and break down the neurons in the brain. Neurosurgeon, Dr. Russell Blaylock in his book, *Excitotoxins: The Taste That Kills* explains that "Aspartame may trigger clinical diabetes." For more information go to www.russellblaylockmd.com or dorway.com.

> **"The ingredients of Aspartame stimulate the neurons of the brain to death, causing brain damage of varying degrees."**
> Dr. Russell Blaylock (Neurosurgeon)

Many scientific studies indicate that systemic Lupus is triggered by Aspartame poisoning. Multiple sclerosis in many cases is methanol poisoning. The neurological problems associated with Aspartame can trigger seizures. It also interferes with dopamine levels, which only worsens the condition for Parkinson's disease.

NutraSweet and Equal are amongst some of the deadliest toxins in our society because they are hidden in so many of our foods, including, children's vitamins, medicines, Kool-Aid, chewing gum and Jell-O. Not to mention that it is found on every table in our restaurants.

Next time you reach for a "sugar-free" product or "diet drink" you might want to reconsider. The research has been done. You can choose to ignore it or use it to promote optimum health. If Americans are ever going to win the war on cancer or any other disease, it will have to start with the discontinuation of putting poisons into our bodies. Look up what Dr. Joseph Mercola has to say about these toxins on his web site www.mercola.com.

Common Symptoms Associated With Aspartame Poisoning

Headaches	Depression	Slurred speech	Fibromyalgia
Vertigo	Anxiety attacks	Chronic fatigue	Brain tumors
Cancer	Epilepsy	Graves disease	Birth defects
Joint pain	Numbness	Rashes	Tinnitus
Loss of taste	Vision loss	Seizures	Retinal problems

Fetal tissue cannot tolerate methanol. Dr. James Bowen calls NutraSweet instant birth control. The fetal placenta can concentrate phenylalanine and cause mental retardation. Aspartame tests on animals showed brain and mammary tumors. After drinking Diet Cokes for ten years we wonder why so many women have to cut their cancerous breasts off and throw them in the garbage.

Why is this deadly poison still in our foods and on the market if it has been proven so lethal? Once again, if we examine it like forensic detectives do a murder mystery, we find the answers. Monsanto, the big manufacturer of Aspartame funds the American Diabetes Association, the American Dietetic Association and the Conference of the American College of Physicians. This is one reason why toxic poisons somehow manage to never get caught. There's big money involved and careers at stake. You scratch my back and I'll scratch yours. When someone is nice enough to donate millions of dollars in your behalf, it somehow helps to magically seal their lips about toxicity issues coming from their products.

Usually, The New York Times plays ball with the big-money boys and doesn't step on too many toes. Surprisingly enough, on November 15, 1996, there was an informative article explaining how the American Dietetic Association receives money from the food industry to endorse their products. This seals their lips in engaging in any criticism of harmful food additives and connects their financial link to Monsanto.

Soft Drinks

If you desire to be healthy, then you must become a label reader. If there are things in your food and drinks that you don't know about or can't pronounce, then it might be a wise idea not to put it in your mouth. For example, in some diet drinks we find polyethylene glycol as an ingredient. This is used in anti-freeze in automobiles and as an oil solvent.

Phosphoric acid is found in most soft drinks. The phosphorus in the acid upsets the body's calcium-phosphorus ratio and dissolves calcium out of the bones. How many people do you know with arthritis who drink their cokes on a daily basis? The phosphoric acid also interferes with hydrochloric acid in the stomach causing digestive problems. Digestive problems are common for those who gulp down soft drinks with their lunch.

Aspartame, sugar and corn syrup are common ingredients in soft drinks. The large amounts of sugars found in these drinks can induce hypoglycemia or hyperglycemia, both which lead to diabetes. The sugar gives you a quick burst of energy, then fizzles out and leaves you sluggish. To get recharged, you reach for another soft drink to start the cycle over. This over taxes the adrenal glands and once the sugar-high burns off you are left feeling tired and worn out.

Aluminum cans are common containers for soft drinks. The acid in the drink eats away at the aluminum so that every time you drink a soft drink you ingest trace amounts of aluminum. Aluminum is very toxic and builds up in the body. It interferes with proper brain function and has been linked to Alzheimer's disease.

Most soft drinks are very acidic with a pH of about two. Remember that our ideal pH should be 6.8-7.0. So if we are continually drinking acidic, carbonated beverages throughout the day, how do we expect our pH to be in a healthy range? It won't, and that is one reason we have so much disease in this country. Soft drinks should be avoided or reserved for only special occasions as a treat.

> **Soda (soft drinks) is the number one acid producing substance ingested into the body. Thus the country's number one killer is really soda!"** Johnnie Strickland, M.D.

Birthing

Dr. Lewis Mehl of the University of Wisconsin Infant Development Center researched some 2,000 births. Half of the births took place at home and the other half in the hospital. The study reported that there were thirty birth injuries among the hospital born children and none among those born at home. Fifty two of the babies born in the hospital required resuscitation, while only fourteen of those born at home. Six hospital babies suffered neurological damage, compared to one born at home.

A hospital is where sick people go. Why would a healthy pregnant woman want to go where sick people are to have a healthy baby? Think of all the sick people coughing with infections and those germs. No doubt there are millions of germs circulating through the heating and cooling system's duct work blowing in on you and your brand new baby. Is this what we want to expose our brand new infants to on the first day of life?

The first mistake doctors make when a woman is in labor is laying her flat on her back. The woman should be up and walking or in whatever position feels most comfortable to her. Lying flat on her back makes unnecessary work for the woman's body. She has to bring the baby uphill, against the force of gravity. Using gravity to assist the birth, squatting is a very natural and effective way to deliver.

The next mistake is made when the doctor breaks the water. Labor should start on its own and it will when the mother's body and the unborn child is ready. When the doctor goes in and breaks the water, Mother Nature is out of control and the doctor is in control. Think about it. The pregnant woman's body was intelligent enough to grow a new life, do you think it somehow gets confused at the end and is all of a sudden not smart enough to know when to break the water and let the baby come down the birth canal?

Childbirth should be as natural as possible to ensure good health and wellness for your baby. Robert A. Bradley, M.D., in his must read book for pregnant couples, *Husband Coached Childbirth,* explains how most doctors interfere with the natural birthing process that leads to unnecessary pain and suffering. With the help of the husband, Dr. Bradley has delivered over 23,000 babies and concludes that only three percent need cesarean sections and another three percent require medicated births. The remaining ninety-four percent should deliver fine with the husband doing most of the work. The doctor is there as a lifeguard in case further assistance is needed. Dr. Bradley's statistics are astounding when compared to how many women are coaxed into drugging themselves up in hospitals and going into surgery for a C-section in order to pull the child out. Coming through the birth canal is a natural stressful experience for the child to go through.

In the U.S., thirty-five percent of births end up with doctors pulling the child out by C-section. That is saying that one-third of our women are abnormal and are not capable of a natural God-designed vaginal birth. This is ridiculous, especially if you look at Third World countries where the masses can't afford surgery. Strangely, women there seem to deliver babies fine. The problem is once again money. The doctor makes a whole lot more by performing a C-section and then of course it is done when convenient for him so he can schedule you and the baby around his schedule instead of him being available when you and your child are ready. That way, he doesn't miss the golf game or the weekend on the lake, because he has taken control and decided when the baby will be born. He breaks the water, does the C-section and is on his way. It's nice for him but the mother and child are forced into the most beautiful and sacred moment in life before they are ready.

Hospital Birth vs. Home Birth

> "The safest place for a healthy mother to have her baby is not in a hospital, but at home. …I tell all healthy women, including my own daughters, that they should refuse to have their babies in the hospital." Robert Mendelsohn, M.D.

Our first child, Dallas was born in the hospital. My wife, Bethanne was in labor for about thirty-six hours. When her contractions got intense, we went to the hospital. As soon as we walked in they immediately made her get in a wheelchair and would not allow her to walk. She was upset because she knew walking was good when in labor. They took her to a room and made her lie down on her back. She was only dilated two centimeters. They convinced her to get an epidural for the pain. The doctor came in and broke her water. Later on, she began pushing and the nurse could see the baby's head. She called for the doctor and he didn't come. The nurse told her not to push anymore. Bethanne argued that she felt she needed to push. The whole thing was ridiculous and about fifteen minutes later the doctor casually came in, taking his own time.

After all that, Bethanne's temperature and the baby's heart rate were escalated a little. They wanted to start with drugs and Bethanne said she didn't want a drug to lower her body temperature. The doctor then suggested, "Well maybe you should find yourself a new doctor if you don't want to follow my orders." They sent another doctor into our room to convince us that baby Dallas needed the drugs even if Bethanne refused to take them. This doctor said over and over, "Your baby could die!" We asked that they wait for the results to come back from the lab to see if something was actually wrong before they gave her the drugs. They used scare tactics to administer the drugs immediately. When the lab work came back, there was nothing wrong with our baby or Bethanne. After a huge fiasco, we finally made it home.

Two years later Bethanne was pregnant with our second child, Brooklyn and we didn't want another experience like we had at the hospital. We found a knowledgeable and loving midwife who we felt comfortable with helping us experience the miracle of birth. We could feel her love and dedication to helping bring children into the world in a safe and peaceful way. Every month we would go and meet with her and she would do some routine checks. We loved her and she loved us. We were on the same team, whereas in the hospital we dealt with arrogant, insensitive strangers who were just there to do their job and pick up a paycheck.

About three in the morning Bethanne said, "The baby's coming, I can feel it." I called Karen, our midwife, and she said that she was on her way. Bethanne walked, kneeled, sat and did whatever her body told her to do. If she was hungry, she ate. If she was thirsty, she drank. She started feeling the urge to push just a couple of hours into the labor and with one push baby Brooklyn was born into my arms. Karen was right beside me the whole time, coaching me to deliver my own baby. We let baby Brooklyn lie on Bethanne's chest and nurse for about a half-hour and after the placenta detached by itself I cut the cord. Karen then asked everyone to step outside the room except me, my wife and our new baby. We sat there bonding with our child and basking in the intense love and the miracle of birth. It was beautiful, the most sacred and awesome experience I have ever had.

After Brooklyn was asleep, I told Bethanne to get some rest. She replied, "I'm not tired." She took a shower, got dressed and we went outside for a walk. Our third child, Rockman was born at home also. We were actually eating dinner at a restaurant when the contractions came on strong. We went home and called our midwife. Karen came over about ten p.m. A little after one a.m. my son was born and once again, I was a proud father. There were no drugs used and my wife and son did wonderfully. Family and loved ones were in our home that night to experience the birth of our son. After he was cleaned up, everyone came into the room to see him and we quietly sang happy birthday to him. That is how it should be when we come into this world and more importantly, that is how it should be when we leave this world. We should be surrounded by family and friends, not a bunch of strangers in a hospital where sick people are.

After having experienced home births and hospital births, Bethanne says there's no way she would ever go back to the hospital when she could have the baby in the comfort of her own home surrounded by loved ones.

> "After working in hospitals for most of my life, I can assure you that they are the dirtiest and most deadly places in town. ... 5% of all hospital patients contract new infections that they didn't have when they arrived." Robert Mendelsohn, M.D.

Protein

How much protein does your body require in order to be healthy? The average American consumes 90 to 120 grams of protein per day. Let's see what some of the experts say. According to extensive research on protein, Dr. Ragner Berg, a world famous Swedish nutritionist, whose works on nutrition are used as text books in medical schools says that 30 grams of protein in the daily diet is a generous allowance. Dr. Siven from Finland reports 30 grams of protein a day as well. Dr. Chittenden concludes that athletes and soldiers require 30-50 grams of protein per day for maximum physical performance. Dr. Eimer showed that an athlete's performance improves after switching from a 100-gram a day animal protein diet to a 50-gram a day vegetable protein diet. Dr. Hegsted of Harvard University concludes that 27 grams of protein a day to be the correct amount. The Japanese expert, Dr. Kuratsune, reported that 25-30 grams of protein a day is sufficient for good health.

> "There is little evidence that muscular activity increases the need for protein." The National Academy of Science

Scientific research has proven that protein combustion is no higher during heavy exercise than under resting conditions. As a matter of fact, physical performance in sports and people who perform heavy physical work do better on a low protein diet. John Robbins, author of *Diet For A New America,* explains how Dave Scott won the grueling Ironman Triathlon an amazing six times, on a vegetarian diet. The world record for the twenty-four-hour triathlon, which consists of swimming 4.8 miles, cycling 185 miles, and running 52.4 miles in a single day, is held by Sixto Lenares who is a vegetarian. He does not eat meat, dairy or eggs. Where does he get the protein to have all the strength and stamina to perform such tough competitions? It's time to reveal the forbidden secret of health. That secret is; all fruits and vegetables contain protein.

Robert Webb holds the world record for climbing Mt. Shasta in the least amount of time. In order to climb Mt. Shasta in Northern California, it takes the average mountain climber eight hours to go from the 8,000-foot level to 14,164-foot summit. People who make the climb in five hours are considered to be in outstanding shape. Only elite athletes can make the climb in less than three hours and they are considered super-human. Robert Webb made the climb in 1 hour and 39 minutes! The next best time is 2 hours and 24 minutes. Even more impressing than that is that Mr. Webb set another world record in 1998. He climbed Mt. Shasta six consecutive times and set the world's record for the most elevation gain in a 24 hour time period. All of these climbs were done at over 8,000 feet in elevation and he soared over 36,000 feet in 24 hours! Out of those 36,000 feet climbed, 24,000 were above the 10,000-foot mark. Have you tried exercising at 10,000 feet elevation before?

So what's the big deal, Mr. Webb is an awesome mountain climber right? Mr. Webb also happens to be a colon cleansing health enthusiast who eats whole living foods, which he believes, gives him his strength and stamina. Fruits, vegetables, nuts, seeds and whole grains are your best sources of protein. It seems to be the popular belief that you need milk and meat for protein. Why do Americans believe this? Because the meat and dairy industry pay big advertising fees to make sure that we do. They need you to believe that lots of protein builds healthy bodies. You know the dairy industries slogan, "Milk it does a body good." The truth is that protein is found in almost all foods and it is almost impossible for you not to get enough of it.

Where Do Cows Get Protein?

If you look at a cow or a massive Brahma bull, what do they eat to get so big? They eat plant-like material such as alfalfa, grasses, corn and grains. How much milk does an adult cow drink? None, of course. Well then, how does she get protein to produce milk for her calf? Obviously, she gets all the protein she needs from a vegetarian diet. What about her calf who gains a pound of body weight per day? What does it eat? Mother's milk, and it contains less than three percent protein for that calf to double its body weight every few months. What does this tell us about protein consumption?

Some will argue that cows and humans are different and that it isn't a fair comparison, so we will look at a baby human. What is the newborn baby fed? It should be mother's breast milk exclusively for the first six months to one year, according to health experts. Now, how much protein is in mother's milk? Less than 2%, usually 1.6 percent and that child doubles in size in a short amount of time. So, if a child, who doubles in body weight every six months has a diet consisting of less than two percent protein, how much do non-growing adults require? Not near as much as the media wants you to think. Most adults are looking to lose, instead of gain weight.

What's the strongest animal in the world? Pound for pound, a gorilla is king. Gorillas are ripped and chiseled and have massive physiques that would intimidate any NFL football player. A gorilla has a digestive system very similar to humans. As a matter of fact, if you take the intestinal tract from a gorilla and a human and lay them side by side, you cannot tell which one is which. How long do they live? They live about 140 years. What do they eat? They consume fruits, vegetables, grains, nuts and seeds. Where do they get all the protein to build massive muscles containing tremendous amounts of strength? Gorillas don't eat steak, chicken, milk, eggs, cheese and protein muscle-gainer powder-5000. They eat a vegetarian diet. A little piece of information that was probably never taught to you is the fact that protein is found abundantly in Mother Nature's perfect whole foods. Green vegetables, fruits and grasses contain protein and it is easily absorbed and digested by the body, especially when compared to cooked animal meat.

High Protein Diets – Not So Healthy

A friend came to me excited about losing forty pounds of weight. He proceeded to tell me about how he cut carbs out and enjoys eating bacon, sausage and eggs for breakfast. He eats meats for lunch and more meat for dinner. By eating lots of meat and cutting out breads, pasta and sugar, he is losing weight. It is true that high protein diets will help you lose weight, however, there is a price to be paid.

Eating a high protein diet places a tremendous burden on the digestive system to break all that meat down. Not to mention all the nitrates, phosphates, steroids and other harmful chemicals put in as preservatives and fed to the animals so that they grow bigger in a shorter amount of time. As mentioned earlier, meats are high in purines which break down into uric acid. These acids accumulate in the joints. In order to buffer the acids, the body will use up its sodium, calcium, potassium, magnesium and iron reserves thus leaving you depleted. These acids are what cause inflammation, joint pain, gout and arthritis. It also causes the pH to be very acidic, which creates the terrain for all diseases to thrive. Remember, an alkaline terrain is where good health grows and an acidic terrain favors disease.

High protein diets create a negative calcium balance in the body which leads to arthritis. In other words, the more protein we eat, the more calcium is lost through the urine than is absorbed by the body from our food. This is why most arthritic people are heavy meat-eaters and dairy product consumers. The body uses up its mineral reserves to buffer the acids created by the high protein diet. When this happens, bone density decreases and osteoporosis sets in. Your mainstream medical doctor never addresses this cause, but you can bet your bottom dollar he has a bag full of prescriptions ready to prescribe to treat the pain. Lots of money is made by maintaining the arthritic condition but never healing the cause. Like one client told me, *"The cortisone shots made me feel better but once they wore off the intensity of the pain kept getting worse and worse. I knew that this was not the answer to health."* Once he came in and we addressed the cause and got his body more alkaline, his arthritis was gone like bumblebees in winter.

People who are on the high protein diets to lose weight are setting themselves up for disease. You may lose forty pounds, but gain sore stiff joints and eventually battle cancer and heart disease. If we want to lose weight, we would be wise to get on a high vegetable diet. If you don't have blood sugar issues, you can eat all the fruits and vegetables you want and you'll lose weight. What causes us to gain weight is when we eat all these foods along with breads, pastas, processed foods, dairy and meat.

Mother Nature's foods are cell builders. You'll lose weight and feel great. You can't overeat with fruits and vegetables. How many carrots can you eat in one sitting? Once you eat what your body needs nutritionally, you lose the desire to eat more. Your body will let you know when you've had enough and you won't feel bloated like you can easily do with cooked, processed foods like breads, pasta, dairy and meat. Even with sweet fruits like apples or grapes, you can only eat until you are satisfied and then your body will let you know when you've had enough and you stop eating before you feel full and bloated. This is how our bodies were designed to receive nutrition.

The following case study is an example of what happens to the body when an athlete consumes a high protein diet for many years. The doctor told him there was no cure for arthritis and that pain medication and steroid injections were the only treatments available. After changing to an alkaline diet and getting his pH to a 7.0, Leon was feeling eighty-five percent better in two months.

Case Study – December, 2007

I'm a 60 year old Tool and Die Maker (machinist) by profession. For most of my life I have been very involved in athletics and fitness training. I am a 2nd degree Black Belt in Yoshukai Karate and was an instructor for 1 ½ years. I have also been an avid runner most of my life, running at least five miles a day.

Going to the gym every morning at 4:30 to train keeps me in shape but has taken a toll on my joints. For most of my life I have been in tip-top shape, able to do 500 pushups and sit-ups without stopping. This I would do every day. When I was in my prime I could do 200 consecutive pull-ups. I would spend four hours a day training in the gym.

In 2003 I tore my meniscus in my left knee kicking. Then in 2005 I had my left shoulder scoped. I had torn the rotator cuff completely loose and also the bicep tendon. In 2006 I was attacked by a cat and had to have surgery on my right arm and wrist. The cat bite got infected and actually did nerve damage to my arm and caused me to lose some of the cartilage in my wrist. I had a lengthy recovery and did not heal well. My injuries forced me to stop training. In 2007 I had my right knee scoped. I felt like my body was falling apart and my joint pains were becoming unbearable. Then I hit another brick wall, pleurisy in my left lung, not to mention my sinus trouble that had been plaguing me for the last 20 years.

My chiropractor, Dr. Hudgins has helped me get off the steroid drugs I was taking for my sinuses. She recommended I see Dr. Reed Sainsbury, a naturopath, for my other complaints.

I was taking Darvocette for pain but that wasn't enough so I started taking 6 to 8 Aleve on top of that every day for joint pain. In the past I had been on Dyclophenac, Celebrex, Loritabs and massive amounts of Tylenol and aspirin. I was living on pain medication.

When I went to see Dr. Sainsbury he did a CEDSA exam and identified what was causing my joints to be in so much pain. He checked my pH and found that I was very acidic and taught me that my high protein diet was killing me and preventing me from healing. He told me that if I wanted to get well I would have to get off the acidifying meats and get on an alkaline-vegetable diet. I was willing to do anything to get rid of this pain.

He found that my body had a tremendous amount of pesticides built up in my kidneys and liver, not to mention the pain medication-drug residue. He told me I was low on essential fatty acids and had a lot of calcium build-up in my body. He gave me some supplements to detoxify and nourish my body.

Once I got started on the detox program and began to juice vegetables everyday (Dr. Oz's green drink) my pain began to subside. The silver dollar-sized calcium deposit (carbuncle) on my foot has shrunk down to the size of a nickel since I've been on this program and all of my pain is gone. It's been two months now and I am feeling 80 to 90% better! I have come off all of my pain medication! I have turned things around and feel like a new person. I am amazed at how fast my body is healing. No drugs, no surgery, but lots of alkaline vegetables, herbs and nourishing supplements.

A. Leon Smith
Guntersville, Alabama

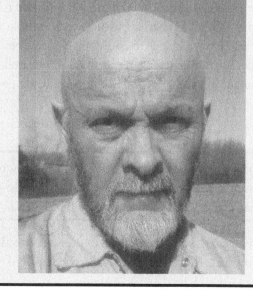

Mother Nature's Healers

Alfalfa is one of the most complete foods on the planet. It is actually higher in protein than beef. Alfalfa is 18.9 percent protein, beef is 16.5, eggs are 13.1 and milk is 3.3 percent. Alfalfa has been used for thousands of years to cure disease. It cleans, builds, strengthens and rejuvenates cells back to health. It is loaded with vitamins, minerals, amino acids and enzymes that are alkalizing agents to help neutralize acids that cause inflammation and pain. It has been used to heal just about every disease and is extremely beneficial for arthritis and gout. As a matter of fact, if you have arthritis and started today eating only fresh fruits and vegetables along with large doses of alfalfa, arthritis would disappear like ice cubes in the Arizona desert.

Wheat grass and barley greens are two more of Mother Nature's greatest healers. If we incorporated these greens into our diets, then the body's nutritional needs would be met and toxins could be eliminated. When cells are nourished and cleansed, then the disease environment disappears, inflammation subsides and healing occurs.

Bee Pollen is another complete nourishing food that is capable of sustaining life and healing disease. It is made from the flowering plant. Every little grain contains a powerhouse of nutrients. Scientists have discovered that the male sperm cells of flowering plants contain a miracle concentration of nearly all known nutrients. It is said that bee pollen contains the secret "ambrosia" eaten by the ancient gods to acquire eternal youth.

Bee pollen researchers conclude that bee pollen fights cancer. William Robinson, M.D., of the U.S. Department of Agriculture demonstrated that bee pollen added to food could prevent or slow down the growth of cancerous mammary tumors in a unique strain of mice bred to succumb to such tumors. Further research showed that existing tumors were reduced in size in the mice that were given bee pollen. The USDA published a report by the National Cancer Institute in 1948 that bee pollen has a pronounced effect on malignant mammary tumors. Other scientific studies reveal that bees sterilize the pollen they harvest with a secretion that is anticancer.

According to French researchers, an antibiotic element has been identified in bee pollen. When salmonella and other harmful bacteria are exposed to bee pollen, it is destroyed. Could bee pollen be used as a natural antibiotic? Has Mother Nature already given us the greatest antibiotics?

Where to Start?

> **Approach impossible goals by breaking them down into possible increments. Or, to put it another way: how do you move a mountain? One rock at a time."** John W. Travis, M.D.

At this point you may be convinced that you have the ability to take control of your health and be healed. However, this can be very overwhelming if you don't know where to begin.

To start out we recommend getting a complete CEDSA evaluation. You can find out exactly what toxins are in your body and what deficiencies you have. You will find out why you have the symptoms you have and what you need to regain your health. If you do not have a CEDSA exam to determine your individual needs, then you are playing a guessing game and the supplements may or may not work. You deserve more then a guess. You deserve to know. Your health is your wealth and you are worth it.

> "The journey of a thousand miles begins and ends with one step."
> Lao Tsu

Health Tips

- Keep in mind that an acidic pH will cause almost any disease you can name to thrive in your body. Remember that your body is alkaline by design and acidic by function. If we want to heal, we must get the pH more alkalized. Your body will function best when the pH of the saliva is in the 6.8.-7.0 range. This changes the terrain of the body and is an unfriendly environment for almost every disease, especially cancer.

- If we stop feeding disease, it cannot prosper. Fasting can cure disease because the body will metabolize garbage within. When we fast, cells start an automatic house cleaning party and toxins come out. That is why some people develop headaches when they fast; toxins are being released. Once the toxins come out, we feel better. The body will heal when it has correct nutrition. Many diseases are a result of malnutrition. Every cell in your body needs sodium and potassium in order to be healthy. Most of us are depleted and the result is dis-ease.

- Pain and symptoms occurring on the left side of the body are usually a cry indicating a sodium deficiency. The best foods to replenish depleted sodium levels are; spirulina, celery juice, alfalfa, okra (not fried), carrots, cabbage, spinach, strawberries, beets, cucumbers, plums, powdered whey, raw goat's milk, chicken and turkey gizzards.
  When we talk about sodium, I don't mean the junk you buy from the store to sprinkle on French fries. I'm talking about organic sodium that Mother Nature puts in plant-foods. Sodium found in fruits, vegetables and herbs are absorbable at the cellular level. It is the fuel your body needs.
  Table salt is produced by heating sodium chloride up to approximately 1500 degrees to solidify the salt crystals. Additives are used as anticoagulants so the salt will pour under moist conditions. This man-made product is not completely soluble in water or the blood stream and it can adhere to the arteries.

- Problems on the right side of the body are warning signals that the cells are in desperate need of potassium. The best emergency rescue workers to get potassium levels up are; bee pollen, alfalfa, burdock, potatoes, oranges, tomatoes, bananas, kelp, apricots and dates.

- Be aware that conventional methods of checking the blood for nutritional deficiencies are many times inaccurate. The body does everything in its power to keep the blood in homeostasis. When the blood chemistry changes, we have very serious deficiencies and we are way late to the rescue. CEDSA exams can identify nutritional deficiencies before we develop a serious problem that shows up in blood work in the lab. Don't wait until your engine blows oil everywhere to take it to the mechanic to be serviced. Remember, **"AN OUNCE OF PREVENTION IS WORTH A POUND OF CURE."**

> **"Orthodox medicine has not found a cure for your condition. Luckily for you I happen to be a quack."** Author unknown

Chapter 11
HEALING SECRETS YOUR DOCTOR NEVER TOLD YOU

ACNE
- Most acne is caused from toxins built up in the liver, spleen and or sluggish bowels. Get the bowels moving 2-3 times a day. Cascara sagrada, senna, aloe vera and psyllium are good for the bowels.
- Many times with acne we find the lymphatic system to be sluggish. Dandelion, nettles, burdock and red clover are good lymphatic, liver and spleen cleansers.
- Hormonal issues can also be a factor. Evening primrose oil can help.
- Acne in teenagers can sometimes be a potassium and zinc deficiency.
- Niacin and vitamin A can be beneficial.
- Essential fatty acid deficiency can trigger acne. Flaxseed oil, borage oil or black currant oil are good.
- *I recommend Alpha E Spleen, Omega Complete & KLS Plus*

ADD/ADHD
- Get off junk food (sugar and chemicals). Most ADD kids are sensitive to sugar. Don't skip breakfast. Start the day off with a healthy breakfast (eggs or omelet with vegetables, rolled oats, buckwheat pancakes, millet, plain yogurt, raw nuts etc.) to stabilize blood sugar levels throughout the morning. You can't feed a child sugar-laced cereals and other junk foods and expect them to sit still and concentrate all morning long in school.
- Check for food allergies and heavy metals.

- Supplement the diet with minerals, amino acids, essential fatty acids and B vitamins.
- The adrenal glands may be out of balance. Norepinephrine can be very effective.
- Check for blood sugar issues. Chromium is good.
- Thyroid dysfunction may be a factor. Kelp is important.
- Dopamine is nature's Ritalin.
- Phosphatidyl serine can be very beneficial.
- ADD kids usually have an inability to break down fats. Supplement their diets with digestive enzymes. Lipase is the enzyme that breaks down fats.
- GABA, valerian, kava, passionflower and chamomile help calm and relax.
- Ginkgo is good support for the nerves and brain.
- *I recommend intraMAX, Dopamine, Calmazon & Diadren Forte*

AIDS

- Una de Gato (Cat's Claw) is good to help stop viruses from replicating and help balance the immune system.
- *I suggest Cat's Claw, Immu Boost, Thymo Plus & Alpha E Spleen*

ALLERGIES

- Many allergies are caused by a toxic liver and intestinal tract.
- Do a colon cleanse and get the bowels moving 2-3 times a day.
- Do a liver cleanse. Milk thistle, dandelion, nettles and barberry are good liver cleansers.
- An imbalance in the digestive system can be a big factor. Take enzymes.
- The stomach needs potassium and zinc in order to produce hydrochloric acid to break down foods correctly. Undigested foods cause acidosis. When we are acidic we become highly sensitive and allergic.
- Sodium deficiency can trigger many allergies. Spirulina, alfalfa and celery juice are high in sodium.
- Stop eating dairy. Milk and dairy products are mucous forming. Mucous causes many allergies.
- CEDSA testing can identify other allergens (inhalant or food) that can be desensitized.
- The sycosis miasm can be causing increased activity in the organs and glands thus creating allergies.
- Many times you crave what you are allergic to.
- Bee pollen and royal jelly can be beneficial.
- *I recommend Myrrh Plus, Cat's Claw, Hista Plus, Uniphenol & Diadren Forte*

a
- Check for heavy metals, especially aluminum poisoning. Get silver dental fillings removed and replaced with composite materials. Locate a dentist who follows the Huggins protocol for a safe and effective extraction. For more information go to www.drhuggins.com and www.IAOMT.COM.
- Garlic, chlorella, cilantro and parsley binds to metals, thus helping the body to detoxify.
- Increase circulation, especially to the brain. Ginkgo biloba, ginseng, capsicum, rosemary and gota kola are good.
- Phosphatidyl serine and lecithin can be beneficial.
- Acetylcholine can help with memory and mental alertness.
- *I suggest Detox HM, Circu Plus, Gota Plus, Dopamine & Phosphatidyl-Serine*

ANEMIA

- Eat more raw fruits and vegetables. Bananas are good. Juice green vegetables and beets. Kelp, nettles, dandelion, comfrey, yellow dock, parsley, alfalfa and blackstrap molasses are good.
- Make sure zinc levels are balanced. A zinc deficiency will cause the body to reject iron.
- Vitamin B-12 is important.
- Iron has a positive charge and so does the lining in your intestinal tract. Like repels like, so iron and other positive-charged minerals may pass through the digestive system without being absorbed if the hydrochloric acid levels are low in the stomach. When the stomach produces sufficient amounts of acid, then this allows iron to bind with a protein. The protein is absorbed and carries the mineral piggyback into the later stages of digestion and into the blood.
- Liquid Iron by Natrol is a good supplement for anemia.
- *I recommend Ferro B Plus C, Scrofulara Plus, Alpha E Spleen & intraMAX*

ANGINA

- Magnesium is the mineral that nourishes the heart. When we get low in magnesium, we have chest pains.
- Vitamin E has proven very valuable.
- L-Carnitine, L-Arginine and coenzyme Q10 can help.
- *I recommend MG/K Aspartate, Cardi Plus & Hawthorne Plus*

ANXIETY
- Many times there is a magnesium/potassium deficiency causing the nervous system to be out of balance. Valerian, passion flower, chamomile and kava are good.
- Serotonin levels may need balancing. Norepinephrine can help especially with children.
- GABA can help calm and relax.
- B vitamins are important.
- The sympathetic and parasympathetic nervous system is like a teeter-totter that needs to stay balanced for health.
- Emotional issues from the past can throw the body out of balance into a chaotic frenzy creating anxiety. A CEDSA exam can pinpoint the source of the anxiety.
- *I recommend Valeri Plus, GABA & MG/K Aspartate*

ARTHRITIS
- Rheumatoid arthritis may be triggered by allergies, Lyme disease and heavy metal poisoning. Cat's claw is good to balance the immune system and stop viruses from replicating.
- Most arthritis is caused by an imbalance in the digestive system.
- Your diet needs to be mostly fresh fruits and vegetables. Test for allergies to make sure you are not allergic to citrus juices. Some do well to limit citrus to only once a week.
- Get your pH more alkaline, 6.8-7.0. Juicing fruits and vegetables nourishes the body, flushes acids out and alkalizes the body. Carrot, celery, and red beet juice are very effective for melting stiffness away. Raw potato juice helps arthritis. Alfalfa, comfrey, carrot tops, beet tops, wheat grass, and any other edible greens are healing foods for inflamed joints. Dr. Oz's green drink can help. Take (2 cups spinach, 2 cups cucumber, 1 head of celery, ½ inch or 1 teaspoon fresh ginger root, 1 bunch parsley, 2 apples, juice of 1 lime and juice of ½ lemon. Combine all ingredients in a juicer. This recipe makes 28 to 30 ounces or 3 to 4 servings.
- A majority of arthritis is caused from eating too much meat. High protein diets cause arthritis because they create an acidic condition in the body. The body draws upon sodium, calcium, potassium, magnesium and iron to neutralize or buffer the acids. This leaves the body depleted of minerals and without sufficient organic plant-sodium, crystallization takes place.
- Knots on the fingers, spurs and gout are warning signals by the body to get sodium into the cells. Sodium (from vegetables, not table salt) keeps the joints limber and movable.
- Supplement with enzymes and hydrochloric acid so you break your foods down and get nutrition to the cells.

- Most arthritic people have indigestion, so they take acid blockers like Prilosec, Zantac etc. These only make arthritis worse because they shut down the secretion of digestive juices in the stomach.
- Do a colon cleanse so that the small intestines can absorb nutrients.
- Get off meats and dairy products. The more milk you drink the more calcium deficient you'll become. Pasteurized milk, like meat, drains the body of alkaline minerals. It takes more calcium to digest it then it gives back. Milk does not do a body good. It does it a lot of harm unless you can get it raw from a farmer.
- Iodine controls calcium in the body and nourishes the thyroid. Get the thyroid gland balanced. Calcium, magnesium, phosphorus, vitamin D, manganese, sodium and potassium are important. Take large amounts of alfalfa, comfrey and bee pollen. They are loaded with nutrition.
- Arthritis pain on the left side of the body can be caused from a sodium deficiency. Take spirulina. It is rich in sodium. Juicing celery is very beneficial.
- Arthritis pain on the right side of the body can be caused by a potassium deficiency. Take bee pollen, burdock and alfalfa. They are rich in potassium.
- Cod liver oil is good.
- Lecithin will dissolve calcium deposits in the body.
- Orthophosphoric acid will help dissolve calcium plaquing in the arteries, kidney stones and bone spurs. It will lower blood viscosity so it shouldn't be used with blood thinner medication. It is also good for swelling.
- *I recommend Alpha Green II, Arnica Plus, Liga Plus & Alpha Gest III*

ASTHMA
- Weak adrenal glands will trigger respiratory issues. The adrenals need pantothenic acid, potassium and sodium. Royal jelly is high in pantothenic acid. Alfalfa is rich in potassium and sodium.
- Licorice root is good for the adrenals.
- Lime juice is good.
- Bee pollen can help. Mullein and ginger are all good for the lungs.
- Lobelia is a bronchial dilator. It helps you breathe easier. It also helps relax the body and is antispasmodic.
- Asthma may be allergy induced.
- Get off dairy products.
- The psorinum miasm may be a factor.
- *I recommend Mullein Plus, Licro Plus, Pneumo Plus & Adrena Plus*

ATHLETE'S FOOT
- Is a form of ringworm caused by the fungus Tinea pedis. In order to clear fungal (yeast) forms out of the blood stream, we must change the terrain of the body and get it alkaline. Fungals thrive in an acidic atmosphere. Thyme oil, tea tree oil, pau d' arco, garlic, oregano, caprylic acid, grapefruit seed extract, olive leaf extract and colloidal silver are all antifungal.
- Tea tree oil can be used topically to help kill nail fungus.
- A good probiotic (acidophilus) is important.
- Get off sugar, breads and pasta. Sugar feeds yeast. Even fruit sugar will feed yeast.
- *I suggest Lapacho Plus, Alpha Statin, Alpha Green & Alpha Dophilus*

AUTISM
- Detoxify the body of heavy metals, especially mercury.
- Vaccinations contain mercury (thimerosal).
- Supplement the diet with liquid minerals/vitamin supplement. Magnesium and vitamin B-6 are important.
- Ginkgo, dopamine and malvin may help.
- Dental fillings are another big source of heavy metal poisoning. Dr. Rashid Buttar has successfully treated over 500 children with autism in North Carolina. Look him up at http://drbuttar.com.
- *I recommend intraMAX, Detox HM, Dopamine & Universal Complex*

BACK PAIN
- Chiropractic adjustments can help tremendously if you have subluxations or pinched nerves. The adjustments may not hold if you have nutritional deficiencies. Manganese is disc food. Low back pain and headaches are many times caused from a manganese deficiency.
- Massage therapy is effective for relaxing tight muscles that are pulling vertebrae out of alignment.
- Remember, calcium is required for muscle contraction and magnesium is required for muscle relaxation. Many Americans are depleted of magnesium thus not being able to relax, feel good and sleep well.
- Inflamed and toxic kidneys can trigger back pain.
- Backed-up fecal matter in the colon can trigger back pains. Make sure your bowels are moving 2–3 times a day.
- *I suggest Arnica Plus, Liga plus & Alpha Gest III*

BALDNESS (FALLING HAIR)
- You can spend hundreds of dollars on hair care products or you can nourish the roots of your hair so it's shiny, healthy and not coming out in clumps.
- An essential fatty acid deficiency can cause the hair to fall out. Evening primrose oil is good.
- Hypothyroidism can cause hair loss. Take kelp
- Vitamin E and B complex are important.
- *I recommend Omega Complete, Chola Plus & Alpha B*

BLADDER INFECTIONS (CYSTITIS)
- Usually the body is too acidic. Get the pH more alkaline.
- Drink lots of lemon water to flush out the urinary tract and alkalize pH.
- Magnesium is good to help pass any gravel or stones.
- Organic, unsweetened cranberry juice is good to drink. Solidago (golden rod), corn silk, uva ursi, juniper, goldenseal and parsley are good.
- *I suggest Solidago Plus, K/B Plus & Rena Plus*

BRONCHITIS
- Mullein and lobelia are good.
- When we support the adrenal glands we strengthen the lungs. Royal jelly and bee pollen are good.
- The psorinum miasm may be present.
- Get off dairy products and check for other possible allergens.
- *I recommend Mullein Plus, Pneumo Plus & Adrena Plus*

CANCER
- Is a condition when organs, glands and systems are out of balance. Everyone has cancer, however, a properly functioning immune system will destroy cancer cells before they get out of control. When cells begin to mutate and the immune system is unable to stop them, then cancer is diagnosed. Instead of trying to kill, poison or radiate cancer, let's build up and balance the immune system so that it can effectively do what God created it do naturally–seek and destroy cancer cells.
- It doesn't do any good to kill the cancer if the lymphatic system cannot drain the toxins. Detoxify the body, especially the lymphatic system, liver, spleen and kidneys.
- Increase circulation. Ginkgo biloba, ruscus and ginseng are good for circulation.
- Dr. Otto Warburg, Nobel Prize winner proved that cancer cannot live in a high oxygen environment. Increase circulation and we increase oxygen to the cells. Deep breathing exercises are good.

- Rebounding on a mini-trampoline is beneficial. Dr. Morton Walker states that rebounding thirty minutes every day will reduce your risk of cancer by 90%.
- Do some emotional release. What's eating at you? Are you subconsciously looking for an escape route? Cancer patients always have emotional issues on a subconscious level. Anger, resentment and bitterness are common.
- Get the pH of the body more alkaline, 6.8-7.0. Graviola, una de gato (cat's claw) Essiac tea, laetrile, garlic and Haelin (SE 851) are good anticancer agents. Acidosis and sugar feeds tumors. Stop feeding the cancer. Get the body alkaline, change the terrain and cancer cannot exist.
- If it is white don't put it in your mouth with the exception of cauliflower.
- Remove metal, silver (amalgam) fillings from teeth and replace them with composite materials. Locate a dentist who follows the Huggins protocol for a safe and effective extraction. For more information go to www.drhuggins.com and www.IAOMT.COM
- *I suggest KLS Plus, Immu Boost, Alpha Green II, PH Enhancer, SE 851, Circu Plus & intraMAX*

CANDIDA YEAST
- Heavy metals in the body favor the growth of yeast.
- Yeast and fungals thrive in an acidic body just like mold does in a warm, dark, humid bathroom.
- Get off sugars including fruit and honey. Sugar feeds yeast. Stop eating breads, pasta and dairy.
- Oral contraceptives (birth control pills) feed yeast.
- Vitamin B-12 feeds yeast.
- Get the bowels moving three times a day. Take a multi-strain probiotic formula to balance good bacteria in the intestinal tract.
- Most vaginal yeast infections hit people who have been on antibiotics because the antibiotics kill off the good bacteria in the body and allow normal candida yeast to multiply and get in the blood (systemic). Pau d'Arco (taheebo tea), garlic, echinacea, goldenseal, caprylic acid are antifungal.
- *I recommend Lapacho Plus, Alpha Statin, Alpha Dophilus, Alpha Green & PH Enhancer*

CHRONIC FATIGE SYNDROME
- Support the endocrine system, especially the adrenal glands.
- Low energy in the morning is usually a thyroid issue. Kelp is good for the thyroid.
- Low energy in the afternoon indicates sluggish adrenal glands. Magnesium is the spark plug for the adrenal glands. Royal jelly is good for the adrenals. Norepinephrine can be beneficial.

- Lyme disease could be triggering sluggish adrenals.
- Yeast (candida) can cause low energy.
- *I recommend Endo Glan F (Female) or Endo Glan M (Males), Ginseng Plus, Diadren Forte, Sumacazon & Warrior*

CIRCULATORY PROBLEMS
- Ginkgo biloba, ginseng, butcher's broom, cayenne, ginger, garlic and parsley help increase circulation.
- High cholesterol, triglycerides and calcium plaque build-up can restrict blood flow.
- Calcium bonds to heavy metals. This is another culprit that can interfere with circulation.
- Cold hands and feet are common complaints. Magnesium and potassium helps circulation.
- Alpha phosphoric acid dissolves calcium plaquing in the arteries.
- When the pH of the body is acidic and those acids meet calcium, it turns to stone. Blockages in the arteries, kidney stones and bone spurs are results.
- EDTA (chelation) therapy can be beneficial for increasing circulation and detoxifying heavy metals out.
- *I suggest Circu Plus, Chola Plus & Ginkgo Complex*

COLDS
- The common cold is a good old-fashioned house cleaning party. When so much trash and mucous accumulates in the body and the dumpsters (lymph nodes) are so full and inflamed that your cells can't do their jobs, then they have a special clean-up party. The sinuses become inflamed and the mucous is discharged from the nose. Coughing up phlegm is another way to help rid the body of these wastes.
- Any medication you take to suppress what your body is cleaning out is about as foolish as you bringing the garbage sack back into the house after mom just took it out. She doesn't want the stinky garbage in her house and neither do your cells want mucous and garbage interfering with the work they are doing in keeping you alive.
- Make sure your channels of elimination are open. Are you constipated? Get the bowels moving 4 or 5 times a day with herbal laxatives like aloe vera, cascara sagrada, senna leaves etc.
- Do a garlic enema.
- Drink lots of water and hydrate those mucous filled areas of the body. They need water to clean with just like your toilet. It's hard to flush the crap out when there's not enough water.

- Get out in the fresh air and move. Rebound on a mini-trampoline and pump the lymphatic system so the garbage can move out.
- Do a dry brush massage to stimulate the skin. Then lie down and rest.
- When you are sick, it's good to get lots of sleep, but it's also important to go out and get some fresh air, sunshine on the skin and rebound to pump the lymphatic system.
- A hot sauna bath with essential oils (peppermint, myrrh, lavender, eucalyptus and lemon) can help eliminate toxins. Don't pour chlorinated/fluoridated tap water over your hot rocks in the sauna, unless you want a gas chamber!
- Fruits and vegetables should be your foods. Get off dairy products. They are mucous forming foods. Cook homemade vegetable soup with fresh garlic, ginger and onions. Eat three cloves of fresh garlic daily. Garlic is a natural antibiotic.
- The best herbs for colds are; echinacea, cat's claw, astragalus, elderberry, golden seal, ginger, garlic and thyme leaf.
- Colloidal silver, beta glucans, reishi mushrooms, vitamin C and zinc help fight infection and boosts the immune system.
- CEDSA testing will determine what is best for your body at this specific time.
- Colds can also be triggered by nutritional deficiencies.
- Stuffiness in the right nostril indicates a potassium deficiency. The best sources of potassium are; bee pollen, alfalfa and burdock.
- Stuffiness in the left nostril indicates a sodium deficiency. The best sources of sodium are spirulina, celery, watercress, Irish moss and dulse.
- Stuffiness in both nostrils can be helped with royal jelly, which is high in pantothenic acid and nourishes the adrenal glands.
- A sore throat and swollen tonsils can be caused from a sulfur deficiency. The tonsils are the sulfur sack of the body and they help purify the blood.
Eat eggs, onions, garlic and apricots, they are high in sulfur.
- Nasal drip can be triggered by an excess amount of mucous in the pituitary.
Gota kola and wood betony can help.
I suggest Immu Plus, Echinacea Plus, Thymo Plus & Adrena Plus

COLD SORES
- Caused from the herpes simplex virus I.
- L-lysine is very beneficial. Other important nutrients include; vitamin C, vitamin B complex, zinc, calcium, magnesium and acidophilus.
- *I recommend H-S Formula, Cats Claw, Alpha E Spleen, L-lysine and Thymo Plus.*

CONSTIPATION
- First thing upon arising, drink 16 ounces of water and hydrate the body. Just as a toilet cannot flush without water, neither can the bowels move when dehydrated. Many Americans are dehydrated and don't know it. The difference between a prune and a plum is water content.
- Beneficial bacteria (flora) in the intestinal tract is important. Antibiotics kill this "good bacteria" off. Many drugs are constipating, especially pain medication.
- Magnesium is the mineral that helps you relax so that the muscles in the colon can move. Psyllium husk, cascara sagrada, aloe vera and senna are good bowel movers.
- *I recommend Intestinal Formula & Fiber Life*

CRAMPS
- Muscle cramps and twitches are usually caused from calcium and magnesium deficiencies. Calcium allows a muscle to contract. Magnesium allows it to relax. In our high pace lifestyle we get stressed out and burn up our magnesium reserves and then wonder why we can't sleep at nights, have cramps, high blood pressure, constipation, indigestion, hormonal issues etc.
- *I recommend Cal lac Plus & Nerve Formula*

CROHN'S DISEASE
- Heavy metals and parasites can cause inflammation in the intestinal tract.
- Emotions can disrupt this part of the body.
- Mainstream medicine claims Crohn's is incurable. Dr. Jordan Rubin founder of "Garden of Life" cured himself of Crohn's disease. The Primal Defense formula is a blend of homeostatic soil organisms, fermented whole foods and 12 probiotics (good intestinal bacteria). This blend helps restore proper intestinal balance in the gut thus eliminating symptoms. Visit www.TMDiet.com for more information.
- Remove the toxins in the body, change the terrain in which all 100 trillion cells live and give the body the nutrition it needs and it heals.
- Sangre de drago from the Amazon Rainforest is a powerful antioxidant and healer.
- *I recommend Sangre de drago, L/GB-AP, Para Plus & BR-SP Plus*

CUTS
- Cayenne pepper (capsicum) sprinkled on cuts will stop the bleeding.
- Table sugar sprinkled on cuts will also stop bleeding.
- Hydrogen peroxide is a good disinfectant.
- Sangre de drago is a sap you can pour on the cut that fights infection and seals

the cut. Natives in the jungle use it effectively for large cuts when stitches aren't available. It's a very powerful antioxidant and helps knit the skin back together.
- *I recommend Sangre de drago for cuts to stop bleeding & fight infection*

DEPRESSION
- A sluggish thyroid can bring on depression. Kelp is high in iodine that nourishes the thyroid.
- People who take cholesterol medication can get the cholesterol too low and then the body can't manufacture hormones which may cause depression. Cholesterol below 150 is dangerous.
- Essential fatty acids are important.
- St. Johns wort, skullcap, valerian, kava, dopamine, L-dopa, serotonin and norepinephrine can help with depression.
- Postpartum depression is usually a sign of exhausted adrenal glands.
- *I suggest Endo Glan (F) or Endo Glan (M), Kelp Plus, Serotonin & Valeri Plus*

DIABETES
- The adrenal glands, pancreas and liver need support. Increase circulation throughout the body. Ginkgo, ginseng, butcher's broom are good vessel dilators.
- EDTA (chelation therapy) may be beneficial.
- Enzymes, chromium and vanadium are important.
- Stop consuming dairy products and red meat. They are high in fats.
- Juniper berries are good.
- Alpha Lipoic Acid is good support for diabetic neuropathy (stinging, burning, tingling etc).
- See chapter on diabetes for more details.
- *I suggest Diadren Forte, Circu Plus, Ginger Plus II & Cinnamon 6*

DIARRHEA
- The body is cleansing itself of infection. We want the infection to come out, not stay in.
- Stay hydrated. Drink lots of liquids.
- Shepherd's purse will stop diarrhea if needed. Other beneficial herbs include; bayberry, cayenne, chamomile and ginger.
- *I recommend Universal Complex & Alpha Dophilus*

DIVERTICULITIS
- Intestinal cleansing is needed. Psyllium husk powder will help sweep out built up fecal matter that causes inflammation and feeds infection.
- Stop eating meat, breads, pasta and dairy.
- Go on raw fruits and vegetable diet.
- Parasites, heavy metals and emotions can all contribute to diverticulitis.
- Be careful with small seeds and nuts. They can get trapped in diverticuli and cause discomfort.
- *I recommend Verma Plus, BR-SP Plus & Fiber Life*

EAR INFECTIONS
- Get off all dairy products, especially milk.
- Garlic, echinacea and acidophilus helps boost the immune system and fights infection.
- We recommend putting a couple of drops of Wally's Ear Oil in both ears. Warm the oil before dropping in ear. Massage the oil into the skin around the ears. It contains; almond oil, tea tree oil, eucalyptus, garlic, mullein and echinacea.
- *I suggest Otalga Plus, Immu Plus and Acidophilus.*

EDEMA
- Swelling occurs when the lymphatic system becomes sluggish.
- Many times the kidneys are bogged down with toxins. Kidneys regulate fluid levels in the body.
- Drink lots of water. Cells will hoard water if they have been deprived of water in the past.
- The adrenal glands secrete hormones that regulate salt and water balance. Cortisol helps reduce inflammation.
- A lack of potassium can cause swelling.
- Switch from table salt to sea salt.
- Start juicing carrots and celery or Dr. Oz's green drink to get mineral levels balanced.
- *I Suggest Lymphatic Drainer, Solidago, Rena Plus & Alpha Flavin*

> "The greatest crime physicians are guilty of is administering Diuretics (water pills). These pills not only take the fluid out of the body, but also the sodium, potassium, and minerals that might be in the solution, therefore starving the body of essential nutrients!"
> Donald Lepore, N.D.

EPILEPSY
- Heavy metal poisoning is the #1 culprit.
- Remove metals from teeth. Get silver dental fillings removed and replaced with composite materials. Locate a dentist who follows the Huggins protocol for a safe and effective extraction. For more information go to www.drhuggins.com and www.IAOMT.COM.
- Eggs, onions and garlic are high in sulfur. Sulfur helps detox metals out.
- Support the pituitary gland and nervous system. Valerian root, passion flower, skullcap and chamomile can help balance the nervous system.
- Vitamin B-6 can help.
- Magnesium and potassium can be beneficial.
- Serotonin, dopamine and malvin are neurotransmitters that need to be balanced for health.
- Emotional issues can be the root of epilepsy. The RFA process can heal emotional issues and subsequently heal physical ailments.
- The syphilinum miasm is usually detected in epilepsy.
- Phosphatidyl serine can be beneficial.
- *I suggest Valeri Plus, Circu Plus, MG/K Aspartate & Detox H.M.*

EYE DISORDERS (CATARACTS)
- May be a warning sign that the calcium is out of solution in the body.
- Get the calcium levels balanced. Iodine (kelp) helps keep calcium in balance.
- Vitamin E, B complex, vitamin D, vitamin C, vitamin A, zinc, selenium and L-glutathione can be beneficial.
- Heavy metals may be culprits.
- Bilberry, eyebright, bayberry, cayenne, comfrey and golden seal can help.
- *I recommend Bilberry Plus, Kelp Complex & Veno Plus*

FEVER
- Leucotaxis is the body's way of heating up to increase immune function and fight infection. Let a fever run its course, your body is intelligent and knows what it's doing. Do not suppress it with drugs unless temperatures reach 105 degrees.
- Stay hydrated by drinking lots of fluids and stay off of solid foods. Fresh fruit and vegetables juices are good.
- *I suggest Echinacea Plus and Immu Plus*

FIBROMYALGIA
- Usually chronic fatigue, joint pain and rashes are a result of the body being too acidic, accompanied with heavy metals which favors candida yeast.
- Get on a vegetable diet to alkalize the body. Start juicing Dr. Oz's green drink.
- Detox the metals out and clean up the blood.
- Get silver dental fillings removed and replaced with composite materials. Locate a dentist who follows the Huggins protocol for a safe and effective extraction. For more information go to www.drhuggins.com and www.IAOMT.COM.
- Take enzymes to help metabolize interstitial fluids that accumulate in certain areas and cause pain.
- *I recommend Universal Complex, Lapacho Plus, Alpha Green II & Diadren Forte*

FOOD POISONING
- Charcoal helps absorb toxic poisons in the body.
- Garlic and goldenseal are good.
- Drink lots of water to flush poisons out.
- *I suggest taking 6 charcoal tablets every six hours*

GALLBLADDER DISORDERS
- Gallstones can be dissolved with boldo.
- Parasites can cause liver/gallbladder issues. Black walnut hulls, wormwood, cloves, pumpkin seed powder, pink root and male fern cleanse parasites from the body.
- Stop eating pork. Meat from swine is a risky source of contracting parasites.
- Lecithin and flaxseed oil help break down fats.
- See chapter on gallbladder/liver flush for stones.
- *I suggest L/GB-AP, Hydrangea Plus & Beta Plus*
- *(For a gallbladder attack take 50 drops of Hydrangea every 1/2 hour)*

GOUT
- Get off the high protein diet. Stop eating meat and dairy.
- Get on a fruit and vegetable juice diet to get the pH of the body alkaline. Dr. Oz's green drink recipe mentioned earlier in book is good. Eat lots of red sour cherries. They neutralize uric acid.
- Burdock, nettles, dandelion, alfalfa, comfrey and parsley are good to flush out uric acid that accumulates in the joints and causes severe pain and inflammation.
- Take digestive enzymes to metabolize acids in the tissue.
- *I recommend KLS Plus, Arnica Plus, PH Enhancer & Alpha Zyme III*

HALITOSIS (Bad Breath)
- Supplement the diet with enzymes and start breaking down proteins so that the fecal matter stench doesn't come out your mouth when you speak and floor your associates.
- Floss your teeth after meals.
- Get your bowels moving 2-3 times per day.
  I recommend Otalga Plus & Alpha Zyme

HEART ATTACK
- In an emergency heart attack, a teaspoon of cayenne pepper in a cup of hot water has helped save lives.
- Increase circulation. Clean up the calcium deposits and plaque build up in the arteries so that the heart doesn't have to pump so hard to push the blood through the crud. Hawthorne berry, garlic, potassium, magnesium, L-carnitine, L-taurine, vitamin E, vitamin B complex, vitamin C, selenium and coenzyme Q-10 are good.
- All muscles, including the heart, run on potassium. Do not use elemental potassium. Plant derived or potassium aspartate are good.
- Check for the Coxsackie virus. It can cause the heart to malfunction.
- *I suggest Heart Formula, Circu Plus & Cardi Plus*

> "Vitamin C is the cement of the blood vessel walls and stabilizes them. Animals don't get heart disease because they produce enough endogenous vitamin C in their livers to protect their blood vessels. In contrast we humans develop deposits leading to heart attacks and strokes because we cannot manufacture our own vitamin C and generally get too few vitamins in our diet."
> Matthias Rath, M.D. www.dr-rath-research.org

HEARTBURN
- Is usually caused from a deficiency of hydrochloric acid. In order to produce hydrochloric acid the body needs potassium and zinc.
- Supplement your meals with potassium, zinc, hydrochloric acid and pepsin.
- Helicobacter pylori bacteria may be a factor.
- Take 2 tablespoons of apple cider vinegar in water with 1 teaspoon of honey, before each meal. This increases the production of hydrochloric acid.
- A spoonful of buttermilk before meals can be beneficial.
- *I recommend Alpha Gest, Alpha Green II & Sage Plus*

HEMORRHOIDS
- Hemorrhoids form from constipation and a copper deficiency. Like a rubber band that has the ability to expand and contract so should your colon. When it balloons out we call it a hemorrhoid. Copper is the mineral that allows it to expand and contract. Varicose veins and aneurysms are the next step if support isn't provided.
- Take natural laxatives and drink more water to keep the bowels moving easily so you don't have to strain. Magnesium may help relax muscles so you're not so "uptight."
- *I recommend Veno Plus & Chestnut Plus*

HERPES
- Herpes Simplex I usually refers to fever blisters, cold and canker sores.
- Herpes II Progenitalis usually refers to genital infections.
- L-Lysine, cat's claw, echinacea and golden seal can be very beneficial.
- Sangre de drago is effective for healing cold sores.
- *I recommend Cat's Claw, Sangre de drago & Alpha E Spleen*

HYPERTENSION (HIGH BLOOD PRESSURE)
- 115 over 75 is considered normal blood pressure.
- Coffee, alcohol and smoking has been shown to raise blood pressure.
- High blood pressure is usually a symptom of clogged arteries and veins. When a group of cells in your body sends out an S.O.S. signal because they are not receiving enough oxygen and nutrients to stay alive, then the heart and arteries receive the warning and increase blood pressure to get emergency supplies delivered to panicking cells. By decreasing blood pressure with drugs, without addressing the cause, we run the risk of starving cells to death. There is always a reason the body does something. Working with the body and not against it almost always results in improved health.
- Increased blood pressure can be caused from a calcium and magnesium deficiency. Magnesium helps dissolve calcium deposits restricting blood flow in arteries.
- Potassium regulates heart muscle action and arterial blood pressure.
- Essential fatty acids and vitamin C can help. Fish oil and flaxseed oil are good.
- Cadmium and lead poisoning from cigarette smoke and even second hand smoke can cause elevated blood pressure.
- Allergies can cause the arteries to swell up and narrow.
- Toxic kidneys can cause fluid levels in the body to be high.
- Avoid all animal proteins. Eat three cloves of garlic and lots of celery daily.
- Garlic, cayenne, goldenseal, hawthorne and ginseng can help normalize blood pressure.
- *I suggest Cal lac Plus, Circu Plus, Hawthorne Plus & Rena Plus*

HYPOTENSION
- Low Blood pressure many times is caused from weak adrenal glands.
- *I recommend Adrena Plus & Norepinephrine*

HYPOGLYCEMIA
- Low blood sugar can be caused from weak adrenal glands.
- Licorice, juniper berries, ginger, ginseng and cayenne can help.
- Chromium and vanadium are important for the pancreas to function correctly.
- *I recommend Diadren Forte, Ginger Plus I & Cinnamon 6*

HYPOTHYROID
- Kelp is high in iodine, which nourishes the thyroid gland. A deficiency can cause goiters. Iodine must piggyback on protein to get to the thyroid, so make sure your hydrochloric acid levels are up and you are properly digesting your foods.
- Selenium, zinc and L-tyrosine are important contributors to a healthy functioning thyroid.
- Pesticides, chemicals and heavy metals accumulate in the glands and need to be detoxified in order to achieve balance.
- *I suggest Thyro Plus & Kelp Complex*

IMPOTENCE
- Suma, maca, ginseng, sarsaparilla, damiana, saw palmetto, yohimbe, oat straw, kola nut and ginger help nourish the reproductive organs.
- Calcium, magnesium, zinc, vitamin E, flaxseed oil, amino acids and selenium are important.
- The inability to achieve an erection could be caused from poor circulation bringing blood to the muscles of the penis. Circulation support includes; gingko, ginseng, cayenne, ginger and garlic.
- *I recommend Prosta Plus, Circu Plus, Male Formula & Endo Glan M*

INDIGESTION
- Supplement your diet with hydrochloric acid, pepsin and enzymes so you can break your food down.
- Potassium and zinc are needed so the stomach can manufacture hydrochloric acid.
- Chew your food 30 times before swallowing. Don't drink liquids with your meals. Wait 30 minutes before or after a meal to drink liquids.
- Support your adrenal glands with pantothenic acid.
- Follow proper food combining chart.

- Peppermint can be beneficial.
- Take 2 tablespoons of apple cider vinegar in water with 1 teaspoon of honey, before each meal. This increases the production of hydrochloric acid.
- *I recommend Alpha Gest, Sage Plus & Alpha Green II*

INFERTILITY

- Suma and maca help nourish the reproductive organs and are high in amino acids which play a big role in proper glandular function.
- Yarrow is good to balance the endocrine system where hormones are manufactured. Other glands out of balance could be causing infertility.
- Dong quai, wild yam, chaste tree berry, evening primrose oil, zinc, vitamin E, vitamin C, calcium and magnesium are all beneficial.
- *I recommend Female Formula, Sumacazon, Ovary Uterus Plus & Endo Glan F*

INSECT BITES

- Poisonous snake and spider bites need immediate medical attention. Consult your doctor.
- Echinacea, "king of the blood purifiers" will neutralize poisons in the blood. Take two dropperfuls every 15 minutes for several hours to help detoxify venom out of the body.
- *I recommend Echinacea Plus*

INSOMNIA

- Magnesium and potassium can help relax the body so that you can sleep.
- Valerian root, hops, lobelia, passion flower, chamomile and skullcap can help you sleep.
- Melatonin and serotonin can be beneficial.
- Heavy metals can throw the nervous system out of balance causing you not to be able to sleep.
- Tryptophan and GABA can help you relax and sleep.
- Sluggish adrenals can cause insomnia.
- Do not take naps during the day and force yourself to get up and do something all day long so you are tired at night. Work a job or stay busy with a hobby. Lying on the couch all day long will cause you not to sleep well at night.
- *I recommend Nerve Formula, MG/K Aspartate & Melatonin*

KIDNEY DISEASE
- The kidneys filter toxins out of the blood and regulate fluid levels in the body.
- Goldenrod, uva ursi, parsley, corn silk, juniper berries, horsetail, burdock and gravel root are all good kidney flushers.
- Magnesium helps dissolve kidney stones.
- Orthophosphoric acid can dissolve stones as well.
- Emotions can play a big role with kidney problems.
- *I recommend Solidago Plus, Rena Plus & K/B Plus*

LIVER DISORDERS
- Your liver performs over five hundred functions in the body. Your health and vitality depends largely upon your liver. No one can be healthy without a clean, well-functioning liver.
- Burning in the feet, allergies, headaches & arthritis can be caused from a toxic liver.
- Avoid alcohol, vaccines, coffee, tobacco, white bread, margarine, foods cooked in oils, drugs, chlorine and fluoride. These substances are very hard on the liver.
- Hepatitis – inflammation of the liver is usually caused by a virus.
- The best herbs for cleansing and strengthening the liver are; milk thistle, dandelion, nettles, burdock, barberry, Oregon grape, red root and yellow dock.
- *I recommend Dandi Plus, Hepachol, Omega Complete & Beta Plus*

LUPUS
- Sodium and potassium levels in the cells need balancing. Take alfalfa, bee pollen and spirulina.
- Support the thymus gland.
- Essential fatty acids are important.
- Candida yeast and heavy metal poisoning could be factors. Many times Lupus is a build up of too many toxins causing the body to attack itself.
- *I suggest Thymo Plus, Universal Complex, Cat's Claw, Detox HM & Alpha Green*

MENIERE'S DISEASE
- Ringing in the ears, dizziness and nausea are symptoms usually caused from the lymphatic system not draining properly.
- Nettles, dandelion, solidago, echinacea, calendula, cat's claw, garlic and cayenne are good lymphatic drainers.
- Vitamin C (Citrus bioflavonoids) can help.
- Poor circulation may be a culprit. Ginkgo, butcher's broom and ginseng are good.

- Allergies may be a factor.
- *I suggest Circu Plus, Universal Complex, Alpha Flavin, Adrena Plus & Thymo plus*

MENOPAUSE
- Support the endocrine system so that the glands can produce the hormones you need in the correct proportions.
- Natural progesterone cream containing wild yam is good.
- Black cohosh, chaste tree berry, angelica, dong quai, licorice, hops, vervain, damiana, evening primrose, selenium, black currant and borage oil can be beneficial.
- *I recommend Female Formula, Evening Primrose Oil, Endo Glan F & F.H.S.*

MIGRAINE HEADACHE
- Many times migraines are caused from constipation and too many toxins in the blood stream. This causes inflammation and puts pressure on the capillaries, thus creating pain. Get the bowels moving 2-3 times a day so toxins have a way out of your body, instead of recirculating in the blood putting pressure on the capillaries thus causing a headache.
- A toxic liver can trigger headaches. Do a liver cleanse.
- The pituitary and thyroid glands being out of balance can create hormonal imbalances that trigger these headaches. Manganese and kelp are good.
- Manganese is the mineral that nourishes the anterior pituitary which can help relieve headaches. It also nourishes discs in the back. Many times back pain and headaches are caused from a simple manganese deficiency.
- Sodium deficiency can trigger headaches. Take spirulina and drink carrot and celery juice.
- Pain behind the left eye may be a zinc deficiency, while pain behind the right eye and the temple may be a cry for iron.
- Nettles, kelp, yellow dock, beets and green vegetables are high in iron.
- Vitamin B-6 and niacin can be beneficial.
- Blood sugar issues can trigger headaches. Get off carbohydrates and sugars.
- Tryptophan (amino acid), the precursor to serotonin, can help.
- *I recommend Pitui Plus, Circu Plus, Alpha Flavin & Gota Plus*

MONONUCLEOSIS
- Is a viral infection usually caused by the Epstein Barr virus.
- Cat's claw, echinacea and pau d' arco are good for the immune system.
- Homeopathic remedy "Infection E.B." is good.
- *I recommend Echinacea Plus, Lapacho Plus & Alpha E Spleen*

MORNING SICKNESS
- Pregnant women who experience morning sickness are usually suffering from a sodium deficiency. That little fetus growing inside of them is robbing sodium from mother, leaving her depleted. Get your sodium levels up. Drinking freshly squeezed carrot and celery juice daily is very beneficial, ensuring that both mother and child get the nutrients they need. Dr. Oz's green drink is very beneficial as well.
- The best foods to replenish depleted sodium levels are; spirulina, celery juice, alfalfa, okra (not fried), carrots, cabbage, spinach, strawberries, beets, cucumbers, plums, powdered whey, raw goat's milk, chicken and turkey gizzards.
- Ginger can help with nausea.
- *I suggest intraMAX & Alpha Green*

MULTIPLE SCLEROSIS
- Heavy metals, especially mercury, can be a culprit.
- Get silver dental fillings removed and replaced with composite materials. Locate a dentist who follows the Huggins protocol for a safe and effective extraction. For more information go to www.drhuggins.com and www.IAOMT.COM.
- Evening primrose oil, lipoic acid, magnesium, potassium and B vitamins are important.
- Malvin, pyrole, serotonin, dopamine, and norepinephrine may help.
- The syphilinum miasm may be a factor.
- Get off artificial sweeteners, like aspartame, found in diet soft drinks.
- *I suggest Nerve Formula, Gota Plus, Circu Plus, Evening Primrose Oil, MG/K Aspartate & Detox HM*

NOSEBLEEDS
- A warning sign that the capillaries are weak and fragile.
- Bruising easily and gums bleeding, when brushing your teeth, are other indications that more Vitamin C (citrus bioflavonoids) are needed to strengthen tissue integrity.
- Camu camu from the Amazon Rainforest is the world's highest concentration of vitamin C. It contains 30 to 60 times more vitamin C than an orange.
- Cayenne and yarrow can help. Calcium and magnesium levels may be low.
- *I recommend Alpha Flavin & Cal lac Plus*

OBESITY
- A sluggish thyroid is a common culprit when weight is an issue. Kelp is high in iodine which nourishes the thyroid gland.

- Deal with the emotions that are causing you to hold on to the weight. What are you trying to "protect" yourself from? Weight gain can be a self-defense mechanism on a subconscious level.
- Chickweed, hoodia and apple cider vinegar can help.
- Do not skip breakfast. Eat 5-6 smaller meals during the day to keep your metabolism burning calories. Eat healthy foods such as fruits, vegetables and raw nuts.
- Drink lots of water throughout the day and 16 ounces upon arising.
- Get the bowels moving 2-3 times a day.
- Stop consuming artificial sweeteners, especially diet soft drinks. They cause you to crave carbohydrates and retain fluids. Use stevia for a natural sweetener.
- Do not eat after 6 p.m. Read chapter on losing weight.
- *I recommend Thyro Plus, Sumacazon & Kelp Complex*

OSTEOPORSIS
- Is usually caused by the sycosis miasm which causes the parathyroid gland to be hyperactive. This pulls calcium from the bones, leaving them fragile.
- See Arthritis section for more information on getting the body alkaline.
- *I recommend intraMAX, Alpha Green, Arnica Plus, Liga Plus & PH Enhancer*

PARKINSON'S DISEASE
- The syphilinum miasm can affect the nervous system.
- Calcium, magnesium and potassium deficiencies can be causes.
- An out of balance parathyroid gland can trigger blood/calcium levels to be abnormal producing "the shakes."
- Bone meal and B-vitamins can be beneficial.
- Phosphatidyl serine can help.
- Heavy metal poisoning is almost always a culprit. Get silver dental fillings removed and replaced with composite materials. Locate a dentist who follows the Huggins protocol for a safe and effective extraction. For more information go to www.drhuggins.com and www.IAOMT.COM.
- Gingko, cayenne, valerian root, ginseng, passion flower, kola nut, rosemary, lobelia, L-dopa, dopamine and hops can be beneficial.
- *I suggest Nerve Formula, Circu Plus, Gota Plus, L-dopa, Cal lac Plus & Phosphatidyl Serine*

PINK EYE (CONJUNCTIVITIS)
- Sangre de drago mixed in a saline solution and dropped in the eye will clear out infection and reduce inflamed membranes.

- Eyebright, goldenseal and colloidal silver may be beneficial.
- *I recommend Echinacea Plus, Sangre de drago & Immu Plus*

PNEUMONIA
- Weak adrenals always affect the lungs. Royal jelly is good for the adrenals.
- Mullein and lobelia are good for the lungs.
- Echinacea, garlic and colloidal silver fights infection.
- Eucalyptus helps loosen lung congestion.
- *I recommend Mullein Plus, Echinacea Plus, Pneumo Plus & Adrena Plus*

POISON IVY/OAK/SUMAC
- Homeopathic remedies; clematis, graphites, mezereum, rhus tox and croton tiglium are effective.
- Burdock, jewelweed and aloe vera can help.
- *I recommend Poison Ivy, Echinacea Plus, Alpha E Spleen & Immu Boost*

PREMENSTRUAL SYNDROME
- PMS symptoms usually indicate that the endocrine system is out of balance.
- Progesterone is made in the ovaries and adrenal glands.
- Magnesium deficiency can cause an imbalance of hormones.
- Suma, maca, dong quai, chaste tree berry, wild yam, damiana, black cohosh, licorice, hops, manganese and yarrow are good.
- Testosterone helps increase sexual desire for both females and males.
- *I recommend Female Formula, Endo Glan F, Evening Primrose Oil & Ovary Uterus Plus*

PROSTATITIS
- When the prostate gland swells, it can cause a constant need to urinate.
- Flaxseed oil, juniper berry, saw palmetto, ginseng, yohimbe, sarsaparilla, zinc, vitamins A and E, lecithin, calcium and magnesium are all beneficial.
- According to the University of Arizona's medical school, (JAMA Dec. 25, 1996) selenium supplemented at 250 mcg/day will reduce ones risk of developing prostate cancer by 69%.
- *I recommend Prosta Plus, Circu Plus, Male Formula, Flaxseed Oil & Endo Glan M*

PSORIASIS
- Many types of skin conditions are caused from toxins built up in the liver and spleen.

- Flush the toxins out and the skin clears up.
- Dandelion, burdock, echinacea and nettles are good.
- Evening primrose oil is good.
- Kelp is high in iodine, which keeps the skin from getting dry.
- *I recommend KLS Plus, Trifolo Plus, Alpha E Spleen & Omega Complete*

SCHIZOPHRENIA
- Avoid all animal protein. Get on a high vegetable and fruit diet.
- Zinc and vitamin B-6 is important.
- Hypoglycemia is almost always involved with schizophrenia. Support the adrenals, liver and pancreas.
- Dopamine can help.
- Niacin has been proven to be extremely beneficial by Dr. Abram Hoffer, who has treated over 5,000 cases with an 80% success rate. Usually 1,000 mg. to 3,000 mg. of niacin in the form of niacinamide given with each meal works well.
- *I suggest Alpha B, Diadren Forte & Chola Plus.*

SHINGLES
- Shingles (Herpes Zoster) is caused by the varicella-zoster virus, the same virus that causes chickenpox.
- Vitamin C and vitamin B are important.
- Cayenne, lobelia, echinacea and cat's claw are good.
- *I recommend Echinacea Plus, Immu Boost, Immu Plus & Alpha E Spleen*

SINUS CONDITIONS
- Toxins built up in the liver can trigger allergies and sinus issues.
- Parasites, causing an imbalance with the ileo-cecal valve, can trigger sinus issues.
- Thyroid and adrenal glands can be another factor. If the discharge from the nose is a thick green color, then the thyroid is usually sluggish. When the adrenal glands become exhausted, we are tired and may be allergic to citrus fruits.
- Vitamin B-5 (pantothenic acid) is needed. The best source is royal jelly.
- Stuffiness on the right side indicates the need for potassium, while stuffiness on the left side means a sodium deficiency.
- Alfalfa, bee pollen and spirulina are high in sodium and potassium. Echinacea and vitamin B-12 can help.
- Peppermint, eucalyptus, melaleuca, rosemary, golden seal, echinacea and lemon oil can help open sinuses. For tough guys, who want to put some hair on their chest, try a straight shot of ground horseradish.

- Quercetin can be beneficial.
- *I recommend Myrrh Plus, Hista Plus, Adrena Plus & Royal Jelly*

SMOKING
- Eat small frequent meals with slow-releasing carbohydrates combined with proteins to help stabilize blood sugar levels.
- Niacin (vitamin B-3) helps reduce nicotine cravings. If you experience flushing or tingling from taking niacin switch to niacinamide.
- Supplement your diet with vitamin C, chromium, lecithin, calcium, magnesium and a B complex.
- *I suggest intraMAX, Chola Plus & Alpha B*

> **"One puff of a cigarette lets loose a trillion free radical molecules in the smoker."** Hyla Cass, M.D. – UCLA School of Medicine

SORE THROAT
- Gargle with warm salt water. Salt kills bacteria. It is one of the oldest germ fighters around.
- Gargle with and drink a hot lemonade. To make a hot lemonade, squeeze the juice of a lemon in a glass of hot water and add 3 Tbsp. of apple cider vinegar and 1 Tbsp. of raw honey. Add 4 dropperfuls of una de gato (cat's claw), Arcozon or Echinacea to make it a powerful infection fighter. You may also add 20 drops of Sangre de drago to "turbocharge" your immune system. Stir and sip. Gargle before swallowing.
- Eat three cloves of fresh garlic daily. Garlic is a natural antibiotic.
- Eat eggs, onions and apricots. They are high in sulfur. The tonsils are the sulfur sacks of the body. Tonsils help purify the blood and become inflamed when low in sulfur.
- *I recommend Una de Gato w/ Honey Vinegar, Sangre de drago & Echinacea Plus*

STROKE
- Most strokes occur when an artery becomes blocked and oxygen and nutrients cannot circulate to certain areas of the brain, thus causing the death of brain cells.
- Increase circulation to the brain. Circulation support includes; ginkgo biloba, ginseng, butcher's broom, cayenne, ginger, gota kola, oat straw, rosemary, garlic and parsley.
- A stroke on the right side of the body is usually caused from a potassium deficiency. Bee pollen, burdock and alfalfa are high in potassium.
- Strokes on the left side can be caused from a sodium deficiency. Spirulina, celery,

- watercress, Irish moss and dulse are high in sodium.
- Soybean lecithin can help.
- *I recommend Veno Plus, Gota Plus, Circu Plus & Chestnut Plus*

TINNITIS
- Sluggish adrenal glands can trigger ringing in the ears.
- Magnesium, manganese and Vitamin C (bioflavonoids) can help.
- Circulation support can be helpful. This includes; ginkgo biloba, ginseng, butcher's broom, cayenne, ginger, gota kola, oatstraw and rosemary.
- *I recommend Alpha Flavin, Adrena Plus & Gota Plus*

ULCERS
- A simple ulcer test is performed by taking 2 capsules of protease on an empty stomach. If burning or discomfort occurs within 10 minutes this is an indication of ulcers.
- Sangre de drago is a powerful antioxidant that heals ulcers.
- Raw, freshly made cabbage juice several times a day is beneficial for duodenal ulcers.
- Raw, freshly made potato juice is great for gastric (stomach) ulcers. Drink cabbage or potato juices immediately after juicing because the medicinal value disappears the longer it sits.
- Wheat grass, alfalfa, chlorophyll, spirulina, parsley, camu camu, marshmallow root, gota kola, papaya leaf, prickly ash bark, licorice root, sage, and aloe vera will help heal ulcers.
- *I suggest Sangre de drago, Gastro, Alpha Green, BR SP Plus & Black Radish Complex*

VARICOSE VEINS
- Varicose veins are many times caused from a copper deficiency. Copper is the mineral that allows tubing in the body to stay pliable.
- *I recommend Veno Plus, Chestnut Plus and Alpha Flavin*

VERTIGO
- Dizziness occurs many times because of sluggish adrenal glands. Licorice, kelp and ginger support the adrenals.
- Royal jelly is high in pantothenic acid, which is good for the adrenals.
- Vitamin C from citrus bioflavonoids can be beneficial for chronic fatigue and vertigo.
- B vitamins are important.

- Increasing circulation can help. Support includes; ginkgo biloba, ginseng, butcher's broom, cayenne, ginger, gota kola, oat straw, rosemary, garlic and parsley.
- *I recommend Adrena Plus, Alpha Flavin, Circu Plus & Brain Formula*

Healing Poisoned Medicine

Health Evaluation

Place number next to the symptoms which apply to you:
Use (1) for MILD symptoms (2) for MODERATE symptoms (3) for SEVERE symptoms

GROUP ONE

___ "Nervous" Stomach   ___ Mentally alert, quick   ___ Cold sweats often
___ Dry mouth, eyes, nose   ___ Extremities cold, clammy   ___ Fever easily raised
___ Pulse speeds after meals   ___ Heart pounds after retiring   ___ Neuralgia-like pains
___ Keyed-up – fail to calm   ___ Acid foods upset
___ Are your symptoms made worse by emotional stress?

GROUP TWO

___ Perspire easily   ___ Digestion rapid   ___ Joint stiffness after rising
___ Muscle-leg-toe cramps   ___ Vomiting frequent   ___ Circulation poor, sensitive to cold
___ Eyelids swollen, puffy   ___ Difficulty swallowing   ___ Subject to colds, asthma, bronchitis
___ Indigestion soon after meals   ___ Constipation, diarrhea
___ Are your symptoms made worse by physical stress?

GROUP THREE

___ Afternoon headaches   ___ Heart palpitates if meals   ___ Crave candy or coffee in
___ Get "shaky" if hungry   missed or delayed   afternoons
___ Faintness if meals delayed   ___ Awaken after few hours   ___ Abnormal craving for
                                  can't get back to sleep   sweets or snacks

GROUP FOUR

___ Bruise easily   ___ Swollen ankles   ___ Hands & feet go to sleep easily,
___ Sigh frequently   ___ Muscle cramps   numbness
___ Breathe heavily   ___ Shortness of breath   ___ Tendency to anemia
___ Opens window in rooms   ___ Dull pain in chest or   ___ Tension under breastbone or feeling
___ Susceptible to colds/fevers   radiating into left arm   of "tightness"

GROUP FIVE

___ Dry skin   ___ Biliousness (constipation, headaches)   ___ Laxatives used often
___ Skin rashes frequent   ___ Greasy foods upset   ___ History of gallbladder
___ Bitter metallic taste in   ___ Stools light colored   attacks or gallstones
    mouth in mornings   ___ Pain between shoulder   ___ Sneezing attacks
___ Bowel movements painful   blades
    or difficult

GROUP SIX

___ Lower bowel gas several hours after eating
___ Burning stomach sensations, eating relieves
___ Coated tongue
___ Indigestion ½ - 1 hour after eating; may continue for 3-4 hours
___ Gas shortly after eating
___ Stomach "bloating" after eating

GROUP SEVEN

(A)
___ Pulse fast at rest
___ Nervousness
___ Can't gain weight
___ Intolerance to heat
___ Highly emotional
___ Flush easily
___ Night sweats
___ Inward trembling
___ Heart palpitates
___ Insomnia

(C)
___ Low blood pressure
___ Failing memory
___ Increased sex desire
___ Headaches
___ Decreased sugar tolerance

(E)
___ Hot flashes
___ Headaches
___ Dizziness
___ Increased blood pressure
___ Sugar in urine (not diabetes)
___ Masculine tendencies-female

(B)
___ Impaired hearing
___ Decrease in appetite
___ Ringing in ears
___ Constipation
___ Mental sluggishness
___ Headaches upon arising, wear off during the day
___ Slow pulse, below 65
___ Increase in weight

(D)
___ Bloating of intestines
___ Abnormal thirst
___ Weight gain around hips or waist
___ Sex desire reduced or lacking
___ Tendency to ulcers, colitis
___ Increased sugar tolerance
___ Menstrual disorders
___ Delayed menstruation

(F)
___ Low blood pressure
___ Chronic fatigue
___ Weakness, dizziness
___ Tendency to hives
___ Arthritic tendencies
___ Perspiration increases
___ Crave salt
___ Brown spots on skin
___ Allergies – asthma
___ Exhaustion –muscular/nerves
___ Respiratory disorders

GROUP EIGHT

(Female Only)

___ Painful menses
___ Premenstrual tension
___ Very easily fatigued
___ Depressed feeling before
___ Menstruation excessive and prolonged
___ Painful breasts
___ Menstruate too frequently
___ Vaginal discharge
___ Menopause, hot flashes, etc.
___ Menses scanty
___ Acne, worse at menses

GROUP EIGHT (cont.)

(Male Only)

___ Tire too easily
___ Urination difficult
___ Night urination frequent

___ Pain on inside of legs or heel
___ Feeling of incomplete bowel evacuation

___ Prostate trouble
___ Leg nervousness at night
___ Diminished sex desire

GROUP NINE

___ Chronic cough
___ Pain around ribs
___ Shortness of breath
___ Chest pain

___ Difficulty breathing
___ Coughing up phlegm
___ Coughing up blood

___ Bronchitis (frequent)
___ Infections settle in lungs
___ Sensitive to smog

GROUP TEN

___ Frequent urination
___ Rose colored (bloody)
___ Dripping after urination
___ Difficulty passing urine

___ Cloudy urine
___ Rarely need to urinate
___ Strong smelling urine
___ Frequent bladder infections

___ Painful/burning when passing urine
___ Urination when you cough or sneeze

GROUP ELEVEN

___ Throat infections
___ Poor wound healing
___ Slow to recover from colds or flu
___ Chronic lung congestion
___ Post nasal drip

___ Gets boils or styes
___ Swollen lymph glands
___ Catch colds or flu easily
___ Breathe through mouth
___ Swollen tongue

___ Bumpy skin on back of arms
___ Inflamed or bleeding gums
___ Hyperactivity
___ Food sensitivity or allergies

KEY

Group One **Sympathetic Nervous System** – People who are Sympathetic Dominance are in high gear. They burn up their mineral reserves, especially magnesium and potassium. Many of these people are on diuretics, which flush out minerals, thus worsening the condition.

Group Two **Parasympathetic Nervous System** – Those who are Parasympathetic Dominance are usually always in slow gear and have difficulty "getting in gear." They need extra phosphorus. Lecithin is high in phosphorus.
- Understand that the sympathetic and parasympathetic nervous systems need to be balanced like a teeter-totter for optimum health.

Group Three **Pancreas** – Regulates sugar metabolism. Diabetes and (hyper) or hypoglycemia are common symptoms. Normal glucose levels are 70-110. Stay off dairy products and red meat. Supplement your diet with enzymes. Ginger and licorice can help.

Group Four **Cardiovascular System** – If you experience pain, you may need heart support. Magnesium, L-carnitine and L-taurine are good for the heart. If there is no pain, then you probably need circulatory support. Ginkgo biloba, ginseng, butcher's broom and flaxseed oil are good for circulation.

Group Five **Liver and Gallbladder** – Relates to digestion and the breakdown of fats. Parasites can be a factor causing symptoms. Stones can form and cause symptoms. The best herbs are dandelion, milk thistle, globe artichoke, turmeric, boldo and Oregon grape.

Group Six **Digestion (Gastro-Intestinal Tract)** – Gas and bloating usually indicates the need for more enzymes. Heartburn and burning in the stomach indicates the need for more hydrochloric acid. For ulcers we use wheat grass, barley greens, alfalfa, chlorophyll, spirulina, parsley and marshmallow root. An intestinal cleanse may be needed to blast through built up fecal matter.

Group Seven
    A   **Hyper-thyroid** – Need more calcium.
    B   **Hypo-thyroid** – These people usually carry most of their weight from the waist up. Kelp is needed. Check body temperature. Temperature should be between 97.8 and 98.2.

<u>C</u>	**<u>Hyper-Pituitary</u>** – Manganese and yarrow are good.	
<u>D</u>	**<u>Hypo-Pituitary</u>** – Weight gain from the waist to the knees. These people have a tendency to carry their weight in the buttocks, hips and thighs. Manganese and yarrow are beneficial.	
<u>E</u>	**<u>Hyper-Adrenal</u>** – Pantothenic acid found in Royal Jelly, bovine adrenal concentrate and licorice can help.	
<u>F</u>	**<u>Hypo-Adrenal</u>** – These individuals usually experience fatigue, dizziness when standing up too quickly and respiratory issues. They have a tendency to gain weight in the midsection or belly. Support includes pantothenic acid, adrenal concentrate, licorice and ginger.	

Group Eight

<u>Reproductive System (Female)</u> - Yarrow, black cohosh, blue cohosh, dong quai, zinc and amino acids can help.

<u>Reproductive System (Male)</u> – Flaxseed oil, juniper berries, saw palmetto, ginseng and yohimbe are good.

<u>Group Nine</u> **<u>Respiratory System</u>** – Respiratory symptoms may be caused from weak adrenal glands. Mullein, myrrh, ginger, althea and nutmeg are good.

<u>Group Ten</u> **<u>Kidneys and Bladder</u>** – Golden rod, uva ursi, juniper berry, corn silk, parsley and horsetail are good. Orthophosphoric acid dissolves kidney and bladder stones.

<u>Group Eleven</u> **<u>Immune System</u>** – Echinacea, una de gato (cat's claw), elderberry and garlic are good.

Did You Know…

1. Watermelon seeds are great for kidney problems, high blood pressure and stress.
2. Sesame seed milk is wonderful for gaining weight.
3. Eggs have lecithin, which balances cholesterol levels in the body.
4. A sluggish thyroid, many times, is a cause for high cholesterol.
5. Black pepper irritates the liver. Use cayenne.
6. Years ago, poor people in India and Russia, who couldn't afford to go to the doctor, ate garlic to stay healthy. Garlic is considered "Russian penicillin." Research has proven that garlic stimulates natural killer cells, which are our main defense against cancer. Garlic with purplish skin is the best.
7. Goiter is caused by a lack of iodine. Take Kelp.
8. Sugar leaches calcium from the bones.
9. Charcoal-grilled meats contain large amounts of tar and are unhealthy. Headaches are common after eating barbeque.
10. 80% of women who take "the pill" (contraceptive) are deficient in Vitamin B-6.
11. Sodium feeds the adrenal glands. Sluggish adrenal glands can cause low blood pressure, low blood sugar etc.
12. Carbonated drinks block calcium absorption in the body.
13. Bananas are the only food containing the neuro-transmitter serotonin.
14. A lactating woman's milk from the right breast has a predominate potassium composition, while the left breast has a high sodium composition. The baby may prefer one side to the other based upon which nutrients he or she needs most at that particular time.
15. A natural form of birth control, according to American Indians, is to eat wild yam roots every day. After eating those for two months, conception will not occur. When Indians wanted to become pregnant, they simply stopped eating wild yam roots.
16. Marijuana burns the adrenal glands out leaving you feeling tired all the time.
17. Bee Pollen is an excellent supplement for athletes, because it contains so much nutrition and gives strength and stamina.
18. Eating 5 almonds a day will prevent cancer according to Edgar Cayce.
19. Cellulitis is primarily blocked lymphatic fluid in the tissue.
20. Decaffeinated coffee is worse than natural coffee because of the chemical additives.
21. The only difference between chlorophyll (the green lifeblood of the plant) and human blood (hemoglobin, the protein of red blood cells) is one molecule. The metallic atom in a molecule of human blood is iron, while that of chlorophyll is magnesium. Chlorophyll is a powerful healer.

Healing Poisoned Medicine

Chinese Meridian Clock

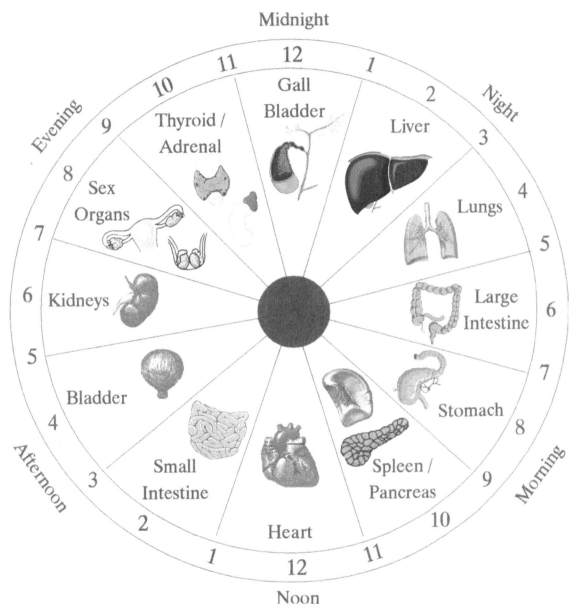

    The above organs and glands are most active at these times. If you have symptoms that occur like clockwork, then there may be a connection. For example, a client of mine told me that every night at 2:15 A.M. she wakes up. On the chart we see that 2 A.M.. is when the liver is most active. We gave her some liver/digestive support and now she sleeps the whole night through without waking up.

Reed T. Sainsbury

A Recipe for Dis-ease

1. Take prescription and nonprescription drugs.
2. Take antibiotics.
3. Get vaccinations & flu shots.
4. Have your dentist put silver (amalgam) fillings in your teeth.
5. Have root canals done in your mouth.
6. Remove your gallbladder.
7. Drink city tap water.
8. Work a night job.
9. Hate your job.
10. Never take a vacation.
11. Take one aspirin every day. It causes leaky gut syndrome.
12. Remove your tonsils, adenoids & lymph nodes.
13. Cut your uterus out (Hysterectomy).
14. Be angry at others.
15. Eat processed foods out of packages, wrappers & boxes.
16. Use a microwave.
17. Stop breastfeeding your child before the age of 6 months old.
18. Take diet pills.
19. Drink coffee. 208 acids have been identified in one cup of coffee.
20. Smoke cigarettes.
21. Hold a grudge.
22. Drink soft drinks.
23. Use fat free and sugar free products.
24. Worry about things you can't control.
25. Eat when you're not hungry.
26. Try to control others.
27. Hate the way God has created you.
28. Believe in bad luck and that you are a poor victim.
29. Feel like a failure.
30. Be serious and never laugh or joke.
31. Eat charcoal-broiled meats.
32. Believe that life is hard and then you die.

You may say, "Well, I do a lot of those things on the list and I am fine." Great, feel blessed that your body is amazing at dealing with trash, but remember that you reap what you sow. We live in a cause and effect world. What comes around goes around.

> **"We who have no time for our health today, may have no health for our time tomorrow."** Anonymous

Health Books for Seekers of Wisdom

1. Cleanse & Purify Thyself by Richard Anderson, N.M.D.
2. Confessions of a Medical Heretic by Robert S. Mendelsohn, M.D.
3. Vibrational Medicine by Richard Gerber, M.D.
4. An Alternative Medicine Definitive Guide to Cancer by Burton Goldberg
5. There is a Cure for Arthritis by Paavo O. Airola, N.D., Ph.D.
6. How To Get Well by Paavo O. Airola, N.D., Ph.D.
7. The Ultimate Healing System by Donald Lepore, N.D.
8. The Cancer Answer by Albert E. Carter
9. You can Heal your Life by Louise L. Hay
10. The Makers Diet by Jordan Rubin, N.M.D.
11. Rare Earths Forbidden Cures by Joel D. Wallach, N.D., D.V.M.
12. The Cancer Industry by Ralph W. Moss, Ph.D.
13. Whole Body Dentistry by Mark A. Breiner, D.D.S.
14. Natural Health Natural Medicine by Andrew Weil, M.D.
15. Own Your Own Body by Stan Malstrom, N.D.
16. Solved The Riddle of Illness by Stephen E. Langer, M.D.
17. Beating Cancer with Nutrition by Patrick Quillin, Ph.D.
18. A Promise Made, A Promise Kept: One Son's Quest For The Cause And Cure of Diabetes. By James Chappell, D.C., N.D., Ph.D., M.H.
19. What Your Doctor May Not Tell You About Menopause by John R. Lee, M.D.
20. Back to Eden by Jethro Kloss
21. Politics in Healing by Daniel Haley
22. Power VS. Force by David Hawkins, M.D., Ph.D.
23. How To Raise A Healthy Child In Spite Of Your Doctor by Robert Mendelsohn, M.D.
24. Male Practice How Doctors Manipulate Women by Robert Mendelsohn, M.D.
25. Bypassing Bypass by Elmer Cranton, M.D.
26. Rockefeller Men: Medicine and Capitalism in America by Richard Brown
27. What Your Doctor Won't Tell You by Jane Heimlich
28. Excitotoxins: The Taste That Kills by Russell Blaylock, M.D.
29. Feelings Buried Alive Never Die by Karol K. Truman
30. The Biology of Belief by Bruce Lipton, Ph.D.
31. The Secret by Rhonda Byrne
32. Molecules of Emotion by Candace B. Pert, Ph.D.
33. The Antibiotic Paradox How Miracle Drugs Are Destroying the Miracle by Stuart B. Levy, M.D.
34. Death by Modern Medicine by Carolyn Dean, M.D., N.D.
35. Selling Sickness by Ray Moynihan and Alan Cassels
36. Racketeering in Medicine The Suppression of Alternatives by James P. Carter, M.D., Dr. P.H.
37. Overdosed America The Broken Promise of American Medicine by John Abramson, M.D.
38. It's All In Your Head by Hal A. Huggins, D.D.S.
39. The Truth About the Drug Companies by Marcia Angell, M.D.
40. Health at the Crossroads by Dean Black, Ph.D.

Chapter 12
THE ENERGY IN EMOTIONS

Healing the Cause of Cancer

> **"If cancer or any other illness returns, I do not believe it is because they did not 'get it all out,' but rather that the patient has made no mental change."** Louise L. Hay - Author of You Can Heal Your Life

A few years ago Jan came to our clinic. She had cancer, Multiple Myeloma and had exhausted her insurance, spending over $300,000 on chemotherapy treatments. Naturally she began to worry about how she was going to afford further treatments because her doctor told her the chemotherapy was the only thing keeping the cancer from spreading to other parts of her body. On the other hand, it was leaving her exhausted and unable to work.

Jan knew that the chemotherapy wasn't correcting the cause of her cancer, it was only treating her symptoms. She heard about our clinic and made an appointment. When she came to see us the neuropathy in her legs was causing her a tremendous amount of discomfort from the cell-damaging drugs she had been taking. The numbness, tingling and low energy levels made it difficult for her to work even part time.

We wasted no time. The first thing we did was a CEDSA exam. The evidence of why cells were mutating pieced together like a puzzle. As with all cancer patients, we found poor circulation, her pH to be acidic and a miasm. Heavy metal poisoning also showed up as a contributing factor. We put Jan on a program to detoxify her for the miasm and heavy metal poisoning. We also put her on circulation support, pH alkalizing green cell foods, herbal drainer formulas, and some natural cancer killers like graviola, cat's claw and a fermented soy product called Haelin.

All of the physical ingredients mentioned above are important, but they do not work effectively until we remove the mental/emotional cactuses growing inside that feeds cancer subconsciously. Weeding your garden effectively requires pulling the weeds out and getting the roots. We all know that, if you don't pull a weed out by its roots, it will grow right back. Only a fool clips the tops off with scissors. Just as weeds will grow right back if the roots are left, so will cancer come back if the mental/emotional blueprint is not healed that nourished it to grow in the first place.

> "All disease originates in the mind. Nothing appears on the body unless there is a mental pattern corresponding to it."
> Joseph Murphy, Ph.D.

Jan did what was suggested and came back for a follow-up appointment to work on clearing out the emotional issues. What we found feeding this cancer was ancient history. When she was nineteen years old she got pregnant before she was married. Jan came from a very religious family and doing such was frowned upon to say the least. In order to escape the embarrassment and shame of having an illegitimate child, she had an abortion and never told a soul. Well, thirty six years later Jan is diagnosed with cancer and this emotion of "guilt" is eating her alive. Deep down inside she felt guilty and unworthy of God's blessings, especially good health. Cancer was the way she subconsciously felt that she could bear the cross of guilt and serve justice for the abortion she had.

> "Releasing resentment will dissolve even cancer." Louise L. Hay

We went through the RFA (emotional release) process and Jan was able to understand a little more about herself, forgiveness and love. Guilt, hurt and pain can melt into nothing through the power of love. Once Jan comprehended and felt that she was forgiven and that she no longer needed to carry that cross of guilt, her body chemistry changed. She walked out of our office that day healed emotionally, mentally and spiritually. The chains of guilt no longer held her in bondage and with that freedom her immune system was balanced and charged strong enough to overcome the cancer.

Now Jan works twelve hours a day, six days a week and her co-workers can't believe it. She went from being diagnosed with cancer to chemotherapy treatments and was given a death sentence by her oncologist if she chose to quit her treatments. When she announced that she was stopping the chemotherapy everyone expected her to die, especially her doctor. Obviously, her doctor didn't understand what was causing her cancer and what to do so that she could heal.

Jan believes that had she chosen to continue to follow her oncologist's program to kill, kill, kill cancer with poisonous chemotherapy without ever addressing the cause of it, then she would have died. The body can only tolerate so much poison before it gives up, especially when there are unhealed emotional issues feeding it on the subconscious level. Remember, a great portion of your health is determined on a subconscious level.

> "I feel that all disease is ultimately related to a lack of love, or to love that is only conditional, for the exhaustion and depression of the immune system thus created leads to physical vulnerability. I also feel that all healing is related to the ability to give and accept unconditional love."
> Bernie Siegel, M.D. - Author of Love Medicine & Miracles

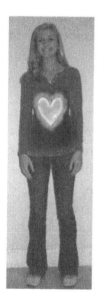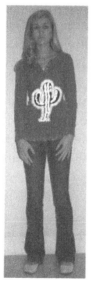

You can't expect healing to occur on the physical level when the emotional level is filled with thorns of anger, guilt, hate and fear. When these dark, dis-ease producing emotions are resonating within, healing is blocked. The intelligence that instructs the cells of your body cannot send out healthy energetic frequencies, if feelings of guilt, fear and anger are flowing through you. How do you expect to create health and healing from those signals? You can't. It just doesn't work. It's like trying to produce fire from water. The elements are not conducive to each other. They create friction and will not flow. On the other hand, gasoline will produce fire because the elements are conducive to one another. Love, peace and forgiveness are conducive to vibrant health and healing.

> "We are the only creatures on earth who can change our biology by what we think and feel." Deepak Chopra, M.D.

Reed T. Sainsbury

Healing Power of the Mind

When I was twenty-one years old, I developed terrible allergies. My nose was constantly stuffed up and having to breathe through my mouth was nothing short of pure misery. The only time I got relief is when I would run or workout intensely. I was miserable.

I went into see my medical doctor because something was obviously out of whack and I thought, since he was a doctor, he could fix what was wrong. The nurse spent about three minutes checking my blood pressure, weight etc. Then the doctor came in and asked, "What's up?" I proceeded to explain how I was miserable from not being able to breathe through my nose. He asked if I had any nasal discharge in which I replied, "No, it's like someone poured cement in my nose and it's totally sealed off." He immediately wrote a prescription for two drugs. He spent a whole two minutes with me and, not having insurance, I had to pay over a hundred dollars for the office visit. The two prescriptions cost well over two hundred dollars.

I took the drugs and experienced fatigue, constipation and headaches, and still got no relief from my allergies. Three weeks later I went back to tell him that it wasn't working, so we went through the same procedure again and he prescribed some different drugs. Of course, I was again billed more than $100 for the five-minute office visit. For some people that's no big deal, but when you are a college student working construction for seven dollars an hour, that is an out right rip-off. My two full days of hard labor in the 100-degree heat didn't even cover his two minutes it took him to write the prescription.

The second round of drugs also failed to clear up my problem, so this time my doctor pawned me off to his tag-team partner. His partner was an ear, nose and throat specialist. I went to the specialist and he disappointed me by not jumping off the top rope in a ring, wearing a sparkling uniform with a cape and mask hollering how he was going to kick the crap out of my allergies. He X-rayed my nose. We looked at the X-ray together and he pointed out that my left nostril was smaller than the right and told me, "We could do surgery and widen the nasal passage of the left nostril but there's no guarantee that it will help your nose clear up." What a joke! You've got to be kidding me? I mean, come on, if you look at every other body part and measure you'll probably find one arm longer then the other, one leg a little off, fingers etc. That was the final straw, I looked him square in the eyes and said, "You doctors have no idea what's causing my allergies and so you're just guessing as to what might help. I can't afford your guessing games." I told him I was through and walked out. I poked my head back in the door and asked, "I don't have insurance. Just out of curiosity, how much would the surgery that might help cost?" He turned his nose up and sniffled, "You don't want to know."

I realized then that as sure as Hulk Hogan's punches and kicks to his opponents' heads are phony, so are the guessing games doctors play with their drugs. There is no testing performed to find what is wrong, or how it got that way. They simply are suppressing symptoms with harmful chemicals and anxiously awaiting the opportunity to carve on you like a Thanksgiving turkey. That is not health!

I wanted to heal my stopped-up nose and I knew there was a cause and the doctors failed miserably in even attempting to find it, let alone eliminating it. Common sense kept badgering me with the question, *"If you don't know the cause how are you going to cure it?"*

After my doctor's drugs failed to clear my sinuses, I tried visiting health food stores. I talked to nutritionists and bought a lot of herbs and vitamins, but once again to no avail. I was still unable to breathe and finally declared to my mom one night that I would pay anything if I could just breathe. In that moment of misery, disappointed in my doctors failure to help me, and not willing to go through surgery, I vowed to myself that I would find the cause of my allergies. I wanted to know what was causing my nose to feel as if a cement truck had backed into my bedroom at night and filled each nostril solid. I had no idea how, but I knew I had to study health, not disease, to find the solution.

Divine Guidance from on High

One cold, snowy day in the winter, I was studying for a college exam. Something within told me to turn on the radio, but I ignored it. I had another strong premonition to turn the radio on, but rationalized that I couldn't. I had to study or else I would fail the exam. On the third time, I finally turned the radio on to hear Dr. Jack Stalkwell's K-Talk program with his guest, Max Skousen, talking about how to heal allergies. I immediately knew that the teacher had appeared if I, the student, was ready.

It is important to understand that everything in life is energy. We either attract or repel certain situations to us. I highly recommend you watch a documentary movie called *The Secret*. For more information go online to thesecret.com.

Max announced that he would be speaking at a local hotel in a few days. I made it a priority to attend his lecture, and it's history from here. I live in a different world now. My allergies are healed and I have never experienced clogged-sinuses since. Max used a technique called the RFA process, which I went on to learn and still use to this day. RFA stands for Relaxed, Focused, Attention. It's a way to heal emotional issues that are causing physical ailments like allergies. Kinesiology or muscle testing is used to identify what is causing the illness.

> **"The visible world is the invisible organization of energy."**
> Heinz Pagels

Kinesiology

Kinesiology or muscle testing received scientific attention through the works of Dr. George Goodheart and later Dr. John Diamond. Max demonstrated that muscle testing was effective for identifying which nutritional products would be beneficial for each individual through a strong or weak muscle response. For more information on kinesiology, I recommend reading *Power vs. Force* by David R. Hawkins, M.D., Ph.D.

How does kinesiology work? Our body sends out very minute electrical currents, which flow from the brain to the thousands of muscles. If the mind is speaking truth, it is in harmony and the electrical signal goes out unimpaired. But if the mind is not telling the truth, it creates conflict, making some degree of static and confusion, so that the electrical current is not sent out with the same strength and therefore causes a weakness in muscular response. If doing a muscle test with an arm, the muscles become weaker to some degree. Through muscle testing we can identify what is causing a person's illness. We can also use it to determine which products are good for you and which ones are not. It, in effect, acts as a human lie detector.

> "Your subconscious mind is all-wise. It knows the answers to all questions. However, it does not know that it knows."
> — Joseph Murphy, Ph.D.

Many allergies are caused by traumatic experiences that have occurred in life. Through the RFA process (Relaxed, Focused, Attention), I learned that my allergies were caused by something that happened when I was in the second month of my mother's womb. Since a baby in the womb is a magnet to its mother's feelings, he or she feels everything mother does and those feelings are permanently recorded in the subconscious mind. Once we make a decision with feeling and attach a meaning to it, then we create a story which usually results in some form of ill health.

The RFA process took about an hour and a half and we completely healed my allergies in one session. My allergies are gone and to this day remain a thing of the past. My allergies were not caused from a physical problem, although my symptoms were physical. They were caused from an emotional one and once we released the negativity stored in my subconscious, healing occurred. My many prayers were finally answered and I have been eternally grateful ever since. I can breathe now through my nose. I didn't need a bunch of drugs or surgery. I didn't need herbs, minerals or any other remedy. What I needed was an emotional, subconscious detox. Once we released the negative programming in my subconscious mind, my physical body functioned properly without allergies. We healed the cause.

> "From the bitterness of disease man learns the sweetness of health."
> Catalan Proverb

The Subconscious Mind

Have you ever closed your eyes and began to think about something and the next thing you know, your body is experiencing the very thing you were thinking? For example, imagine yourself trapped in a snowstorm, lost in the woods and freezing. If you concentrate hard enough, you can actually decrease your body temperature enough to produce goose bumps. Tibetan monks in China can spend the night meditating in the high mountains where the temperature drops way below freezing, wearing only a sheet and stay perfectly warm.

Have you ever smelled something so rotten and vile that it made you gag or possibly even vomit? Most of us have. If you close your eyes and really concentrate, you can probably bring those old memories up and re-experience them.

> "The mind is so powerful that it can create an experience to support any belief. Then we believe the experience proves the belief, not knowing that the belief created the experience." Krishnamurti

The power of suggestion is real. People who are hypnotized can do some amazing things. Suggest to someone that they are allergic to dust and you are now going to hold some in front of them. Instead you hold a cup full of paper clips and they begin sneezing uncontrollably. What do you think caused the individual to sneeze? Was it the paper clips or the suggestion? What we learn from these examples is that the cause of many symptoms are in the subconscious mind.

Since our right brain (subconscious) has total recall of every feeling we have ever felt, many of us have issues from the womb, birth and early childhood. The left brain, the one we rationally think with, forgets all the time, but the right brain never forgets. Once we make a decision with feeling, subconsciously, it becomes our reality.

We are the result of everything we have ever believed. Our beliefs act as a filter of logic through which we see the whole world. We go through life and never let anything through this filter that is inconsistent with our beliefs. Sometimes our beliefs and prejudices can be ridiculous and inconsistent with reality.

> "The miracle-working powers of your subconscious mind existed before you and I were born, before any church or world existed."
> Joseph Murphy, Ph.D.

The RFA process gets a person relaxed and focused. Our subconscious mind is like a large library of feelings and information. It can be accessed at any time. When I went through the RFA process, we found the cause of my allergies. The cause was a feeling of not being wanted and loved by my mother.

Muscle testing revealed something traumatic occurred in the second month, when I was just a fetus in mother's womb. I felt that my mother, who already had four children, didn't really want me. I felt that she didn't love me and then made a subconscious decision that I was right, "momma doesn't love me." So twenty-two years later I was venting the hurt of not being wanted through the form of an allergy (stopped-up nose). The amazing thing about this whole ordeal was that it was only a story I created and wasn't true, but I was believing it, so it became my reality.

> **"Everything you can imagine is real."** Pablo Picasso

The truth was that my mother did love me and wanted me but I made a decision subconsciously that she didn't and it was affecting my health. It doesn't matter what is real; it only matters what you believe because that is what becomes your reality. Let me help you understand this by asking you the following question.

> Is Cinderella a real story?   ___YES   or   ___NO

If you answered "YES" you are correct. It is a real story. You can go to any library, school or video store and get the book or movie and watch or read it. It is a real story that someone wrote. It is told throughout the world.

Now, if you answered "NO" Cinderella is not a real story, you are right too. Of course it's not true. There never was a lady named Cinderella who lost her slipper at the ball. It was a fictitious story all made up in a writer's mind and then he wrote the story in a book and published it. Millions of people have read the made up fairy tale and enjoyed it.

My Cinderella story was that my mother didn't love me. That became my reality. Was it a true story? Yes and no. It was true to me and I played it out as if it were true for twenty-two years. Did I have any evidence that my story was true? No, you could never find a kinder, unselfish, loving person than my mother. Consciously, I knew my mother loved me, however, my subconscious mind had been made up and no matter how great and loving she was, I still felt unloved and unwanted subconsciously.

> "Many illnesses which are manifestations of chakra imbalances are the results of faulty data on old memory tapes which have been recorded and programmed into the unconscious mind during early portions of the individual's life. These tapes have been unconsciously playing back messages told to them by others or falsely thought by themselves, which are no longer appropriate to present-day circumstances." Richard Gerber, M.D.

Most of our lives are a series of events that we attach stories to give feelings meaning. Once we create these meanings with emotions we have our reality. In our minds, with intense emotions, we make something true or false, right or wrong, good or bad, regardless of what the actual reality may be. Ten other people in the same situations may tell a totally different story depending upon their programming in life.

> "Man keeps looking for a truth that fits his reality. Given our reality, truth doesn't fit." Werner Erhard - Founder of the Landmark Forum (formerly known as "est")

"For as he thinketh in his heart, so is he." Proverbs 23:7 The apostle Peter got quite a lesson in this when Christ told him to walk out on the water to meet him. The law of gravity argues that it is impossible for man to walk on water, but Christ taught *"If ye have faith enough you can move mountains."* The real mountains to move in life are not the ones in nature, for they are beautiful and perfect, but the jagged peaks in your mind, the ones you have created out of hurt, pain, guilt, anger and fear. These are the mountains that must tumble in order for you to achieve optimum health, freedom and peace.

> "All that we are is the result of what we have thought."
> Buddha 563-483 B.C.

After several months, college classes let out for Christmas break and I left "to be home for the holidays." A few days after I was home my mom and I were sitting in our living room. As we sat there, I asked her if anything traumatic happened when she was pregnant with me. She paused for a moment and then shook her head and said, "When I was about two months pregnant with you, I went to my doctor and since I already had four children, he suggested the possibility of not having any more. He made it clear that abortion was an option if I wanted it." I asked her how that made her feel, and she said it made her sick to know that she had trusted this doctor, who suggested this, to deliver her babies. She was angry and frustrated and felt compelled to find a new doctor.

I then told my mom how amazing that story was. I told her about healing my allergies through the RFA process and that muscle testing indicated that something traumatic occurred in the second month in the womb. I understood that I, the baby in mom's womb, had picked up and felt the anger and frustration she had towards that doctor and made a subconscious decision that, *"My mom was upset and that it must be my fault."*

> **"The doctor who can cure one disease by knowledge of its principles may, by the same means, cure all the diseases of the human body; for their causes are the same."** Benjamin Rush, M.D.

RFA CHECKLIST

Factors Which May Be Affecting Your Health and Freedom

- _____ Easily embarrassed and self consciousness
- _____ A feeling of shame about hidden secrets
- _____ Fear of abandonment
- _____ Intense fear of speaking before a group
- _____ Irrational fear, such as height, water, freeways, germs, untidiness, claustrophobia, flying or others
- _____ Chronic depression
- _____ Tendency toward extreme gullibility
- _____ General lack of ambition
- _____ Difficulty in knowing or asking for what you want
- _____ Fear of intimacy
- _____ Deep hurt because of having been molested or raped
- _____ Deep distrust of the opposite sex
- _____ Insatiable need of approval
- _____ Difficulty in making up your mind
- _____ A need to control or manipulate others
- _____ Constant procrastination
- _____ Dyslexia
- _____ Physical conditions, such as asthma, hay fever, migraine headaches, frequent colds, arthritis, etc.
- _____ Hypertension, chronic pain, etc.
- _____ Sexual impotence (male)
- _____ Sexual frigidity (female)
- _____ Uncontrollable, spontaneous body movements (ticks)
- _____ Deep sense of unworthiness
- _____ Feeling of financial insecurity or bondage
- _____ Persistent jealousy
- _____ Addictions to alcohol or drugs
- _____ Compulsive over-eating
- _____ Feeling of being too fat
- _____ Sleeping problems
- _____ Sensitivity to certain foods
- _____ Intolerance to certain people, music, subjects, situations, places, sounds
- _____ Times of severe loneliness
- _____ Chronic fatigue
- _____ Deep resentment for having been offended, exploited or misunderstood
- _____ Feelings of being overwhelmed
- _____ Persistent feelings of being unloved or unappreciated
- _____ Deep dissatisfaction with your job, career, home, spouse, church, etc.
- _____ Frustration in not having a meaningful life, not doing what you want to do
- _____ Difficulty with remembering or concentration
- _____ Constantly comparing yourself to others
- _____ Feeling like a victim of other people or circumstances
- _____ Others

Case study – March 2005

For most of my adult life I suffered with terrible allergies; dust, pollen, animals, etc. I was particularly sensitive to cats, which was a nightmare for me because I love cats. And yet I could not get near them without a full-blown allergy attack, with red, itchy, watery eyes, constant sneezing, severely runny nose, and difficulty breathing. If you have ever suffered from severe allergies, you know that it affects your whole life.

Over the years I have tried almost every allergy medication there is, prescription and over-the-counter. They would relieve the symptoms for a little while, but they never went totally away and I didn't like the way they made me feel. Natural remedies and homeopathic formulas made me feel better without the side effects, but nothing ever worked long.

Then one day I found the most adorable little gray kitten that had been abandoned. Even though I knew it would trigger an allergy attack, I had to bring it home anyway. I started on herbal remedies and supplements right away, hoping that this time it would be okay. But it wasn't. The attack was so severe that I could barely even breathe.

I didn't know what to do. I know it sounds silly, but I really, really wanted this kitten. So, in desperation, I asked Dr. Sainsbury to help me.

I went in for an appointment and through the use of a method called RFA, he used guided imagery to help me get to the emotional root of my condition and figure out the cause of my allergies. Once the cause was discovered, he helped me release the negative emotions I was holding on to that kept causing the allergies, and he gave me some mental tools to use to help keep me from slipping back into old patterns.

The whole process took about an hour and when I came out of his office, my allergies were completely gone! Sounds crazy, I know! But I literally went into his office sick as a dog, and left feeling completely well.

However, the real test came when I went home and let my kitten sleep in my lap. I had absolutely no symptoms at all!!! None! From that moment on, I have never had any allergy problems at all. There was a time or two that I was afraid they might be coming back, but I used the techniques that Dr. Sainsbury showed me and it has never happened.

That was about 3 years ago and I am still allergy free. I have a cat that stays in the house all of the time and I never have any symptoms at all.

Thank you Dr. Sainsbury for giving me my life back!
Karen Carswell, Rainbow City, Alabama

KEY CHARACTERISTICS OF THE SUBCONCIOUS (RIGHT BRAIN)

1. The right brain has total recall.
2. It is not logical, instead it just knows – right or wrong, it knows.
3. It cannot tell any difference between an imagined experience and a real one.
4. The right brain gets us into trouble, but it also is the place in which we can heal.
5. Once a decision is made with feeling, it becomes the rule of attitude and action from then on until it is recognized and changed.
6. Although the left brain or conscious mind doesn't have a clue about what is going on in the right brain or subconscious mind, the right brain knows everything going on in the left brain.
7. Since the left brain works with cumbersome language and figures, it works about the speed of sound. However, the right brain operates at the speed of light, doing 90% of the work.
8. All of our feelings, including our upsets, come from our right brain.
9. We are never upset for the reason we think. The immediate problem almost always triggers some issue from the past. Many issues are traced back to early childhood.
10. All of our manual skills come out of the right brain.
11. We never do anything really well until we can do it without thinking.
12. The right brain is the subconscious, not the unconscious. It is very conscious by sensing things. The RFA process brings the subconscious to the conscious.

> "The mind is a complete library of everything that has ever happened to us. This library is called programming."
> Valerie Seeman Moreton, N.D.

In order to understand why people behave the way they do, it is crucial to understand that your mind is programmed for survival. Its job is to protect you and it does this through three crucial decisions. The first decision is to always keep you safe. The mind also works to protect you by always being right. And finally it works so that you will be accepted by others. So, next time you have a misunderstanding or argument, try to put yourself in the other

The Five Lies of Your Mind

1. It claims to know why others are doing what they are doing.
2. It claims to know what is happening at a distance.
3. It claims to know what is going to happen in the future.
4. It claims to know what is to your advantage.
5. It claims to know what ought to be different than what is right. now.

person's shoes. The mind of that individual is working perfectly to keep him or her safe, right and accepted.

A key to being happy and at peace is understanding that the mind is not you, but a servant or a counselor. You are a human being that has a body and a mind. You program your mind and your mind controls your body. At the count of three wiggle your right big toe. One…Two…Three… See how amazing you are? When your brain instructs the muscles to move they obey perfectly. When it comes to healing, your mind directs, your body restores and spirit heals.

Your body has form like the hardware of a computer. The mind is like the software, containing all the information you have ever programmed into it. But the computer (hardware and software) is useless until you plug it into the wall to receive the electricity that brings it to life. Even though you cannot see electricity, it is very real, and the part it plays is paramount. Your spirit is the energy (electricity) that brings your body and mind to life.

You have a body and you have a mind, but you are not what you have. For example, you have a house and you have a car, but that is not who you are. You have a shirt, socks and shoes, but that is not who you are. We are spirit. We are not what we have, we are who we are, eternal spiritual be-ings with a judgmental, fear-based mind always fighting to regain a nondisturbed state we once knew in the womb.

It is important to remember that your mind functions in the past from past experiences or either in the future, in made up possibilities. Both are illusions. Who you really are is spirit, and spirit functions in the present moment or the now. Now is an eternal place, outside time.

> **"The power of the visible is the invisible."**
> Marianne Moore - American Poet

Most of our lives are dominated by fear. Let's take a test. Within the last month, how many times did you allow your mind to torment you with these fear-based questions? These are the three tormentors of the mind.

Fear-Based Questions

1. Did I do the right thing?
2. Am I doing the right thing?
3. Will I do the right thing?

The RFA process has been created to heal our negative programming. The RFA is not hypnosis. It is an emotional release, created to understand, forgive, love and heal by identifying the illusions of your conclusions in your mind. Many of those conclusions are in the subconscious, creating negative feelings so you don't even know they exist.

Most of us are walking around in adult bodies, but the fears from childhood steer us in the direction to go and we don't even realize it. We are still playing out traumatic experiences from when we were younger and they are very much affecting our lives. Almost everyone has some degree of subconscious fear in their survival programming.

> **The Battle Within – Two Fears We Fight**
>
> 1. I am not loved or accepted.
> 2. I am not good enough

Our minds function in opposition to who we are; spirit. At some point in life, most of us make a decision that "something is wrong with me." This illusion we choose to believe creates struggle in life.

Here is an example for parents. Can you stop loving your child right now? Of course you can't. What about if they are disobedient to your commandments? Most parents have unconditional love for their children. That doesn't necessarily mean that you like and approve of all of their decisions when they are breaking the law and getting in trouble, but regardless of what they choose you love them and want them to be happy. You love them because love is the very essence of who you are. Your spirit or electrical energy of your aliveness is made of love. You are light, love, energy and spirit. You have been created in the image of God, but your mind works out of fear. The natural man or our mind working out of fear is an enemy to God.

The NEED to Be Happy

> "Most people are searching for happiness. They're looking for it. They're trying to find it in someone or something outside of themselves. That's a fundamental mistake. Happiness is something that you are, and it comes from the way you think."
>
> Wayne Dyer, Ph.D.

Our minds function on need. We need for things to be better or different. Our minds are greedy and needy and, if not controlled, can create misery. Many of us allow our minds to play out this need for things to be different by changing jobs, relationships, homes, hobbies, automobiles or friends, but we never quite get complete satisfaction. Once we change something, it's just a matter of time before the need compels us to change again. As we continue our search for happiness, we never find it because happiness can never be found outside of one's self. Happiness is only found within.

> "…The kingdom of God is within you." Luke 17:21

We are what we give away. If you want to be happy, give happiness to others. Serve your neighbor and forget yourself. Stop feeling sorry for yourself and all of your problems and go out and help someone because you choose it. Go cut their grass, or find something you can do for them that they'll appreciate. Spend an hour at a retirement home or a hospital every week for a month and be a friend to someone. You may feel grateful for all that you have when you see others who are less fortunate than yourself and suffering. This is a magic success formula for depression. When we stop focusing on our wants and needs and start giving to help someone else out, magic occurs. What we give comes back to us like a boomerang, a hundred fold. It seems like a paradox, but the more you give, the more you have. And always remember, you only have what you give.

> "A candle loses nothing of its light by lighting another candle."
> James Keller

If you want to be miserable, hate everyone and everything. Dwell upon all the times you felt others did you wrong. Hold a grudge and seek revenge. Just go around hating them all day long and guess what? It won't affect them one bit, but you'll be as miserable as you can be. Why? Because you get what you give.

Love Heals

The first step in healing is to love yourself. Some people are sick because deep down inside they hate themselves. We all have a shadow side. In a sense, we each are our own version of Dr. Jeckel and Mr. Hyde. Many times we are intolerant of any bad we see in ourselves and we cannot forgive any imperfection. How many times do you say or do something stupid and then feel bad about it? If you beat yourself up over it for the next ten years, the internal bruises are hidden from your physical eyes, but reveal themselves in the form of guilt. Do you like who you have been in the past? Just because your past is over does not mean that it's not still with you.

Many good people we have worked with cannot forgive themselves for things they have felt were wrong and judged to be bad. Sometimes another person is involved and this feeling that they must be punished for doing something "unacceptable" is many times a culprit in dis-ease. To be healed or as Christ said, "Be made whole," is to come back to who you really are – wholeness. Healing comes from the word whole, just as the word holy.

> **In my counseling I have found that practically everyone (on a subconscious level), does not love themselves. They do not accept themselves nor trust themselves. Most of these same people don't even like themselves. Interestingly enough, they all think they like, love, accept and trust themselves. But sub-consciously, they do not feel it."** Karol K. Truman Author of Feelings Buried Alive Never Die

Healing the inner child, or traumas from the past, can melt allergies, fears, phobias, dyslexia, ADD, OCD etc., like frozen butter in the hot sun. I have witnessed miracles in my office. Once you release the hurt, pain, anger, etc., then proper energy flow is re-established and organs, glands and systems begin to work again. It is awesome.

Mirrors in Life

When you see someone do or say something that really bugs you; usually it is something you hate about your own self. People in life are our mirrors. If there is something you can't stand about someone, something that just really irritates you when they say or do it, then you are sensing or feeling something in that person that you don't like about yourself. Seeing them is a reflection of yourself. You can only see in others according to what you can relate to inside.

People who hate others really hate a part of themselves and that is why some things are not working for them in life. Things don't seem to work because love, joy and peace only come from within. No thing or person can give that to you. They can certainly help you see it and experience it, but ultimately it comes from within. You are the source!

If you find yourself saying you hate someone, then there is a lack of love. Most people believe God is the creator of all. If He creates all, then he created you, me and the guy you hate just the way He did and just the way He didn't. To say you hate someone is in a sense a way to hate God's creations. Stop resisting what is. Accept God's creations for what they are.

> **"I used to be a truth seeker until I realized I AM that which I AM seeking."** James Chappell D.C., N.D., Ph.D.

Peace comes when we accept everyone and everything just the way they are and just the way they aren't because that is the way God created them. That doesn't mean you go out and support everything you believe is wrong like prostitution, drug abuse and murder. What that means is you step back and give others the space they need to be who they choose to be and stop fighting against who they choose. Allow them to be who they want to be just as you are free to be who you choose to be. Stop resisting what is. Flow with the process of life and be at peace with others, even if you disagree with who they choose to be. They may be saying the same thing about you that you are saying about them. Christ taught, take the beam out of your own eye before judging others. In other words, let others be who they choose to be.

How many times do you drive down the road nice and relaxed, enjoying the day as you travel to your destination, when suddenly a reckless speeding car cuts in front of you and several other drivers? Obviously, the speeding driver is disgusted with slow moving traffic. You begin talking about how rude and dangerous he is and how you hope he gets pulled over and ticketed. You holler, "Slow down before you cause an accident you idiot."

The next morning you wake up and get ready for work. Everything that can go wrong does so. Before you know it, you rush out of the house worrying about how late you are going to be for work. You speed out of the driveway trying to make good time and to put the icing on the cake to your crappy morning, you hit another obstacle, old people going ten miles an hour under the speed limit just "pooping along" as if there's no tomorrow. Their casual morning drive has traffic backed up for miles. You begin hollering for them to get moving and at the next break in traffic you punch the pedal to the metal to get around them. You say to yourself, "Obviously they are retired and have nothing to do today." In order to avoid hitting oncoming traffic, you dart in front of the slow moving car and give them your best look of disgust and maybe a finger-gesture depending upon how mad you are.

The old people begin cussing you for being the dangerous, reckless, uncaring driver who needs a ticket to be taught a lesson before you kill someone. They are complaining about you just as you were complaining about the driver yesterday. How many of us are hypocrites? We like to point our finger and make others wrong but given the same circumstances we may do the same thing we can't stand about others. Life is interesting. Our perceptions have a tendency to change according to our own experiences.

How many adults see young teenagers make stupid and foolish decisions in life but are oblivious to the stupid things they themselves did when sixteen? We are all here to experience life in its fullness. Our judgmental mind claims to know "what ought to be." This, many times, creates a need to control and a need to be right, which is another form of fear.

Most contention within religious institutions and families stems from a member making someone else wrong for something they did or said. Instead of being able to accept the individual for who they are, they want to make them wrong. Remember, as soon as you blame someone or something for how you feel, you turn that blame into "energy in motion" which equals emotion. Anger and resentment are automatic by-products of blame. What do you blame on your family, spouse and friends?

> "A man may fail many times, but he isn't a failure until he begins to blame somebody else." Anonymous

The natural man is an enemy to God because his or her mind struggles at accepting others for who they are and who they are not. Since you paint the masterpiece in your mind of the reality of the world you live in, you always get to be right by making someone else wrong. Our minds think we know why people do and say the things they do, but they are only perceptions. Usually those perceptions, formed from fear-based programming create a tremendous amount of friction in life.

Most of us would rather be right than happy, even if it means being miserable. The survival mechanism of the mind is a need to be right. The majority of us pay that price to be right. We may be miserable and unhappy in our relationships, but at least we get to be right. For example, if we have made a decision that a certain individual is unreliable then we will create situations to prove ourselves right about him or her being unreliable. Remember, you only find what you are looking to see. Is the glass half full or half empty? Perception creates the world in which you live.

> **Everyone is doing the best he or she can under the circumstances. If you don't understand how they could do this, then you don't understand their circumstances."** Virginia Satir

Placebos: A Factor in Your Healing

The mind of man can make him sick or well. In medicine when patients get better from ingesting a sugar pill, that they believe is medicine, we call that the placebo effect.

Everyone knows that surgery either helps or it doesn't, right? An interesting study was published in the 2002 New England Journal of Medicine on patients who had severe, debilitating knee pain. At Baylor School of Medicine, Dr. Bruce Moseley knew that knee surgery was beneficial for his patients. Well Dr. Moseley wanted to investigate his surgeries to identify which part of the surgery was giving his patients the most relief. So he divided his patients into three groups. In group number one, he shaved the damaged cartilage. In the next group, he flushed out the knee joint, removing anything thought to be causing inflammation. Both of these two groups received standard procedures. In the last group, he performed "fake" surgery. He sedated the patients, made three standard incisions and behaved exactly as if he were doing a real surgery, but did not shave or flush anything out of the knee. After about 40 minutes, the time the normal procedure takes, Dr. Moseley sewed up the incisions just the same as a real knee surgery. All three groups were then given the same postoperative care, including an exercise program.

The results left Dr. Moseley baffled. All three groups improved. The real head-scratcher was that the placebo group improved just as much as the other two groups! Dr. Moseley concluded, *"My skill as a surgeon had no benefit on these patients. The entire benefit of surgery for osteoarthritis of the knee was the placebo effect."* Members of the placebo group were seen playing basketball and other athletic activities that they were unable to do before their "fake surgery." Two years went by before the placebo patients were finally told the truth. Tim Perez was a placebo surgery patient who used a cane before the surgery and is now able to play basketball. His response was, *"In this world anything is possible when you put your mind to it. I know that your mind can work miracles."*

> **"Doctors should not dismiss the power of the mind as something inferior to the power of chemicals and the scalpel. They should let go of their conviction that the body and its parts are essentially stupid and that we need outside intervention to maintain our health."**
> Bruce Lipton, Ph.D.

Are you ready to heal or do you subconsciously like the payoff you receive by being sick? Does the thought of family, work and friends expecting too much from you, if you were healthy, fill you with fear? Would more responsibility be heaped upon your shoulders than you feel you could bear? Does the thought of being perfectly healthy bog you down with a nagging headache and have you scared stiff with arthritis? If you were healthy, could you carry the load of jumping to your feet to help all those who ask favors or is the thought of it all a pain in your neck? Does your worry and concern for family members and friends choosing to do things that you perceive to be bad or wrong have you all uptight and constipated? Do you sometimes feel they are a pain in the butt? Maybe there's more truth to those thoughts than you know. Perhaps if you were healthy, there would be no excuse for failure in certain areas of your life? Maybe people would expect too much from you? Fear is a disease that manifests itself with physical symptoms. It has been said that the thoughts we choose to think are the tools we use to paint the canvas of our lives.

> **"Disease will never be cured or eradicated by present materialistic methods, for the simple reason that disease in its origin is not material. Disease is in essence the result of conflict between soul and mind, and will never be eradicated except by spiritual and mental effort."**
> Edward Bach, M.B., B.S., D.P.H., - Creator of Bach Flower Remedies

A forty-two year old disabled and severely arthritic male came into the office and pleaded for help. He was in so much pain he could hardly walk. In our first appointment, we found out why he was sick. Addressing the cause of his arthritic state, we found it to be an emotional/mental issue. Subconsciously, he was afraid to face the world as a healthy able man fully responsible and capable to earn a living for his family. His only skills were in construction doing manual labor. He hated construction work. Fear resonated throughout his body at the thought of sweating in the 100-degree heat everyday to earn a living, not to mention a few traumatic experiences he had in the past with some co-workers. Their jokes and persecution made him feel rejected and he made a decision that he never wanted to be in that type of situation again. Subconsciously, he figured out a way to escape the misery of having to go to work every day and deal with a job. His arthritis gave him a scapegoat, a way out so his wife had to work and he could stay at home in his comfort zone and not have to face a bitter, cruel and merciless world, as he perceived it.

This fear was the real cause of his arthritis. It was this resistance to face a dreaded job for the rest of his life, filled with unfriendly people and an unwillingness to step forward, that was causing his joints to deteriorate. Sure, his body was malnourished and toxic, but his mind was the main cause of him not being well.

> **"If you think something outside yourself is the cause of your problem, you will look outside yourself for the answer. Look within and BE HEALED!"** Valerie Seeman Moreton, N.D.

Statistically speaking, more people die from heart attacks on Mondays than any other day of the week. Why? Because they hate their jobs. The subconscious mind figures out a way to get out of work, a way to escape the hell that they perceive has them trapped. When strong emotions resonate within, then the body chemistry changes.

The computer system called your brain that controls your physical body has more power then most realize. If something inside of you won't let you quit, if you are a fighter with a desire to heal then you can. Faith is powerful. If you believe you can't then you are right too. This is the great secret in life. Whatever you believe becomes your reality. Jesus Christ told us that greater things than the healing he was performing we would do also. This book is filled with examples of miracles that happen today, and you can experience that awesome power that you have been endowed with since birth, but you have to want it. When the student is ready, the teacher appears.

> **"Whether you think you can or think you can't; either way you're right."**
> Henry Ford 1863-1947

God has given you dominion over the elements of the earth. There is a way to heal. But remember, faith without works is dead, so get ready to go to work, because nothing ever worth having comes easy. By the way, "the will of God" is usually used as a cheap excuse when we want to blame someone or something and escape responsibility. In reality, the cause of dis-ease is a violation of His natural laws or to say it simply, disease is a natural result of an unnatural lifestyle.

The World We Create with Thoughts

> "The environment you fashion out of your thoughts, your beliefs, your ideals, your philosophy, is the only one you will never live in."
> O.S. Marden

The average human has about sixty thousand thoughts a day. Thoughts become things. A thought has a frequency that can be measured. We choose the thoughts that we dwell upon, which form our feelings, which lead to our beliefs. Then, we make decisions and act according to our feelings. This creates our experiences. Our personalities are nothing more than the sum of our thoughts and feelings of the past.

Whatever you think, you will become. Whatever you dwell upon is where you direct your energy. If you spend your time thinking about how lonely you are and how you'll never meet anyone to connect with, you're probably not going to meet that certain someone. Just as water will take the shape of any object you pour it into, so will the direction of your life flow, according to the guidance of your thoughts. Dwell upon the good in your life and let go of negativity. Start focusing on what you want, not what you don't have. Act as if you already have it and you'll attract it to you.

> "In our laboratory experiments we have found that the act of thinking releases an energy which we can store in the lattice system of a cut quartz crystal. These patterns of thought vibrations are stored and oscillate like a magnetic field.... When one pulses one's thought, that energy ... has the power of a laser."
> Marcel Vogel, Ph.D. - IBM Scientist for 27 years (1917-1991)

William James, the father of American psychology, taught that the subconscious mind has the power to move the world and that it is one with infinite intelligence and boundless wisdom.

I have the capability to sit here and think and, within fifteen minutes, I can be the saddest, most depressed person in the world. All I have to do is start dwelling upon everything I don't have. When I start focusing on everything negative that has ever happened to me, I can produce dark, negative feelings. I don't recommend doing this. It creates dis-ease. Nonetheless, I can create that if I choose. Just as I can produce depression with thoughts, I can go to the other end of the spectrum and focus on all that I have been given. By focusing on every good thing that I've been blessed with, I plant the seeds of gratitude that grows a tree of happiness.

As you read this page there are people suffering in car accidents, dying of cancer, starving to death, paralyzed from the neck down, drowning, lost in the woods, being burned, being robbed, freezing to death in snowstorms, hunched over the toilet sick as a dog etc. If you are able to read this book, then most likely you aren't experiencing any of those terrible things at the present time. You have a lot to be thankful for and are blessed. Realize that your situation could always be worse. An attitude of gratitude produces health.

> **"We become that upon which we put our attention. "...God if thou seest God, dust if thou seest dust."** Anonymous

Many people born in third world countries live in adobe houses with dirt floors and have no running water. Some are illiterate and have never had the opportunity to attend school. They use outhouses that drain into the same rivers where they get water. Some have never worn a pair of shoes in their whole life. Many of the men stay hunched over, swinging a machete chopping sugarcane twelve hours a day in 110-degree heat, earning about five dollars a day. If you were forced to experience this type of life for a while, you would be very thankful for the abundance you have been given. To have clean running water to drink and bathe with is something most of us take for granted. Carpeted floors in beautiful homes that are heated and cooled to our specifications are unimaginable to most third world's citizens. Most of us have delicious foods to eat and cars to drive wherever and whenever we want. We are spoiled rotten compared to the rest of the world. Some may say that we have it too good. We can lie on our couch and complain that we are depressed or bored while others are busy trying to harvest, catch or earn just enough so they can eat.

> **"What we sow or plant in the soil will come back to us in exact kind. It's impossible to sow corn and get a crop of wheat, but we entirely disregard this law when it comes to mental sowing."**
> Orison Swett Marden

Freedom is a Choice

When we begin thinking and feeling grateful for all our blessings, then the mind programs our physical body for health. Release and let go of negative thoughts and feelings. Don't suppress them, experience them when they come and then release them. Replace them with an attitude of gratitude and thank your Creator for the opportunity to live and experience all of life in its fullness.

Outer freedom may be a gift, but inner freedom must be chosen. This is done by being thankful for our experiences in life, especially those which are not to one's taste. The person who is free to be sick can enjoy health. The one who is free to be lonely can enjoy a companion. If you are free to be broke, you can enjoy money. A person who is free to die can enjoy living.

> "A thought held long enough and repeated enough becomes a belief. The belief then becomes biology." Christiane Northrup, M.D.

Weight Gain – An Emotional Issue

Tears of joy are considered nontoxic. But tears of anger are loaded with proteins and are said to be more poisonous than snake venom. A woman who was raped twenty-six years ago had been holding on to anger, fear and hurt. This cactus of negative emotions was growing within her causing thorns to manifest themselves in the form of cysts, cancerous tumors and obesity. It happened a long time ago and there is nothing we can do to change the past. However, she, as so many of us do, was reliving the trauma everyday through her thoughts and stored emotions. What good was it doing to hate that man who raped her? It in no way punished him for hurting her. The only person being hurt was herself. She had to forgive and let go in order to change the terrain so that good health could exist.

What we found, through the RFA process, was that her obesity was created as a defense mechanism to protect her from ever being sexually assaulted again. She made a subconscious decision that if she was fat and ugly, then no man would ever want her again and this would keep her safe. We also found out that her cancer was a subconscious decision to commit suicide. The cancer provided her with an excuse to check out of this cruel world that she was tired of living in and feeling unsafe. These crosses were too much for her to carry. She was at the giving up point.

> **"An angry man is full of poison."** Confucius

Just as tomato seeds fail to germinate on a tar-paved highway, neither does health flourish in a garden of thorns riddled with hate and anger. Dark emotions resonating within, only produce chaos and dis-ease. If we don't forgive, then we aren't forgiven.

Many problems in the male and female organs develop out of unforgiveness with an intimate partner. When we feel we have been hurt by a spouse or significant other, then many times, those emotions cause dis-ease in the reproductive area.

As a priceless, loved son or daughter of God, you are worthy of unconditional love. Sometimes, the guilt people hold on to, cloud that love and they lose touch of who they are. They don't feel worthy of love. We are the ones who shut ourselves off from it. Our Creator loves us with no exceptions. It does not matter what we have done, we are always accepted and loved by our Maker. Just as a loving parent forgives a child of making a mess in their room, so does our Father forgive us of making messes in our lives.

> **"We must take responsibility for the way we feel. The notion that others can make us feel good or bad is untrue. Consciously or-more frequently-unconsciously, we are choosing how we feel at every single moment."** Candace B. Pert, Ph.D.

You can't sit on the couch all day watching soap operas where people are lying, cheating, seeking revenge and expect to go out and have awesome relationships. Turn the trash off and stop feeding your mind negativity. Get out in the community, church, school etc., and make a difference. Do something and be someone. Live your life to the fullest. Be anxiously engaged in a good cause. Stop complaining and be part of the solution, not part of the problem. Give up playing the blame game by making someone else wrong. Create a new possibility of something great.

> **"The universe simply gives us whatever we believe."**
> Carol Tuttle Author of Remembering Wholeness

The following handout was given to me long ago and the author is unknown. It has been a powerful script that helps release negativity so that you can live life to the fullest. I have changed a few things from the original script.

Letting Go

To let go doesn't mean to stop caring; it means I can't do it for someone else.

To let go is not to cut myself off; it's the realization that I can't control another.

To let go is not to enable, but to allow learning from natural consequences.

To let go is to give others the space to choose what they want, which means the outcome is not in my hands.

To let go is not to try to change or blame another; I can only change myself.

To let go is not to care for, but to care about.

To let go is not to fix, but to be supportive.

To let go is not to judge, but to allow another to be a human being.

To let go is not to be in the middle arranging all the outcomes, but to allow others to affect their own outcomes.

To let go is not to be protective; it is to permit another to face reality.

To let go is not to deny, but to accept.

To let go is to stop being right and making others wrong.

To let go is not to nag, scold, or argue, but instead to search out my own shortcomings and correct them.

To let go is not to adjust everything to my desires, but to take each day as it comes and cherish myself in it.

To let go is not to criticize and regulate anyone, but to try to become what I dream I can be.

To let go is to stop playing small and start making a difference.

To let go is to be part of the solution, not part of the problem.

To let go is not to regret the past, but to grow and live for the future.

To let go is to fear less and love more.

Maybe it is letting go of a rebellious child, or a burden or sorrow, losing a loved one, or learning to live with a heartache which we cannot let go. Read this over and over. Let it go deep within and start releasing negativity. You will find that letting go of your load will release a peace within you which will allow your spirit to soar…to be free. Give it completely to God and let a work be done within you…where the need is anyway.

> **"You constantly tear down or build up your health according to the nature of your thinking."** Catherine Ponder

Love

Love is light. Love and light are energy. Love is the light and energy in all creation. Love is the magnetism that holds every atom together in the universe. Love is what heals illness. Love is the most powerful force in the universe. It is through love that we exist.

When you spiritually mature enough to trust God with all of your heart, might, mind and strength, then you come to understand that everyone in life is doing the very best they can with what they have at this time. Trusting God is when you trust that everything works for your greatest good. When you reach this level of trust, then there is nothing to fear. The war is over, you win. You come home to perfect balance, love and peace.

> **"Reasons aren't real; people make them up to justify what they want to do."** Adelaide Bry Author of est 60 hours that transform your life

True love is not a feeling, it is an understanding. When you understand why people do and say the things they do, then you can forgive and healing takes place. This is love. This is what the RFA process allows you to experience. You cannot take an individual who has had something terrible happen like murder or rape and then force them to forgive the perpetrator without understanding; it very seldom happens. They can say that they forgive with their conscious mind, because they know what they should do, but most likely, deep down there is a rat's nest of hurt, anger, revenge etc. Denial doesn't produce health.

In order to heal, one must understand why the individual did or said the hurtful thing. Understanding is the key to forgiveness. Forgiveness is the key that unlocks the hurt in the heart, so healing takes place.

> **"He who cannot forgive others, breaks the bridge over which he himself must pass."** William Thackery

Every emotion resonates at a certain frequency that can be measured. Through a CEDSA test, we have the ability to scan each individual who comes into our clinic to identify which emotion is resonating in their body, compromising their health.

Emotions – Energy In Motion

Abandoned	Abused	Affair	Anger
Anxiety	Apathy	Argumentative	Bitterness
Boredom	Compulsive	Contradict	Critical
Cynical	Death	Demanding	Depression
Despair	Destruction	Dishonest	Dominating
Doubtful	Dread	Embarrassment	Envy
Fear	Fight	Frustrated	Giving
Greedy	Grief	Grudge	Guilt
Hateful	Hunger	Hurt	Immoral
Impatience	Inadequacy	Indecisive	Infidelity
Irritation	Jealousy	Judgement	Kill
Loneliness	Obsessive	Paranoia	Persecuted
Powerlessness	Pride	Rape	Regret
Rejection	Remorse	Repulsive	Resentment
Resigned	Ridicule	Ruthless	Self Pity
Selfish	Shame	Spiteful	Submissive
Suspicion	Unloved	Upset	Vulnerable
Worried			

> "Don't pass judgment on me until you've walked a mile in my moccasins." Navajo Indian Proverb

Agape Love

The old Greek language had five different words to describe five entirely different kinds of love. In English we just have one word – love.

- ♦ **Eros:** Physical attraction between the sexes, as in the word erotic.
- ♦ **Pia:** Protective feeling of mother for child. Parental love.
- ♦ **Storage:** Family or group affection, attachment.
- ♦ **Philia:** Approval, cherish, adore as in Philadelphia, city of brotherly love.
- ♦ **Agape:** Understanding, light, union and oneness, without separation.

The first four types of love; eros, pia, storage and philia are feelings that happen to us. They all have to do with a feeling of warmth, attachment, enjoyment and being comfortable. Through these we obtain our greatest pleasures, but also experience our greatest emotional pains when the objects of these affections are taken away from us.

> "Feelings control our glands. Glands control DNA. Anything less than feelings of love depresses all body functions, propelling us towards death. Calm, vibrant joyful love vitalizes all body functions, propelling us towards unending life and health."
>
> Richard Anderson, N.M.D.

The fourth type of love is Agape. Agape is understanding, light and compassion. It is a way of seeing rather than feeling. It is understanding that we (spiritually) are one with our source, just as the Father and Son are one.

> "…Is it not written in your law, I said, Ye are Gods?"
>
> Jesus Christ - St. John 10:34

Just as the sun cannot obtain light from an outside source, neither can you obtain love by getting it from something outside of you. All things come from within. We have all the attributes of love, just as a ray of sunlight contains all the attributes of the light that the sun produces.

> "In the deeper reality beyond space and time, we may be all members of one body." Sir James Jeans

EGO

- Your ego is what you think you are. It is not the reality of what you are, but everything you have come to believe is true about you.
- Your reality is not the reality. If it were, it would remain constant and would be the same for everyone.
- You made up this reality, and it changes every moment of every day, so in this way it is a fantasy or an illusion.
- Because you created your reality, you love it, and must defend it at all costs.

> **"What you make, you love, and must protect and defend with everything you have."** Max Skousen 1921-2002

True love is giving someone the space for him or her to choose to be just the way they are and just the way they are not. Love is never in competition with anything, even hate. When someone or thing attempts to enforce authority to protect them, or the institution and all is done in the name of what is "good and right," then we have conflict. Being good and right always co-exists with fear. Anxiety and worry are other names for fear. Agape love is the Greek word explaining the type of love Jesus Christ taught. It does not exist with fear. As John the Beloved proclaimed, *"There is no fear in love; but perfect love casteth out fear: because fear hath torment. He that feareth is not made perfect in love." 1 John 4:18*

> **"Fear defeats more people than any other thing, and it is the fear, not the thing we fear, that causes failure. Face the thing you fear and death of fear is certain."** Ralph Waldo Emerson

Why Relationships Fail

A sparkle in the eye and there's something magic about that person that just makes you want to be with them. Conversation leads to a date, then a need or a want to be with the other person. After dates and being together you "fall in love." Many get married to whom they think they love. Their partner seems to fill all of their needs and when they are apart, they count down the minutes until they can be together again.

After a while of being together and fulfilling each other's needs, stored in our powerful subconscious mind is a mountain of guilt and negative feelings we have been suppressing for most of our lives. In the past when these feelings came up, we shoved them back down like a buoy in the lake, but of course they pop right back up with time. When that doesn't work any longer, we look for someone to blame it on, usually our spouse. By projecting it onto others, we get to blame them and escape responsibility. "It's not my fault we aren't close anymore, you don't treat me like you used to when we were dating," is a typical blamer's reply.

This is our feeble attempt to find love. When we enter a relationship to get something out of it, which most of us do, then we feed each other by repressing guilt and doing and saying the little things to make each other feel good. Over time, usually we get tired of playing the "give to get game." Once a partner concludes that the other can no longer give all that is needed to feed the greed of the ego and keep saying and doing nice things, then the ego says, "another can be found."

Children are Great Teachers

> **"It is not what happens, it is how we react to it."** Louise L. Hay

When children misbehave and you as a parent choose to scream and yell at them to shape up, most of the time it only complicates the problem and thickens the friction. A more effective and peaceful route to take is to stop resisting them being in a bad mood and upset for whatever reason. Put yourself in their shoes. Many times they act up because they are starving for attention. They may get a spanking, yelled at or grounded, but nonetheless, they had your undivided attention for ten seconds.

When children are upset, their feelings need to be validated, not condemned. To simply hold an upset child in your arms and tell him or her how much you love them and that it's all right to feel the way they feel, usually melts contention like a fire does chocolate and marshmallows. Ask them to explain why they are upset and many times they have valid reasons and we adults are the ones to blame for something we did or said. Keep in mind that, when children feel unloved, they misbehave. In other words, children misbehaving is a sign that they don't feel loved. What are we creating by how we choose to interact with our children?

I remember a time my four-year-old daughter was in a terrible mood and everything I asked her to do she replied with a sharp rebellious, "No!" In that moment I had choices. I could have chosen to spank her and demand for her to pick up the toys. I could have threatened to punish her such as no TV, but I didn't. Instead I walked over to her. She had a scowl on her face with her bottom lip curled up in a way that would have scared Clint Eastwood. I picked her up in my arms and asked her what was wrong. She started crying and said, "Nobody likes me." She proceeded to name a few previous events that I was familiar with, but had shrugged off as no big deal. To me the incidents weren't a big deal, but to little four-year-old Brooklyn, it was as if the world was coming to an end. Her reason for being upset was perfectly legitimate when I understood from her four-year old perspective.

I told Brooklyn that I would like to be her friend and asked her if she would help me fix lunch, because I needed a good helper to stir the soup. I knew she liked to help cook and that brought a smile back to her sweet face. After lunch, I asked if she could help me out and pick the toys up in the living room. She replied, "Sure Daddy, I can do that."

> **"Everything you teach you are learning."** A Course in Miracles

It's the small and simple things that bring the great things to pass. In every situation, we have a choice and we choose who we want to be. You are the source. You have the ability and choice to make a difference. Do your choices make the problem worse or better? Are you a poor victim or do you choose to make a difference?

> "Love is the master key that opens the gates of happiness."
> Oliver Wendell Holmes

If love is the key to happiness, then forgiveness of self and others opens the door to peace of mind. We cannot have peace of mind and be angry at something mom or dad said or did five years ago. It needs to be cleared up and healed. If a specific incident pops in your mind right now, then that is what you need to heal. Take a moment right now and think of something someone did or said that you thought was wrong. That is what needs to be healed. You are probably thinking, there is a mountain that needs to be moved. With enough faith and some emotional release, you can move that mountain.

Accepting God's creations, just how He created them, is the first step towards peace. Stop making other people wrong for how God created them. Love them for the person they are. They are not perfect and neither are you, so quit fighting the system. Attempting to change things without first accepting them as they are, just how God made them, is like wearing Chinese handcuffs, the harder you try, the more resistance you create. What you resist, persists.

> "All anger is nothing more than an attempt to make someone feel guilty..." A Course in Miracles

Let me give you another example. Take the sun. You can hate it for being hot, bright and burning your skin to a crisp last time you were at the beach with your shirt off for six hours. If you have ever worked construction, you know how miserable it can be on a black roof in the 100-degree blistering hot sun. After ten hours of roofing, you feel like a big baked potato-cooked! You can cuss and hate the sun all you want, but in reality the sun is what it is. God created it and without it we would die. No plants and food could grow and we would freeze to death. Life would cease to exist without the heat, light and energy of the sun.

Let's shift gears. Someone who lives in Alaska learns to love the sun in the cold winter months. It brings warmth and light to the cold, dark and frozen earth. To be able to see after twenty hours of darkness is liberating. The sun can be beautiful, but to the fair-skinned man in a speedo who falls asleep on the Florida beach in August, it can blister the skin with sunburn so severe that you feel like an egg in a frying pan.

> "Many of my patients have nothing wrong with them except their thoughts." Greek Physician

In order to completely heal something, we must take responsibility for it. People make the mistake of feeling like victims and since so-and-so did such-and-such, they have been dealt a bad hand. They sometimes feel that they were unlucky in life. We can play the blame game all we want but remember, when you blame someone, you are escaping responsibility. As long as you see the problem as an outward force, you are unable to affect it, and therefore not responsible, but the second you own it, become responsible for it, you can do what you choose with it. Remember, you are the source.

> "Conflict cannot survive without your participation."
> Wayne W. Dyer, Ph.D.

Transforming Your Life

When we stop pretending to know it all and humble ourselves enough to look at new possibilities, we are enlightened. God always answers the prayer of the heart, not the prayer of the lips. *"And they come close to me with their lips but their hearts are far from me." (James 1:8 and 4:8)* Most of us are double-minded, meaning we say one thing, but feel and believe something totally different deep down.

The Landmark Forum is a three-day transformational seminar taught all over the world. Forum leaders have a unique way of letting you see yourself from an outside perspective. How many times have you wished for a better job, spouse, home, more money, more happiness etc.? Most of us have some pretty good reasons as to why we don't have what we want. But just as we have addressed throughout this book, everything has a cause. There is a reason why you are the way you are and the Landmark Forum provides the opportunity to comprehend that. What there is to get at the Landmark Forum

> *First I was dying to finish high school and start college.*
> *And then I was dying to finish college and start working.*
> *And then I was dying to marry and have children.*
> *And then,*
> *I was dying for my children to grow old enough so I could return to work.*
> *And then,*
> *I was dying to retire.*
> *And now,*
> *I am dying...And suddenly realize I forgot to live.*
>
> *Anonymous*

is, the world you live in doesn't have to be the way it is right now. You have the power to create something different, if you choose.

Everything we experience in life can be summed up by, "It Is." However, our minds work in opposition to who we really are. So instead of just experiencing life for what it is, we judge everything to be either right or wrong, true or false, good or bad. We attach beliefs and ideals to everything. Then we create stories about everyone and everything in our life. These stories usually clutter our lives so much that we no longer are free to experience the experience of life.

> "One creates from nothing. If you try to create from something you're just changing something. So in order to create something you first have to be able to create nothing." Werner Erhard

The Landmark Forum is not about change. It is transformation with the emphasis put on accepting yourself as you really are. It is not something to make your life more, better or different, but to transform the way you experience life so that the problems and situations you have been trying to change just clear up in the process of living.

Instead of trying to change things in your life, or more accurately said, make them more, better or different, nothing really changes because the source is still the same. When we try to fix things, we are only rearranging what is. In other words, one can't create from something. You can only change it by making it more, better or different. But, when you create nothing, then you are free to create something.

Many of us are trapped in self-defeating patterns that keep us from being truly free. You know what I'm talking about, you probably know someone who seems to always have money problems, can't keep a job or constantly having health problems. Perhaps you have a friend or two that you can read like a book. Do you know someone who has a pattern of dating and marrying abusive men? They seem to keep getting trapped in abusive relationships or some other pattern of misery. No matter how hard they try, it's as if they are caught in a spider web and destined for failure. It seems that the harder they try to make it what they think it "ought to be," the worse it gets.

The past keeps repeating itself and is actually creating their future like a programmed robot continuing the same vicious cycle over and over again. The woman keeps marrying abusive men? Why? How does she manage to do that five times in a row?

Many of us have created a destructive way of being from a traumatic experience of the past. We are not free. Our life is a living testimony of a vicious cycle of stupid mistakes made over and over that causes failure and misery.

How many young girls hate their Dads because they are abusive? Then, they grow up and marry some one just like them because they are subconsciously programmed to attract that type of person to them even though they consciously hate and can't stand those types? Their abusive Dad was the male role model for them in their life and that is what they believe men do. Wouldn't it be great to teach that individual to choose something different by clearing up their past so they can attract a loving, gentle-man who would be a good husband and father?

> "Life is not a dress rehearsal. This is it. RIGHT NOW. You can choose to live it to the fullest or sit on the sidelines and watch it go by."
> Dr. Richard Schulze

I remember a conversation I had with a lady who moved into town several years ago. She was a nice person, but her daughter had made some unwise choices that brought painful consequences. When people started saying things, a vicious war broke out and feelings were hurt. I'll never forget what she said to me. "Every where we go, people are out to get us." I wondered how she couldn't see that it wasn't the fact that people were mean and out to get her, but that they kept creating a vicious cycle to prove themselves right. What were they proving? They were proving to themselves that the world is filled with mean and hurtful people who were out to get them. And guess what? They got to be right. As a consequence, they would pack up and move to a new city every four years or so because the nice people turned out to be mean and hurtful jerks.

Is that a great story or what? It's a real story for them, but 100 percent made up in the confines of their own minds and now they go out, city to city and prove their story right, without ever having the slightest clue as to what they are doing. These people are not free. They are caught in the matrix and can't see out. Landmark education helps us see the traps we are caught in, the rackets we run in order to be right and make someone else besides ourselves responsible for our problems.

> "Loving people live in a loving world. Hostile people live in a hostile world. Same world." Wayne W. Dyer, Ph.D.

Most of us have an X, Y and Z, or in simple terms, something traumatic that happened to us that caused us to be a certain way. For most of us something happened when we were 3-9 years old that made us feel that **"something is wrong (I'm not good enough)."** Most people have the script for their life written in the first five years of living life. Somewhere between the ages of 9-16 something else occurred that made us feel like **"I don't belong."** Usually around high school graduation or age 16-21, most of us had another trauma smack us off balance that made us feel that **"I'm all alone and on my own."** Most people connect these three dots perfectly when they go through the Landmark and it becomes apparent why we are the way we are. Our X + Y + Z creates OUR IDENTITY.

What the forum does is dehypnotize our minds long enough so that we can experience directly just being. This amazing awakening is called, "getting it." Through this experience, we realize that anything we call a problem is a barrier we have created which keeps us stuck in our preconceived opinions, judgements, fears and needs. Transformation occurs when we stop resisting what is. This gives us the space and ability to experience living so that the situations we have been attempting to change clear up just in the process of life itself.

If you have a problem in life, you can either choose to have it and take responsibility for it or choose to be a poor victim and resist it and be at its effect, helpless. A good example is depression. If you are depressed, you can choose to own the depression and be its source and take responsibility for it or you can play the poor me victim game and choose to resist it and be at its mercy.

If you desire to know the truth that will set you free, then start taking responsibility for how your life is and isn't. If you have relationships that stink, it is because you caused them to be that way. This is empowerment. To point the finger and play the blame game gives your power away and makes you a victim. Living a powerful life means that you are the source of the quality of all your relationships. Pain is a given in this life, but suffering is an option. There is no suffering in reality, only in your story.

> "All it takes to make a difference is the courage to stop proving I was right in being unable to make a difference, to stop assigning cause for my inability to the circumstances outside myself, and to be willing to have been that way, and to see that the fear of being a failure is a lot less important than the unique opportunity I have to make a difference." Werner Erhard

Once we stop blaming people and things for the way things are and start taking responsibility and realize that we are source, only then will we begin to live the life we love and love the life we live. The Landmark Forum allows us to experience how our past has been creating our future. Once we transform our way of be-ing then we become empowered to create something different. Perhaps something we want and choose.

Nothing I can explain to you can even begin to touch the surface of what the Landmark has to offer. I challenge you to experience the Landmark Forum for yourself. Don't take my word for it, do it yourself and you be the judge. For more information about seminar locations close to where you live and dates, go on line to www.landmarkeducation.com.

The Power of the Spoken Word

> "In the beginning was the Word and the Word was with God, and the Word was God." St. John 1:1

God created the world and the world was in darkness. He created light by the power of the spoken word. He commanded, "Let there be light," and there was light. As a child of God, YOU have been given dominion and authority over the elements of the earth.

Thoughts are energy. The words we speak are energy. Understand that every single "I'm not …" is a creation. What have you been creating in your life? The power of the spoken word can create health or illness. Our words are like a two-edged sword, cutting positively or negatively.

Always put affirmations in the present tense such as "I am" or "I have." Never use "I am not." Speaking positive affirmations with feeling can be a powerful way to start each day. Rebounding thirty minutes every morning and speaking into existence your goals gives the subconcious mind a blueprint to follow. This is an important step in empowering yourself to create what you want.

> "I believe we create every so-called illness in our body. The body, like everything else in life, is a mirror of our inner thoughts and beliefs. The body is always talking to us, if we will only take the time to listen. Every cell within your body responds to every single thought you think and every word you speak." Louise L. Hay

Positive Affirmations

1. I am calm, relaxed and harmonized with everyone and everything.
3. I let go of fear, anger and the need to be right.
4. I am willing to change. I let go of the past now.
5. I give up the need to prove how smart I am.
6. I accept everyone just the way they are and just the way they are not.
7. I give and I receive. I choose to flow peacefully with the process of life.
8. I love myself and I love others.
9. I let go of struggle, friction and contention.
10. I am happy, healthy, wealthy and successful.
11. I am a magnet to success. Everything I touch is a success.
12. I attract wonderful people into my life who I can serve and who can serve me.
13. I feel I am worthy and deserving of God's greatest blessings and choose to receive them now.
14. Golden opportunities are everywhere and I attract them to me now.
15. I am loving, lovable and loved.
16. I give up being a failure. I am alivement, empowerment, success & fulfilled in all that I do.

17. I can do all things through Christ who strengthens me now.
18. I am worthy and deserving of an abundance.
19. Divine intelligence gives me all the ideas I can use.
20. Infinite wisdom fills my mind like a mighty river.
21. I touch, move and inspire others.
22. I make a difference in all that I do.
23. Every day in every way I am getting better and better and better.
24. All things work for my greatest good.
25. I am eternally grateful for the abundance that is mine.
26. My life is fun and fulfilling.
27. Nothing has the power to irritate me.
28. I am powerful beyond measure.
29. I am whole, complete and perfect.
30. God blesses me beyond my fondest dreams.

> "Nature, to be commanded, must be obeyed." Francis Bacon

For those who are interested in the power of the spoken word, I have a C.D. available. This C.D., "Empowerment For Life" is the end result of thousands of hours of research and experiments. It offers you the secrets to living a life you love. Discover your "power within." Start reaching your goals by speaking them into existence. When you are ready to get serious about reaching your goals call and order this empowering C.D. for $20. Our office phone number is (256) 543-3801.

Winning

> "When you are sick of sickness, you are no longer sick."
> Old Chinese Proverb

Some people in America never get sick of sickness. They accept it, tolerate it, carry it around like a backpack and play it like a game. They mope around with their head hung down with a look on their face that says, "Poor me, my life is hard." They have given up, thrown in the towel and are just trudging along. It reminds me of the handful of kids I went to school with who quit football and wrestling every season because "it's too hard." They weren't willing to pay the price and that is fine. Everyone deserves to choose what they want. But, with no guts, there is no glory and what a shame to waste your precious life and God-given talents like that. So much potential is wasted when all that is needed is a little extra added effort to conquer.

> "If people knew how hard I worked to get my mastery, it wouldn't seem so wonderful after all." Michelangelo

The satisfaction of being crowned a champion after an honest effort is truly awesome. Learning self-discipline, overcoming fatigue and self-sacrifice are characteristics that are developed and used in all areas of life, not just athletics. Sure, some of you do not have a desire to wrestle, play football or compete in powerlifting, however, athletics can help you get the feel for winning and success. Once you understand that most champions aren't born overnight, but through their many failures and losses they learn to overcome adversity in order to succeed. These champion attributes go further than athletics. They carry over in to all areas of life. Through the adversity, we can learn to put forth a little extra added effort to win. It's all about how much you want something. The only difference between a diamond and a plain old piece of coal is time and pressure. Are you willing to pay the price to win the gold medal? Do you want to be a champion mother or father? Winning in sports is great, but winning in life is fulfilling. Winning with your health, your relationships, your work and so forth is what it's all about.

> "Many of life's failures are people who did not realize how close they were to success when they gave up." Thomas Edison

Are you willing to do the things your body needs to heal and not get frustrated and throw up your hands when you have a bad day? Do you love and respect yourself enough to say, "It's worth it. I am worth it, I deserve the best." This is your life, live it to the fullest because the day will come when you will fly on out of here. Do you know what the definition of hell is? Not wanting what you have. Heaven is wanting what you have. If you look back at your life and regret what you did and what you didn't do, you'll feel a sense of regret. Why create that? Live your life to the fullest. Be your dreams. Life goes by too fast not to have what you truly want. You can't live the life you want if you are not healthy.

Reed T. Sainsbury

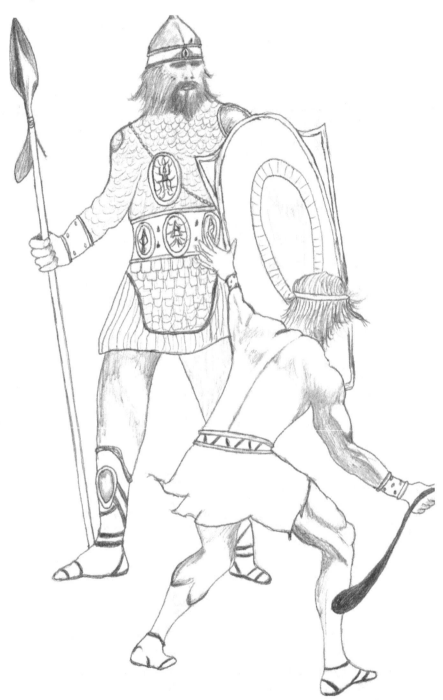

When Goliath came to fight the Israelites everyone cried out in fear, "He is so big we'll never win." David looked at the same obstacle, grabbed his sling, picked up a rock and said, "He is so big, how can I miss?" Attitude determines your altitude.

> "Our deepest fear is that we are powerful beyond measure. It is our light, not our darkness, that most frightens us. We ask ourselves, who am I to be brilliant, gorgeous, talented, and fabulous? Actually, who are you NOT to be? You are a child of God. Your playing small doesn't serve the world. There's nothing enlightened about shrinking so that other people won't feel insecure around you. We are all meant to shine, as children do. We were born to make manifest the glory of God that is within us. It's not just in some of us; it's in everyone. And as we let our own light shine, we unconsciously give other people permission to do the same. As we're liberated from our own fear, our presence automatically liberates others."
>
> Marianne Williamson – Author of A Return To Love

All of us have talents bestowed upon us from on high. To find and magnify those talents is a key to health, happiness and fulfillment. You can't wake up every morning and hate your job and expect to be healthy. Find what you enjoy doing and then find a way to do it and get paid for doing it. This is the secret to good health and a great life. Set that intention for yourself and think about it often. Dwell upon it and engrave that blueprint in your mind. This is called faith.

> "I'd rather be a failure at something I enjoy than be a success at something I hate." George Burns

Every thought you think creates your future. What you feed grows. Choose your thoughts carefully, because what you dwell upon has a magical way of manifesting itself in life. Act as if you already have what you want and be thankful for it. Conceive it and believe it and then you'll achieve it.

> "Far better it is to dare mighty things, to win glorious triumphs even though checkered by failure, than to rank with those poor spirits who neither enjoy nor suffer much because they live in the gray twilight that knows neither victory nor defeat."
>
> Theodore Roosevelt

Conclusion

Two forces exist in this world. One is light and the other is darkness. We are constantly moving towards health and life or disease and death. I hope that you have been empowered through the information in this book. May God bless you beyond your fondest dreams according to your faith and always remember; when the student is ready, the teacher appears.

> "There is an aspect of human physiology that physicians have not yet understood and only reluctantly acknowledge. This dimension of human physiology is the domain of Spirit as it relates to the physical framework. The unseen connection between the physical body and the subtle forces of spirit holds the key to understanding the inner relationship between matter and energy. When scientists begin to comprehend the rule relationship between matter and energy, they will come closer to understanding the relationship between humanity and God."
>
> Richard Gerber, M.D. - Author of Vibrational Medicine

Some will not understand the following message, however, those who are ready will. The great mystery of life is to experience transformation. Does a lowly caterpillar comprehend that the day soon cometh when he gives up crawling on his belly only to receive his wings to soar through the blue sky as a butterfly? Transformation is discovering what you already are.

> "Reality" is what we take to be true.
> What we take to be true is what we believe.
> What we believe is based upon our perceptions.
> What we perceive depends upon what we look for.
> What we look for depends upon what we think.
> What we think depends upon what we perceive.
> What we perceive determines what we believe.
> What we believe determines what we take to be true.
> What we take to be true is our reality.
>
> Max B. Skousen - The Hidden Key to Inner Peace

> "There is no death. Only a change of worlds."
> Chief Seattle 1786-1866

One creates from nothing. If you try to create from something you're just changing something. So, in order to create something you first have to be able to create nothing. To make sure a person doesn't find out who he is, convince him that he can't really make anything disappear.

> "Here is where it is. Now is when it is. You are what it is."
> Werner Erhard

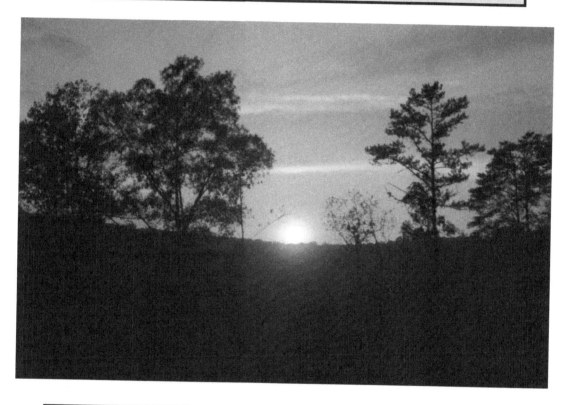

> "If thou canst believe, all things are possible to him that believeth."
> Mark 9:23

Remember; YOU cannot become what you already are.

www.healingthecause.com

Index

A

Acidosis 39, 82, 98, 106, 124, 203, 206, 338, 344
Acne 102, 109, 313, 337, 366
Acupuncture 26, 27, 28
ADD 123, 244, 245, 312, 337, 338, 391
Adrenal glands 71, 74, 105, 113, 121, 294, 301, 306, 325, 338, 341, 343, 344, 346, 348, 349, 354, 360, 361, 363, 369, 370
AERS 247
Agape 402, 403, 404
Alfalfa 74, 143, 206, 330, 334, 335, 336, 338, 339, 340, 341, 346, 351, 356, 358, 361, 362, 363, 368
Allergies 36, 58, 120, 124, 125, 135, 156, 183, 188, 200, 214, 242, 244, 245, 247, 254, 308, 337, 338, 340, 353, 356, 357, 361, 366, 367, 378, 379, 380, 382, 384, 386, 391
Aloe Vera 143, 293, 314, 337, 345, 347, 360, 363
Aluminum 23, 217, 242, 246, 254, 316, 317, 325, 339
Alzheimer's 49, 51, 52, 217, 227, 230, 246, 248, 313, 323, 325, 339
Amino Acids 17, 69, 103, 121, 147, 148, 157, 159, 167, 186, 194, 195, 293, 311, 314, 334, 338, 354, 355, 369
Anderson, Richard 128, 200, 218, 279, 287, 317, 319, 373, 403
Anemia 122, 151, 206, 312, 313, 315, 339, 365
Angina 339
Antibiotics 92, 95, 97, 105, 109, 123, 199, 200, 201, 202, 203, 205, 216, 243, 254, 260, 309, 334, 344, 347, 372
Antioxidants 53, 69, 314
Anxiety 135, 166, 198, 312, 313, 324, 340, 402, 404
Arteriosclerosis 103, 190, 195, 219, 312
Arthritis 23, 34, 38, 47, 56, 57, 60, 70, 78, 94, 125, 126, 127, 152, 154, 181, 195, 197, 199, 204, 205, 209, 210, 215, 216, 244, 247, 249, 282, 283, 286, 293, 312, 325, 331, 332, 334, 340, 341, 356, 359, 373, 385, 394, 395
Aspartame 107, 124, 207, 322, 323, 324, 325, 358
Aspirin 43, 104, 147, 207, 265, 283, 320, 321, 333, 372
Asthma 71, 238, 242, 244, 245, 247, 312, 341, 365, 366, 385
Astragalus 94, 292, 346
Athlete's Foot 342
Autism 229, 230, 238, 240, 241, 243, 244, 245, 247, 252, 254, 342

B

Back Problems 264–268
Baldness 343
Barberry 292, 338, 356
Barley greens 82, 143, 334, 368
Bayberry 348, 350
Bee pollen 143, 206, 296, 334, 336, 338, 341, 343, 346, 356, 361, 362, 370
Bible 65, 76, 100, 179, 280, 288
Bilberry 350
Bioflavonoids 314, 356, 358, 363
Birthing 326
Bitter Melon 293, 302, 303
Black cohosh 294, 357, 360, 369
Black walnut 186, 187, 351
Bladder infection 343, 367
Blood pressure 34, 35, 57, 58, 67, 101, 120, 133, 177, 181, 190, 297, 299, 300, 304, 312, 347, 353, 354, 366, 370, 378
Blood purification 346, 362
Blood sugar 71, 107, 181, 184, 189, 191, 214, 215, 248, 292, 293, 294, 302, 303, 304,

309, 312, 324, 332, 337, 338, 354, 357, 362, 370
Blood type 208, 216
Blue cohosh 294, 369
Boils 100, 109, 367
Bone spurs 195, 210, 293, 312, 341, 345
Borage 54, 337, 357
Breastfeeding 372
Bronchitis 343, 365, 367
Bruising 358
Burdock 217, 336, 337, 341, 346, 351, 356, 360, 361, 362
Burns 102, 153, 325, 370
Butcher's broom 291, 345, 348, 356, 362, 363, 364, 368

C

Cabbage juice 363
Calcium 33, 54, 82, 121, 122, 124, 151, 167, 183, 195, 208, 209, 210, 215, 293, 294, 295, 296, 299, 312, 313, 317, 325, 331, 333, 340, 341, 342, 345, 346, 347, 350, 352, 353, 354, 355, 358, 359, 360, 362, 368, 370
Calendula 356
Cancer 12, 13, 16, 17, 18, 23, 33, 39, 40, 41, 42, 48, 49, 51, 52, 56, 67, 70, 78, 80, 81, 82, 83, 84, 85, 90, 94, 95, 99, 100, 101, 108, 113, 114, 120, 123, 124, 125, 127, 129, 132, 133, 135, 139, 140, 141, 144, 145, 146, 147, 150, 158, 184, 193, 194, 196, 199, 200, 202, 204, 205, 206, 208, 213, 215, 217, 221, 230, 234, 244, 245, 249, 250, 251, 252, 254, 279, 287, 297, 300, 301, 303, 305, 311, 312, 313, 314, 315, 316, 318, 319, 324, 331, 334, 335, 343, 344, 360, 370, 373, 375, 376, 377, 397, 398
Candida (Candidiasis) 20, 124, 201, 202, 203, 204, 300, 308, 315, 344, 345, 351, 356
Cascara Sagrada 215, 293, 337, 345, 347

Cataracts 209, 244, 313, 350
Cat's claw 94, 117, 292, 294, 296, 338, 340, 344, 346, 353, 356, 357, 361, 362, 369, 376
Cayenne 291, 345, 347, 348, 350, 352, 353, 354, 356, 358, 359, 361, 362, 363, 364, 370
CEDSA 20, 21, 26, 28, 29, 31, 32, 47, 50, 53, 54, 94, 101, 105, 109, 111, 120, 121, 122, 124, 156, 157, 182, 196, 286, 299, 309, 333, 335, 336, 338, 340, 346, 375, 401
Celery 17, 183, 206, 211, 335, 338, 340, 341, 346, 349, 353, 357, 358, 362
Cells 9, 10, 11, 12, 13, 14, 16, 17, 18, 23, 33, 39, 40, 67, 68, 69, 70, 74, 76, 77, 81, 82, 84, 85, 87, 91, 98, 99, 103, 105, 106, 108, 112, 115, 116, 117, 119, 121, 122, 125, 140, 142, 147, 150, 151, 153, 154, 155, 158, 159, 161, 162, 163, 164, 165, 166, 167, 168, 169, 170, 171, 172, 173, 174, 175, 176, 177, 178, 179, 183, 184, 191, 192, 193, 199, 204, 205, 208, 209, 217, 218, 219, 220, 221, 225, 249, 291, 292, 294, 296, 297, 299, 300, 301, 302, 303, 304, 311, 315, 317, 318, 334, 335, 336, 340, 343, 345, 347, 349, 353, 356, 362, 370, 375, 377
Chamomile 293, 338, 340, 348, 350, 355
Chappell, James 32, 104, 183, 196, 301, 302, 373, 391
Chelation 16, 221, 345, 348
Chemicals 3, 11, 16, 18, 34, 47, 63, 64, 94, 108, 123, 136, 138, 168, 169, 171, 172, 178, 204, 214, 216, 219, 220, 229, 243, 277, 288, 300, 314, 315, 316, 331, 337, 354, 379, 394
Chemotherapy 16, 18, 38, 40, 41, 81, 82, 83, 84, 108, 135, 139, 140, 146, 150, 205, 375, 376, 377
Chickenpox 95, 242, 250, 361
Chickweed 359

Chiropractic 101, 218, 219, 263, 264, 265, 293, 305, 306, 308, 309, 342
Chlorella 143, 339
Chlorine 12, 215, 315, 319, 356
Cholesterol 34, 35, 46, 59, 67, 102, 103, 120, 133, 167, 181, 183, 188, 189, 190, 191, 192, 193, 194, 200, 208, 296, 299, 302, 303, 304, 312, 345, 348, 370
Choline 121, 294
Chopra, Deepak 9, 377
Chromium 293, 294, 302, 312, 338, 348, 354, 362
Chronic fatigue 94, 135, 181, 228, 304, 306, 308, 312, 323, 324, 351, 363, 366, 385
Cinnamon 107, 206, 293, 294, 302, 303, 348, 354
Circulation 33, 53, 74, 82, 89, 91, 101, 129, 182, 197, 206, 220, 291, 296, 297, 298, 301, 304, 308, 339, 343, 345, 348, 352, 354, 356, 362, 363, 364, 365, 368, 375, 376
Colds 97, 116, 138, 195, 202, 254, 345, 346, 365, 367, 385
Colitis 199, 366
Colon 18, 93, 105, 108, 114, 127, 152, 153, 154, 156, 218, 292, 315, 330, 338, 341, 342, 347, 353
Color 89, 97, 163, 164, 168, 189, 211, 212, 310, 361
Constipation 34, 54, 58, 89, 102, 106, 117, 155, 215, 228, 312, 313, 320, 323, 347, 353, 357, 365, 366, 378
Copper 20, 224, 312, 353, 363
Corn silk 217, 296, 343, 356, 369
Coughs 97
Cramps 228, 312, 347, 365
Cranberry 343
Crohn's 199, 347
Cuts 17, 158, 347, 348, 392
Cyanide 16
Cystitis 343

D

Dandelion 17, 217, 292, 337, 338, 339, 351, 356, 361, 368
Day, Lorraine 81, 94
Dean, Carolyn 38, 44, 65, 74, 284, 301, 322, 373
Dehydration 89, 105, 320
Depression 67, 72, 102, 104, 123, 125, 133, 135, 200, 228, 284, 288, 302, 308, 309, 312, 313, 322, 324, 348, 377, 385, 390, 397, 402, 410
Diabetes 49, 56, 58, 71, 77, 94, 125, 127, 184, 204, 208, 215, 244, 245, 247, 248, 249, 301, 302, 303, 304, 305, 312, 313, 322, 323, 324, 325, 348, 366, 368, 373
Diarrhea 34, 112, 113, 114, 155, 188, 215, 228, 308, 312, 348, 365
Diet 10, 11, 14, 15, 16, 37, 46, 57, 63, 67, 82, 85, 94, 101, 102, 104, 106, 107, 125, 126, 127, 129, 133, 140, 142, 152, 153, 190, 205, 206, 208, 209, 210, 214, 215, 216, 232, 301, 303, 314, 323, 324, 325, 329, 330, 331, 332, 333, 338, 340, 342, 349, 351, 352, 354, 358, 359, 361, 362, 368, 372, 373
Digestion 151, 152, 154, 175, 178, 183, 214, 217, 339, 365, 368
Diverticulitis 349
Dizziness 294, 312, 356, 363, 366, 369
Dong quai 53, 294, 355, 357, 360, 369
Down syndrome 311, 313
Drugs xiii, 1, 2, 3, 5, 7, 8, 9, 10, 11, 13, 14, 17, 18, 19, 21, 22, 23, 28, 33, 34, 35, 36, 37, 38, 39, 42, 43, 44, 46, 47, 48, 49, 51, 52, 53, 57, 58, 59, 60, 61, 62, 63, 64, 65, 67, 68, 69, 70, 71, 72, 74, 75, 76, 77, 78, 84, 85, 87, 90, 94, 95, 98, 100, 104, 108, 109, 113, 114, 115, 117, 120, 121, 122, 123, 124, 126, 127, 128, 129, 132, 133, 135, 136, 139, 141, 146, 147, 148, 149, 150, 155, 156, 157, 158, 183, 190, 191, 192, 193, 194, 199,

200, 207, 213, 220, 221, 222, 223, 231, 239, 242, 246, 271, 273, 274, 275, 277, 278, 282, 283, 285, 286, 287, 288, 289, 297, 300, 301, 303, 305, 308, 309, 314, 319, 320, 321, 322, 323, 327, 328, 333, 347, 350, 353, 356, 372, 373, 375, 378, 379, 380, 385

Dry skin 53, 102, 312, 365

Dyer, Wayne 389

E

Ear 33, 163, 164, 165, 195, 200, 244, 251, 300, 349, 378

Echinacea 17, 28, 94, 117, 148, 292, 294, 296, 344, 346, 349, 350, 353, 355, 356, 357, 360, 361, 362, 369

Eczema 312, 313

Edema 72, 89, 112, 291, 313, 349

Edison, Thomas 9, 11, 12, 80, 413

Ego 403, 404

Einstein, Albert 23, 29, 80, 107, 129

Emotions 99, 102, 124, 205, 220, 293, 320, 347, 349, 356, 359, 375, 377, 383, 386, 395, 398, 399, 402

Endocrine System 50, 52, 53, 74, 102, 104, 212, 293, 295, 344, 355, 357, 360

Enema 345

Enzymes 17, 38, 69, 106, 121, 123, 140, 143, 147, 148, 151, 152, 157, 162, 171, 182, 195, 208, 213, 214, 217, 221, 292, 294, 299, 300, 314, 323, 334, 338, 340, 348, 351, 352, 354, 368

Epilepsy 119, 120, 244, 324, 350

Epstein-Barr 124, 135

Essential fatty acid 17, 52, 147, 159, 184, 314, 333, 337, 338, 343, 348, 353, 356

Est 383, 401

Eucalyptus 296, 346, 349, 360, 361

Evening primrose 52, 143, 184, 293, 337, 343, 355, 357, 358, 360, 361

Exercise 37, 46, 72, 89, 91, 94, 102, 106, 127, 153, 171, 197, 202, 217, 258, 329, 393

Eyes xvi, 13, 18, 22, 45, 58, 70, 159, 163, 164, 165, 170, 176, 177, 209, 308, 312, 365, 378, 381, 386, 390

F

Fasting 127, 153, 189, 217, 218, 335

Fat 58, 85, 103, 105, 152, 183, 184, 186, 190, 219, 296, 302, 303, 304, 323, 372, 385, 398

Fatigue 94, 101, 104, 113, 116, 135, 137, 154, 177, 181, 183, 198, 228, 294, 302, 304, 306, 308, 312, 313, 323, 324, 351, 363, 366, 369, 378, 385, 413

Federal Reserve 280, 281

Fenugreek 293, 302, 304, 305

Fever 55, 112, 115, 116, 120, 147, 238, 254, 350, 353, 365, 385

Fiber 347, 349

Fibromyalgia 94, 132, 135, 201, 204, 205, 210, 254, 315, 324, 351

Flaxseed 143, 184, 291, 295, 337, 351, 353, 354, 360, 368, 369

Flu 1, 19, 23, 95, 97, 98, 109, 135, 202, 216, 233, 238, 246, 248, 249, 367, 372

Fluoride 215, 312, 316, 317, 318, 319, 356

Food xv, 10, 14, 15, 22, 25, 59, 67, 69, 73, 75, 90, 94, 96, 97, 98, 99, 106, 109, 122, 124, 125, 126, 129, 133, 135, 137, 139, 140, 141, 142, 143, 151, 152, 153, 154, 155, 158, 167, 169, 171, 174, 176, 183, 188, 195, 206, 209, 211, 213, 214, 215, 216, 217, 218, 219, 226, 253, 279, 286, 288, 292, 299, 300, 310, 313, 322, 325, 331, 334, 337, 338, 342, 351, 354, 367, 370, 379, 406

Formaldehyde 195, 247, 251, 254, 323

Franklin, Benjamin 32, 80, 114, 314

Free radicals 16, 302, 303

Fruits 67, 85, 94, 106, 125, 140, 143, 149, 183, 204, 206, 207, 208, 209, 210, 211, 213, 214, 215, 216, 218, 289, 300, 313,

314, 329, 330, 331, 332, 334, 335, 339, 340, 346, 349, 359, 361
Fungal 300, 342

G

Gallbladder 22, 101, 108, 109, 152, 157, 181, 182, 183, 184, 185, 186, 189, 196, 217, 218, 292, 293, 309, 351, 365, 368, 372

Garlic 94, 117, 128, 143, 206, 216, 227, 228, 339, 342, 344, 345, 346, 349, 350, 351, 352, 353, 354, 356, 360, 362, 364, 369, 370

Gas 10, 84, 125, 132, 152, 154, 155, 169, 272, 274, 276, 278, 308, 317, 323, 346, 366, 368

Gerber, Richard 25, 29, 373, 383, 416

Ginger 128, 143, 206, 211, 216, 291, 294, 295, 340, 341, 345, 346, 348, 354, 358, 362, 363, 364, 368, 369

Ginkgo Biloba 143, 291, 293, 339, 343, 345, 362, 363, 364, 368

Ginseng 291, 293, 295, 302, 304, 339, 343, 345, 348, 353, 354, 356, 359, 360, 362, 363, 364, 368, 369

Glands 5, 16, 26, 33, 52, 67, 71, 74, 101, 105, 113, 121, 122, 124, 152, 154, 161, 176, 218, 249, 293, 294, 296, 301, 306, 325, 338, 341, 343, 344, 346, 348, 349, 354, 355, 357, 360, 361, 363, 367, 369, 370, 371, 391, 403

Goldenseal 94, 292, 343, 344, 351, 353, 360

Gonads 212, 294, 296

Gota kola 339, 346, 362, 363, 364

Gout 127, 216, 300, 331, 334, 340, 351

Graviola 17, 18, 143, 150, 344, 376

Gymnema Sylvestre 293, 302, 303, 304

H

Hair loss 312, 343
Halitosis 308, 352
Hawthorne 291, 339, 352, 353

Headache 67, 98, 114, 116, 125, 155, 156, 157, 158, 181, 288, 320, 321, 357, 394

Heart 11, 16, 29, 48, 49, 51, 57, 58, 60, 61, 76, 88, 89, 91, 101, 102, 103, 114, 125, 128, 137, 138, 139, 147, 163, 168, 171, 177, 178, 182, 183, 184, 190, 191, 192, 193, 194, 199, 212, 219, 224, 230, 250, 251, 255, 291, 297, 299, 312, 313, 315, 327, 331, 339, 352, 353, 365, 366, 368, 383, 395, 401, 407

Heartburn 58, 113, 120, 152, 153, 182, 228, 288, 322, 352, 368

Heavy Metals 16, 23, 105, 122, 124, 224, 225, 227, 229, 230, 246, 337, 339, 342, 344, 345, 347, 349, 350, 351, 354, 355, 358

Hemorrhoids 353

Hepatitis 231, 238, 245, 246, 247, 248, 254, 256, 300, 356

Herbs 11, 12, 17, 20, 28, 35, 38, 50, 67, 68, 69, 86, 94, 98, 111, 117, 120, 121, 122, 129, 132, 133, 134, 147, 148, 149, 150, 153, 157, 188, 206, 209, 214, 220, 221, 275, 286, 304, 305, 314, 333, 335, 346, 348, 356, 368, 379, 380

Herpes 124, 346, 353, 361

High blood pressure 35, 101, 120, 133, 190, 297, 299, 300, 312, 347, 353, 370

High cholesterol 35, 102, 103, 120, 133, 190, 191, 193, 194, 200, 302, 345, 370

Hippocrates 24, 75, 94, 115, 142, 264

Hives 183, 366

Homeopathy 108, 134, 157, 221, 256, 261, 277

Honey 17, 186, 207, 214, 215, 344, 352, 355, 362

Hops 355, 357, 359, 360

Hormone 51, 52, 53, 103, 104, 320

Horsetail 296, 356, 369

Hot flashes 53, 72, 192, 366

Hydrangea 292, 293, 351

Hyperactivity 243, 244, 312, 367
Hypertension 57, 353, 385
Hypoglycemia 113, 248, 300, 302, 312, 323, 325, 354, 361, 368
Hypotension 312, 354
Hypothyroidism 102, 104, 116, 135, 194, 208, 244, 312, 343
Hysterectomy 34, 372

I

I.G. Farben 69, 108, 276, 277, 278
Immune 56, 74, 77, 78, 80, 81, 82, 84, 85, 88, 89, 90, 94, 95, 96, 97, 98, 99, 115, 117, 140, 153, 154, 159, 172, 192, 196, 202, 205, 208, 216, 218, 219, 225, 233, 242, 243, 244, 245, 246, 247, 250, 255, 260, 261, 262, 291, 292, 294, 299, 301, 303, 312, 313, 318, 338, 340, 343, 346, 349, 350, 357, 362, 369, 376, 377
Impotence 354, 385
Indigestion 106, 152, 181, 182, 188, 200, 308, 341, 347, 354, 365, 366
Infertility 312, 313, 355
Inflammation 29, 33, 58, 91, 92, 94, 120, 127, 154, 184, 192, 216, 265, 300, 312, 331, 334, 347, 349, 351, 356, 357, 393
Influenza 49, 202, 247
Inositol 121, 294
Insect bite 355
Insomnia 187, 228, 293, 308, 312, 313, 355, 366
intraMAX 314, 338, 339, 342, 344, 358, 359, 362
Iodine 103, 104, 121, 122, 194, 209, 293, 312, 341, 348, 350, 354, 358, 361, 370
Iron 122, 133, 151, 168, 169, 208, 209, 269, 312, 331, 339, 340, 357, 370
Irritable Bowel Syndrome 34, 57, 308, 309

J

JAMA 41, 43, 51, 64, 65, 68, 120, 192, 193, 245, 247, 282, 283, 360
Jensen, Bernard 92, 115, 151, 157, 199, 211
Juicing 211, 218, 340, 341, 349, 351, 363
Juniper 217, 296, 343, 348, 354, 356, 360, 369

K

Kava 293, 338, 340, 348
Kelp 53, 101, 103, 104, 143, 194, 206, 293, 336, 338, 339, 343, 344, 348, 350, 354, 357, 358, 359, 361, 363, 368, 370
Kidney 49, 57, 59, 60, 76, 171, 179, 195, 208, 210, 217, 220, 226, 236, 246, 249, 254, 293, 294, 296, 300, 312, 321, 323, 341, 345, 349, 356, 369, 370
Kirlian photography 25
Koch, William 40

L

Landmark Forum 383, 407, 408, 410
L-Arginine 339
Lavender 346
Laxative 206
L-Carnitine 291, 339, 352, 368
Lecithin 339, 341, 351, 360, 362, 363, 368, 370
Licorice 294, 341, 354, 357, 360, 363, 368, 369
Lilly, Eli 57, 59, 230, 245, 274
Lipton, Bruce 10, 51, 63, 75, 98, 113, 203, 373, 394
Liver 8, 9, 35, 36, 46, 57, 58, 63, 71, 74, 77, 78, 107, 108, 109, 111, 112, 123, 124, 127, 143, 152, 154, 156, 162, 163, 181, 182, 183, 184, 185, 186, 187, 188, 189, 190, 192, 200, 217, 218, 220, 286, 292, 293, 301, 303, 309, 312, 313, 321, 333, 337, 338, 341, 343, 348, 351, 356, 357, 360, 361,

368, 370, 371
L-Lysine 294, 346, 353
Lobelia 296, 341, 343, 355, 359, 360, 361
Love 2, 12, 22, 36, 65, 85, 91, 96, 128, 159, 178, 204, 206, 218, 222, 255, 257, 263, 275, 284, 289, 328, 376, 377, 382, 386, 388, 389, 390, 391, 399, 400, 401, 402, 403, 404, 405, 406, 410, 411, 412, 413, 415
Low blood sugar 312, 354, 370
Lupus 23, 94, 120, 198, 201, 244, 249, 254, 313, 315, 324, 356
Lyme 124, 340, 345
Lymphatic 11, 33, 46, 74, 87, 88, 89, 90, 91, 93, 94, 98, 109, 111, 112, 117, 159, 197, 199, 200, 219, 220, 291, 292, 337, 343, 346, 349, 356, 370

M

Magnesium 53, 101, 103, 121, 122, 151, 152, 157, 167, 208, 209, 291, 293, 294, 295, 297, 312, 331, 339, 340, 341, 342, 343, 344, 345, 346, 347, 350, 352, 353, 354, 355, 356, 358, 359, 360, 362, 363, 368, 370
Malnutrition 74, 206, 246, 286, 310, 335
Manganese 293, 312, 341, 342, 357, 360, 363, 369
Marshmallow root 363, 368
Massage 117, 134, 219, 342, 346, 349
Measles 173, 234, 237, 238, 246, 249, 251, 254, 261
Medical Ghost Writing 282
Meditation 212
Melatonin 143, 293, 355
Memory 72, 102, 166, 172, 178, 191, 228, 297, 304, 308, 312, 313, 339, 366, 383
Mendelsohn, Robert 8, 53, 57, 64, 69, 84, 108, 126, 135, 186, 196, 221, 223, 245, 248, 251, 261, 283, 287, 327, 329, 373

Meniere's 73, 74, 356
Menopause 52, 53, 135, 357, 366, 373
Mercury 12, 20, 102, 121, 123, 124, 134, 224, 225, 226, 227, 228, 229, 230, 238, 242, 245, 246, 254, 299, 304, 342, 358
Meridian 371
Microwaves 25, 215
Migraine 19, 155, 156, 357, 385
Milk thistle 217, 292, 338, 356, 368
Minerals xv, 17, 38, 67, 69, 121, 143, 147, 148, 151, 152, 157, 159, 183, 210, 211, 221, 299, 310, 311, 313, 314, 334, 338, 339, 340, 341, 342, 349, 368, 380
Mononucleosis 357
Morning sickness 358
MSG 124, 254
Mullein 296, 341, 343, 349, 360, 369
Multiple sclerosis 19, 23, 56, 225, 226, 313, 324, 358
Muscle cramps 312, 347, 365
Muscle testing 379, 380, 382, 384
Myrrh 94, 292, 296, 338, 346, 362, 369

N

Natural healing xi, 35, 37, 41, 42, 56, 119, 121, 127, 134, 139, 141, 182, 183, 184, 209, 220, 221, 242, 277, 278
Nausea 101, 109, 181, 188, 356, 358
Nerves 33, 162, 176, 177, 218, 264, 265, 293, 306, 320, 338, 342, 366
Nervousness 102, 312, 313, 366, 367
Nervous System 21, 33, 51, 63, 101, 102, 121, 151, 176, 178, 217, 224, 225, 230, 246, 247, 255, 293, 304, 305, 306, 323, 340, 350, 355, 359, 368
Nettle 217, 292, 337, 338, 339, 351, 356, 357, 361
Nopal Cactus 293, 302, 304
Nosebleeds 358
NutraSweet 322, 323, 324

Nutritional 5, 18, 19, 20, 21, 28, 35, 36, 38, 43, 47, 48, 52, 54, 67, 73, 74, 78, 101, 103, 108, 111, 120, 121, 122, 129, 156, 157, 214, 215, 246, 296, 297, 302, 305, 308, 311, 334, 336, 342, 346, 380

O

Obesity 104, 313, 358, 398
Oregon grape 292, 356, 368
Osteoporosis 52, 135, 195, 210, 286, 300, 312, 331
Oxygen 33, 40, 82, 86, 98, 104, 112, 113, 167, 168, 169, 171, 173, 178, 184, 185, 217, 225, 229, 296, 297, 299, 312, 314, 320, 343, 353, 362

P

Pain 1, 14, 33, 34, 59, 60, 74, 76, 78, 87, 88, 95, 110, 112, 113, 114, 120, 127, 135, 137, 155, 156, 157, 162, 177, 181, 183, 187, 197, 200, 216, 217, 219, 264, 265, 266, 267, 268, 286, 306, 308, 309, 313, 321, 322, 324, 326, 327, 331, 332, 333, 334, 335, 341, 342, 347, 351, 357, 365, 367, 368, 376, 383, 385, 391, 393, 394, 410
Pancreas 71, 107, 127, 152, 162, 163, 212, 292, 293, 294, 301, 302, 348, 354, 361, 368
Panic attacks 101, 308, 312
Parasites 20, 96, 121, 122, 124, 183, 186, 189, 196, 218, 293, 300, 347, 349, 351, 361, 368
Parathyroid 293, 294, 359
Parkinson's 324, 359
Parsley 206, 211, 217, 296, 339, 340, 343, 345, 351, 356, 362, 363, 364, 368, 369
Passionflower 338
Pau d' Arco 357
Peppermint 346, 355, 361
Pharmaceutical 16, 17, 18, 21, 38, 40, 41, 46, 47, 48, 52, 56, 57, 58, 64, 65, 69, 70, 72, 75, 80, 81, 108, 114, 132, 141, 144, 145, 147, 190, 192, 194, 221, 223, 236, 253, 256, 271, 273, 274, 275, 276, 279, 280, 282, 283, 285, 287
Phosphorus 313, 314, 325, 341, 368
Pineal 212, 293
Pink eye 359
Pituitary 105, 121, 156, 212, 293, 346, 350, 357, 369
Placebo 51, 57, 239, 393, 394
PMS 102, 312, 360
Pneumonia 49, 242, 360
Poisoning 23, 39, 83, 84, 85, 97, 109, 110, 121, 124, 129, 140, 148, 155, 156, 209, 229, 234, 304, 316, 319, 320, 323, 324, 339, 340, 342, 350, 351, 353, 356, 359, 375, 376
Poison ivy/oak/sumac 360
Polio 234, 235, 236, 240, 242, 245, 249
Potassium 23, 93, 101, 121, 122, 151, 152, 157, 167, 177, 208, 209, 291, 292, 293, 313, 314, 331, 335, 336, 337, 338, 340, 341, 345, 346, 349, 350, 352, 353, 354, 355, 356, 358, 359, 361, 362, 368, 370
Pregnancy 51, 52, 191, 227, 252, 309, 326, 328, 358, 370, 376, 383
Prescription 1, 3, 7, 8, 11, 13, 17, 20, 21, 23, 35, 37, 38, 43, 47, 48, 49, 50, 56, 57, 64, 65, 66, 67, 72, 73, 75, 77, 94, 95, 124, 135, 136, 138, 147, 158, 181, 213, 219, 220, 222, 239, 264, 271, 272, 275, 278, 286, 308, 314, 372, 378, 386
Primrose 52, 143, 184, 293, 337, 343, 355, 357, 358, 360, 361
Prostate 18, 28, 29, 295, 296, 313, 360, 367
Protein 77, 98, 127, 151, 154, 174, 183, 186, 190, 204, 208, 225, 243, 254, 296, 300, 313, 314, 329, 330, 331, 332, 333, 334, 339, 340, 351, 354, 361, 370
Prozac 19, 59, 197, 200, 272, 284, 288, 319,

320
Psoriasis 360
Psyllium 153, 215, 218, 293, 337, 347, 349

R

Radiation 29, 40, 81, 99, 124, 135, 140, 183, 205, 215, 311
Rash 72, 109, 120, 154, 201, 228, 324, 351, 365
Rebounding 91, 93, 106, 344, 411
Red clover 337
Reishi mushroom 143, 346
Reproductive 163, 245, 294, 295, 296, 312, 354, 355, 369, 399
Respiratory 49, 202, 214, 242, 294, 296, 312, 323, 341, 366, 369
Restless leg 120
RFA 350, 376, 379, 380, 382, 384, 385, 386, 387, 388, 398, 401
Rife 40, 41
Rockefeller 10, 69, 108, 190, 276, 277, 278, 281, 373
Rosemary 339, 359, 361, 362, 363, 364
Royal jelly 143, 294, 296, 338, 341, 343, 344, 346, 360, 361, 362, 363, 369

S

Sage 352, 355, 363
Salt 183, 186, 189, 203, 211, 214, 224, 313, 335, 340, 349, 362, 366
Sarsaparilla 295, 354, 360
Saw palmetto 295, 354, 360, 369
Seizure 119, 120, 121, 122, 232, 234, 238, 240, 241, 243, 312, 322, 323, 324
Selenium 313, 350, 352, 354, 357, 360
Semmelweis, Ignaz Philipp 55, 56
Shingles 95, 156, 250, 361
SIDS 227, 232, 233, 240, 241, 244, 248, 312
Sinus 116, 157, 296, 332, 333, 345, 361, 379
Skin 17, 26, 27, 28, 53, 54, 72, 102, 109, 110, 111, 112, 120, 154, 170, 171, 173, 175, 176, 177, 224, 228, 229, 244, 250, 300, 306, 312, 346, 348, 349, 360, 361, 365, 366, 367, 370, 406
Skullcap 293, 348, 350, 355
Sleep 1, 19, 20, 53, 58, 120, 133, 135, 186, 187, 217, 220, 265, 266, 270, 293, 342, 346, 347, 355, 365, 386
Sodium 23, 93, 122, 152, 167, 177, 183, 208, 209, 210, 211, 214, 292, 316, 317, 318, 323, 331, 335, 338, 340, 341, 346, 349, 356, 357, 358, 361, 362, 363, 370
Soft drinks 203, 207, 213, 323, 325, 326, 358, 359, 372
Sore throat 116, 120, 125, 346, 362
Spider bite 355
Spirulina 74, 143, 206, 210, 335, 338, 341, 346, 356, 357, 358, 361, 362, 363, 368
Spleen 74, 101, 107, 109, 111, 112, 154, 162, 163, 169, 217, 291, 292, 337, 338, 339, 343, 346, 353, 357, 360, 361
St. Johns Wort 348
Stress 20, 26, 28, 29, 32, 47, 53, 99, 101, 102, 124, 135, 151, 174, 182, 183, 184, 191, 219, 265, 270, 288, 294, 304, 305, 320, 322, 365, 370
Stroke 49, 51, 125, 132, 135, 156, 169, 190, 192, 362
Subconcious 387, 411
Sulfur 168, 313, 346, 350, 362
Suma 53, 293, 294, 354, 355, 360
Supplements 10, 20, 48, 73, 74, 136, 143, 153, 182, 195, 333, 335, 386
Surgery 1, 15, 19, 22, 28, 33, 48, 63, 72, 76, 81, 83, 90, 92, 99, 103, 128, 134, 181, 183, 184, 186, 188, 190, 196, 198, 204, 222, 286, 287, 288, 297, 306, 308, 327, 332, 333, 378, 379, 380, 393, 394
Sweating 242, 312, 395

T

Tea 143, 207, 342, 344, 349
Tea tree 342, 349
Thyme 342, 346
Thymus 56, 143, 212, 291, 292, 294, 356
Thyroid 20, 21, 101, 102, 103, 104, 105, 121, 133, 183, 194, 200, 209, 212, 227, 293, 312, 338, 341, 344, 348, 354, 357, 358, 361, 368, 370
Tinnitus 312
Tonsils 22, 90, 91, 92, 94, 125, 291, 346, 362, 372
Toxic xiii, 2, 5, 8, 9, 10, 12, 15, 17, 18, 21, 28, 33, 35, 36, 38, 39, 41, 46, 53, 59, 61, 63, 65, 70, 74, 75, 76, 77, 85, 105, 107, 109, 113, 114, 116, 117, 122, 123, 124, 125, 141, 144, 150, 154, 155, 183, 200, 204, 211, 212, 219, 224, 225, 226, 227, 229, 233, 237, 243, 245, 246, 255, 257, 286, 291, 301, 305, 309, 315, 316, 317, 320, 321, 323, 325, 338, 342, 351, 353, 356, 357, 395
Toxicity 108, 117, 124, 154, 224, 225, 228, 231, 300, 312, 325
Toxins 3, 10, 11, 20, 23, 28, 39, 47, 63, 67, 74, 87, 89, 90, 95, 105, 109, 111, 112, 114, 115, 117, 119, 120, 121, 122, 123, 124, 139, 154, 155, 183, 184, 192, 206, 209, 219, 242, 255, 292, 301, 320, 323, 324, 334, 335, 337, 343, 346, 347, 349, 356, 357, 360, 361
Tumor 31, 70, 80, 82, 95, 96, 205, 237, 322, 323, 324, 334, 344, 398
Turmeric 216, 368

U

Ulcer 78, 124, 151, 189, 208, 282, 283, 293, 301, 312, 321, 363, 366, 368
Urinary 296, 304, 343
Uterus 22, 109, 157, 294, 296, 355, 360, 372
Uva Ursi 217, 296, 343, 356, 369

V

Vaccinations 23, 71, 229, 231, 233, 234, 235, 236, 237, 238, 239, 240, 241, 242, 243, 244, 245, 247, 249, 250, 252, 255, 256, 257, 258, 259, 261, 342, 372
Vagina 296
Valerian 293, 338, 340, 348, 350, 355, 359
Vanadium 293, 313, 348, 354
Varicose veins 312, 353, 363
Veins 89, 91, 152, 167, 170, 291, 299, 312, 353, 363
Vertigo 72, 312, 324, 363
Vinegar 106, 143, 203, 206, 207, 352, 355, 359, 362
Virus 40, 80, 95, 97, 124, 135, 234, 236, 249, 254, 346, 352, 356, 357, 361
vitamins xv, 17, 28, 38, 69, 121, 122, 147, 148, 157, 159, 186, 195, 221, 294, 299, 300, 310, 311, 313, 314, 324, 334, 338, 340, 352, 358, 359, 360, 363, 379

W

Wallach, Joel 38, 192, 310, 311, 373
Water 55, 65, 82, 86, 89, 91, 94, 96, 98, 105, 106, 107, 112, 117, 120, 123, 140, 149, 152, 153, 171, 175, 183, 186, 187, 188, 189, 203, 213, 214, 215, 217, 218, 219, 235, 272, 292, 296, 300, 306, 310, 314, 315, 316, 317, 318, 319, 323, 326, 327, 335, 343, 345, 346, 347, 349, 351, 352, 353, 355, 359, 362, 372, 377, 383, 385, 396, 397
Weight loss 58, 101, 104, 105, 106, 302, 312, 323
Wheat grass 17, 74, 82, 139, 140, 141, 143, 334, 340, 363, 368
Whey 206, 211, 335, 358
Wild yam 53, 143, 355, 357, 360, 370
Willow 147
Worms 139, 173, 234
Wormwood 351

Y

Yarrow 53, 293, 294, 295, 355, 358, 360, 369
Yeast 20, 124, 201, 203, 204, 205, 213, 315, 342, 344, 345, 351, 356
Yellow dock 292, 339, 356, 357
Yohimbe 295, 354, 360, 369

Z

Zinc 53, 121, 122, 143, 152, 224, 292, 294, 295, 311, 313, 337, 338, 339, 346, 350, 352, 354, 355, 357, 360, 361, 369

CPSIA information can be obtained at www.ICGtesting.com
Printed in the USA
LVOW02s0528301214
420807LV00004B/4/P